bitter
pills

Medicines and the Third World poor
by Dianna Melrose

First Published in 1982
© OXFAM 1982
Reprinted June 1983

ISBN 0 85598 065 6

Printed by Oxfam Print Unit

Published by OXFAM
274 Banbury Road, Oxford OX2 7DZ.

ACKNOWLEDGEMENTS

This book would never have materialised without the invaluable help of experts, colleagues and friends.

I am particularly grateful to my colleagues David Bull and Adrian Moyes for their unstinting advice and encouragement and for their sense of humour. Special thanks go to David Newell, Julu, Niaz, Saidur and others at OXFAM's Dacca office and to medical advisers, Dr. Tony Klouda and Dr. Tim Lusty. Many colleagues have helped, especially in the Secretarial Services Department, but one in particular has laboured for many hours producing immaculate typescript - my special thanks to Betty Hawkins. Thanks also to Alan Bell for producing the index.

I wish to thank the OXFAM trustees and members of the Field Committees who devoted time and effort to helping with improvements to the early drafts, particularly Dr. William Cutting, Dr. Chris Manning and Michael Rowntree, Chairman of the editorial panel.

For their expert advice and for the many demands made on their time, I especially wish to thank Dr. Humayun Hye, formerly Director of Drug Administration in Bangladesh, Professor Mike Rawlins, Head of the Department of Clinical Pharmacology at the University of Newcastle and Dr. John Yudkin, Consultant/Senior Lecturer in General Medicine, Whittington Hospital, London.

I am grateful to the following for their contributions to our research and to some also for their helpful comments on the early drafts:
Selim Ahmed (Voluntary Health Services Society, Bangladesh); Dr. Raj Anand (Bombay); Dr. F. S. Antezana (WHO, Geneva); Dr. K.M.S. Aziz (International Centre for Diarrhoeal Disease Research, Bangladesh); Dr. K. Balasubramanian (UNCTAD, Geneva); Sharon Banoff and Ritchie Cogan (BBC, London); Dr. Carol Barker (Nuffield Centre for Health Services Studies, Leeds); David Beynon (Pharmaceutical Supply Officer, Madang Department of Health, Papua New Guinea); Dorit Braun; Dr. Pascale Brudon (Geneva); Dr. James Burton and Bill Davies (ECHO, Ewell); Sue Cavanna (Sichili Hospital, Zambia); Dr. Zafrullah Chowdhury (Gonoshasthaya Kendra, Bangladesh); Ralph Cox (DHSS, London); Professor P. F. D'Arcy (Head, Department of Pharmacy, The Queen's University of Belfast); Bharat Dogra (Delhi); Anne Ferguson (Michigan State University, USA); Foo Gaik Sim (Head, Research and Information, International Organisation of Consumer Unions, Penang); Doris Frizel (Bo Hospital, Sierra Leone); Dr. Jaime Galvez-Tan (Philippines); Dr. L. G. Goodwin (Director of Science, Zoological Society of London); Dr. C. E. Gordon-Smith (The Dean, London School of Hygiene and Tropical Medicine); Bob Grose (British Organization for Community Development, Yemen Arab Republic); Dr. Hassani (Director, Norwegian SCF Clinic, Ibb, Yemen Arab Republic); Dr. Andrew Herxheimer (Dept. of Pharmacy, Charing Cross Hospital Medical School, London); Dr. Ann Hoskins and sister Raymi volunteers (British Organisation for Community Development, Yemen Arab Republic); Professor Nurul Islam (Director, Institute of Postgraduate Medicine and Research); Dr. Vida Jelling (ex-VSO); Dr. Juel-Jensen (Oxford University Medical Officer); Dr. Sultana Khanum (SCF Children's Nutrition Unit, Bangladesh); Dr. Sanjaya Lall (Oxford University Institute of Economics and Statistics); Dr. Jane Mackay (ex-VSO); Charles Medawar (Social Audit Ltd., London); Ross Mountain (UNNGLS, Geneva); Linda Nicholls (pharmacist); Professor Georges Peters (Institut du Pharmacologie, Universite de Lausanne); Dr. Ahmed Rhazoui (UNCTC, New York); Dr. B. Sankaran (WHO, Geneva); Dr. Satoto (Indonesia); Dr. Martin Schweiger; Dr. Mira Shiva and S. Srinivasan (VHAI, Delhi); Dr. Milton Silverman and Mia Lydecker (University of California); Dr. Pawan Sureka (Bombay); Ken Temple (ODA, London); Dr. Wanandi (WHO, Geneva); David Werner (Hesperian Foundation, California); the pharmacists at Westlake Ltd. (Banbury Road, Oxford); and Stephen de Winter and colleagues (Belbo Film Productions, Netherlands).

I would like to thank all those representatives of the pharmaceutical industry who have provided help and information, particularly David Taylor (Deputy Director, Office of Health Economics, London); representatives of the Association of British Pharmaceutical Industries and the International Federation of Pharmaceutical Manufacturers Associations; and executives of Beecham, Boots, Ciba-Geigy, Cyanamid, Fisons, Glaxo, Hoechst, ICI, May & Baker UK, E. Merck, Merck Sharp & Dohme, Organon, Pfizer, Rivopharm, Roche, Sandoz, G. D. Searle, Squibb, Upjohn and The Wellcome Foundation.

Finally, special thanks to Helen and Chris for encouragement when I needed it most.

CONTENTS

INTRODUCTION

AS THE BOAT drew into the shore we heard a strange sound from the bank. A woman was crying. We found her with a dead baby in her arms and a collection of medicine bottles beside her. She had spent all her money on these expensive drugs. She could not understand why they had not saved her baby. This Bangladeshi woman had never been told what was obvious to the doctor who found her. The baby had become severely dehydrated from diarrhoea. Her death could have been prevented with a simple home-made solution of water, salt and sugar. No amount of medicine could have kept her alive.

People in remote mountain villages in North Yemen are cut off from the country's very limited health services concentrated in the towns. Drug pedlars, known locally as 'health men', have a ready market. They sell a wide range of sophisticated drugs which can have harmful side-effects. Most of these medicines can only be obtained on a doctor's prescription in Europe and North America. Some have even been taken off the market in rich countries because the possible risks outweigh their benefits. But in Yemen the drug sellers are unaware of the hazards or how the drugs should be used. Most have acquired their training working as hospital cleaners, or behind the counter in a drug store.

On open market stalls in Upper Volta red and yellow capsules of antibiotics are displayed for sale alongside equally colourful sweets. Poor people buy just one or two capsules at a time to treat themselves. They have no idea that antibiotics are not fully effective unless you take a complete course, or that tetracycline, left out in the heat and humidity, can become toxic. But the main hazard from the uncontrolled use of antibiotics is that bacteria build up resistance to drugs. A poor community can find itself with no alternatives to the drugs that no longer work.

In 1980 governments and aid agencies all over the world responded to the plight of the Kampuchean people by rushing in a mass of drugs they had well-meaningly scrambled together. But this jumble of medicines, labelled in dozens of different languages, created chaos. In the absence of a team of multilingual pharmacists to sift through them, many potentially useful and useless drugs alike had to be discarded.

Throughout Asia, Africa and Latin America millions of the poorest have no access to life-saving drugs. But drugs are wasted and misused worldwide. In poor countries those that are most needed are often the hardest to obtain, at least at prices the poor can afford. Where the need is for a limited selection of priority drugs at low prices, manufacturers and retailers come under commercial pressure to sell a mass of wasteful, often non-essential products. In some countries the

1

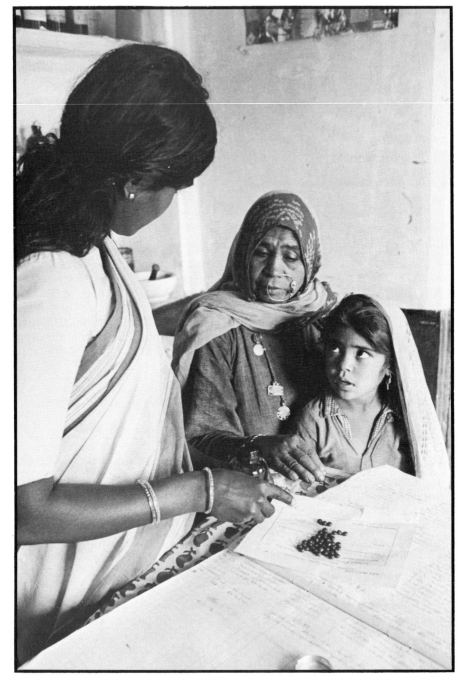

(Credit) Mike Wells.

market is flooded with an assortment of vitamin tonics, cough and cold remedies, and other expensive combination products, when single- ingredient, basic drugs like penicillin and chloroquine are in desperately short supply.

The first-hand experiences of OXFAM colleagues and friends throughout the Third World have made us forcefully aware of the problems. Very few of the poor benefit from the potential of modern medicines. Valuable drugs developed decades ago could be used to prevent unnecessary suffering and death. But through their uncontrolled sale and promotion in many poor countries, medicines often do little good and can be positively harmful.

OXFAM's commitment to the relief of suffering made it our duty to investigate the problems and publish our findings with the aim of pressing for action to benefit the poor. This report is based on the experience of OXFAM field staff, project workers and friends in many very different countries. But what emerges is a striking similarity in the problems worldwide. The report also draws on a wide range of both published and unpublished material in addition to research carried out by the writer in North Yemen, India and Bangladesh.

A doctor in Bangladesh told OXFAM that he is acutely aware of three contrasting but equally tragic situations. There are patients he cannot help who are dying of diseases for which there is no drug treatment. Secondly, the poorest, who cannot obtain treatment or drugs, die of diseases that are curable, and often preventable. Thirdly, and seemingly paradoxically, some poor families make sacrifices and even go without food to buy unnecessary drugs, when the 'medicine' they need is food.

Rich and poor could benefit from new drugs to treat incurable diseases. But only the poor are denied the life-saving drugs available to the rich. This report attempts to unravel the complexities of the medicines issue. The focus throughout is on the needs of the Third World poor.

Chapter 1 assesses the role of medicines in creating better health. Chapters 2 to 6 highlight the special problems in the distribution, production and marketing of drugs in developing countries. Chapter 7 focuses on traditional medicine which remains the major source of health care for most of the world's population. Chapters 8 and 9 describe constructive initiatives to improve health and the supply and use of essential drugs both at project level and on a wider national and international scale. These and the following chapter are concerned both with attempts to rationalise drug policies to benefit the majority and with obstacles to change. Chapter 10 also examines attitudes and policies in the major drug-producing nations and their impact on drug needs and policies in developing countries. Finally, in Chapter 11, we put forward OXFAM's suggestions on action that is urgently needed to benefit the Third World poor.

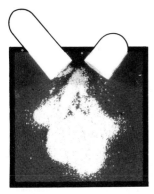

CHAPTER 1

A PILL FOR ALL ILLS?
Medicines and health

FIFTY YEARS ago in the world's poorest countries average life expectancy was only 30 years. At that time the first modern drugs were only just being developed in Europe and America. In the poor world today average life expectancy is 50 years. [1]The poor may live longer now but the evidence suggests that during their lifetime, they are likely both to experience as much ill-health as their great-grandparents, and to suffer from essentially the same health problems. In fact, for the vast majority of the Third World poor, the quality of life has barely improved. For some it has almost certainly worsened. [2]

Do modern drugs offer a solution? Could their use radically improve the quality of life of the Third World poor? Before looking at the potential of modern drugs, we need to take stock of the health problems in poor countries and examine their underlying causes.

DIAGNOSIS OF ILL-HEALTH
Even the most 'reliable' statistics on ill-health in poor countries can be little more than 'guesstimates'. Localised studies can often give a more accurate picture than national statistics. In many countries official figures on causes of death are based entirely on hospital records. But hardly any of the dead end up in hospital, for example, less than 4% in Tanzania. [3] Official statistics also tend to mask the major health problems of the poor. After all, they can only cover patients treated by the health services, whereas WHO estimates that in many Third World countries as many as 70% of the population has no access to organised health care. [4]

So official statistics are almost invariably underestimates of the true incidence of premature death and disease. But there is little doubt about the major health problems in poor countries, or the fact that the poorest are most severely affected. The single most widespread cause of ill-health is malnutrition. [5]

MALNUTRITION
The most vulnerable group in poor countries are young children. Deaths of children under the age of five can account for up to three-quarters of all deaths in the community. [6] According to the United Nations Industrial Development Organisation (UNIDO), of the 15.6 million children under five who die each year,

5

15.1 million are from developing countries, and of these, 12 million deaths could probably be avoided. [7]

The under-fives are especially at risk because they have little resistance to disease, and their vulnerability becomes acute when they are malnourished. Repeated bouts of diarrhoea and other common infections reduce a child's ability to absorb food. The child becomes weak and stops growing and may become severely malnourished. This precipitates a vicious circle of malnutrition and disease that is often only broken with the child's death. A large-scale study of child deaths in the impoverished north-east of Brazil found that measles was the probable cause of half of all child deaths. But three-quarters of these children also showed obvious signs of malnutriton. [8] The problem of malnutrition is not of course confined to those who die. Many are saved from death but are left severely physically and mentally disabled.

Poor nutrition undermines the health of other vulnerable groups in the community, such as pregnant and lactating mothers who can become severely anaemic from the effects of repeated pregnancies. A recent nutritional study carried out in North Yemen found that in one region almost three-quarters of mothers were suffering from anaemia. [9] In most developing countries the basic food intake of a large section of the population is totally inadequate for their health needs. It was estimated in 1980 that at least a third of the people in Mozambique get less calories than they require. [10] In the very poorest countries, such as Bangladesh, where there is tremendous pressure on the land and rapid population growth, there is likely to be a much higher percentage of people undernourished and consequently vulnerable to infectious disease.

COMMUNICABLE DISEASES

People in the Third World today suffer from the same communicable diseases that were widespread in developed countries in the nineteenth century. Many of these illnesses are transmitted by food and water contaminated by disease organisms from human and animal excreta. They include diarrhoeal disease, amoebic and bacterial dysentery, typhoid, cholera, polio and infectious hepatitis, which are all major problems in the Third World. [11]

One Bangladeshi expert on diarrhoeal disease describes it as the major health scourge of Asia, responsible for at least half and possibly as much as three-quarters of infectious disease. [12] In Bangladesh itself, an estimated 60% of children who die under the age of five, die as a result of diarrhoea, and in India it is thought that acute diarhoeal diseases alone take 1.5 million lives each year. [13]

Respiratory infections are major problems throughout the Third World. During the 1970s pneumonia and bronchitis were the main causes of death recorded in Tanzania and Nepal. [14] In some countries TB is a disease of epidemic proportions. A report published in 1981 estimates that each year TB kills half a million people in India alone. [15]

TROPICAL AND VECTOR-BORNE DISEASES

Nearly one thousand million people - a quarter of the world's population - are affected or threatened by tropical diseases. [16] The most prevalent of these include malaria, schistosomiasis, filariasis, trypanosomiasis, leishmaniasis and leprosy.

Of these, malaria is a major killer, each year causing the death of about one million children under the age of 14 in Africa alone. [17] Chagas' disease, a South American form of trypanosomiasis affecting over 10 million people, is also often fatal in children. [18] But the effects of most tropical and vector-borne diseases are severely debilitating and crippling, rather than fatal. One example is onchocerciasis, or river blindness, a form of filariasis transmitted by blackfly, which is endemic in parts of Africa and Latin America. In the upper basin of the Volta River in West Africa about a million people are thought to be suffering from partial blindness caused by worms that grow under the skin where the blackfly have bitten. The disease is progressive and leaves thousands completely blind. [19]

The parasites that cause many of the different tropical diseases attack the blood and vital organs like the liver. They cause painful and debilitating symptoms such as recurring bouts of fever. In common with the mass of infectious diseases, they can perpetuate poverty by their constant debilitating effect. For example, a poor family of subsistence farmers may have their livelihood destroyed if an attack of malaria leaves them too weak to work at critical times of the year, especially when crops need to be planted and harvested.

In many poor communities parasitic diseases are a fact of life for the majority. Many are easily transmitted because of lack of sanitation and clean water supplies. The prevalence of these parasitic diseases is well illustrated by studies from Sri Lanka, Bangladesh and Venezuela showing that over 90% of 6 year olds examined had some form of worm infestation. [20]

URBANISATION AND DISEASE

Finally, industrialisation and the rapid growth of the cities are beginning to change the pattern of ill-health. Over half the population of Latin America now lives in urban areas, and rural people are also migrating to the towns throughout Asia and Africa. Today the urban poor are exposed to infectious diseases from insanitary living conditions in the shanty towns and the new hazards of industrial accidents, pollution and traffic accidents. Even the rural poor bear the brunt of pressures from the consumer society as they are enticed away from local foods and encouraged to consume expensive factory- produced food and drinks and high-tar cigarettes.

The fact that life expectancy is now longer, particularly amongst the affluent minority, means that cancer, cardiac and coronary-artery disease and other major problems of industrialised societies are becoming more significant. But the incidence of these conditions is proportionately minute compared to the mass of nutritional, infectious and tropical diseases, suffered by the poor.

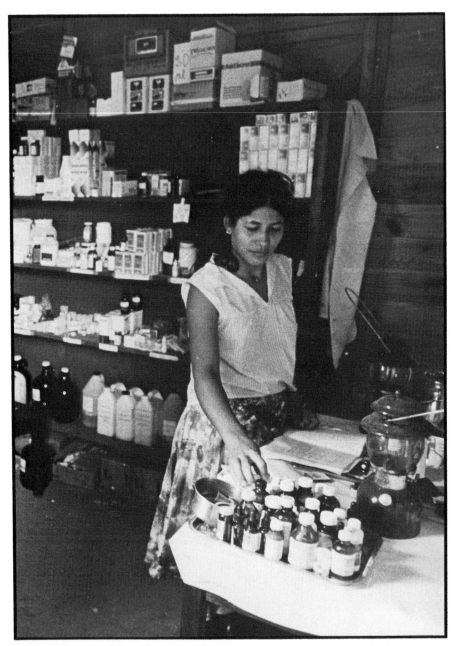

Medicines can represent a major financial burden to poor people. Health centres to provide the necessary drugs and clear instructions on their use are not available to millions of people in the Third World.

THE UNDERLYING CAUSES

The poor suffer disproportionately from ill health. [21] This is as true of the prevalence of disease in the world's poorest countries, as in rich industralised nations. In Britain, for example, the 1980 Black Committee Report, *Inequalities in Health,* showed that the poorest suffer more illness and are more likely to die in infancy than the affluent. [22] In other words, poverty is one major cause of ill-health. As the Indian Council of Social Science Research (ICSSR) and Indian Council of Medical Research (ICMR) state in their 1981 report, *Health for all: an alternative strategy,* " 'Poverty', itself is an extremely tenacious disease. It must be directly attacked to improve the health status of the people." [23]

But, as the ICSSR/ICMR report points out, in India, a country that is modernising and industrialising fast, "... although there is some evidence to show that the percentage of people below the poverty line may have declined, there is no doubt that their absolute numbers have increased substantially". [24] It is OXFAM's experience that, in many developing countries, the distribution of wealth is becoming more concentrated in the hands of a small minority, whilst the mass of the poor sink deeper into the poverty trap. [25]

Poverty means different things in different societies, but above all it means powerlessness. In the words of Dr. Klouda, OXFAM's medical adviser in Tanzania, "The existence of the poor has almost no effect on the national goals, and the poor have no power or voice to influence village thinking, let alone national thinking. The nation rewards those who actively contribute to its success." [26] Powerlessness means that the poor have only a limited ability to improve their health by obtaining more food, or changing their physical environment. As a result, they are trapped in semi-permanent hunger and squalid living conditions.

Powerlessness means, for example, that the growing minority of relatively well-paid factory workers, many in the Third World's new free trade zones, are in no position to protect their health by demanding safer working conditions. There is chronic unemployment and underemployment in both urban and rural areas, and in most countries wages are extremely low in relation to the cost of basic necessities. Inflation, particularly rising food prices, has a direct impact on nutrition, because the poor have to spend a very high proportion of their income on food. [27] For example, a doctor reports that in Ghana in 1979, at a time of rapid inflation, a labourer's basic daily wage "would have just covered the cost of carbohydrate for two adults and two children, with no allowance for protein, rent, clothes or other essentials". [28]

Many poor families have so little purchasing power that their health has been endangered by the growth of the money economy. In Tanzania, for example, a detailed study of the nutritional status of people in the Southern Highlands in 1977 found that the highest nutritional levels were in families that had stayed outside the money economy and still depended on subsistence farming. [29] Commenting on this study, Dr. Klouda points out that "money introduces a new method of obtaining status or acceptance". [30] Moreover, the pressures of

9

modernisation and consumerism have made an impact even in remote rural areas. They have created new aspirations that can often only be satisfied at the expense of buying food. [31]

The food intake of families dependent on subsistence farming can, however, be dangerously low because of their inability to produce enough food. Marginal farmers are particularly vulnerable to drought and floods. Very few can get advice on how to improve poor, overworked soil or legal aid if forced off their land. They may have no access to credit to buy seeds or water supplies to irrigate their land. [32]

The availability of water can be critical for food production and conseqently for nutrition. Lack of water is also a major factor in the spread of infectious disease. Skin infections and communicable disease are rapidly transmitted, when families have no easy access to water for washing. [33] Moreover, the poor are particularly vulnerable to water-borne diseases, because many have to rely on unsafe water for drinking. In North Yemen, for example, only 4% of households had clean piped water in 1978. [34] In India, although 80% of the urban population has been provided with a protected water supply, out in the rural areas, only one village in ten has safe drinking water. One village in five lacks even basic water facilities. [35]

In most developing countries there is a chronic shortage of sanitation facilities and sewerage, particularly in the rural areas, where even simple latrines are virtually unknown. In Bangladesh, for example, no more than 6% of households throughout the country had sanitation facilities in 1977. [36] The Third World poor almost invariably live in overcrowded housing. In North Yemen the Government has estimated that nearly half the population live in one- room housing. [37] Living conditions in the Third World's sprawling urban slums are particuarly unhealthy, as people are forced to live alongside open drains and refuse tips.

The problems of lack of food and unhealthy living conditions are compounded by ignorance, apathy and fatalism, generated by a lifetime of powerlessness and deprivation. The oppression of millions of poor women is an important factor in perpetuating ill-health. In some societies girls have even less access than boys to elementary education with the result that over 90% of women are illiterate. [38] Their low status can mean that adult males come first in sharing out a family's meagre diet, to the disadvantage of women and children. Mothers may have little understanding of hygiene or the nutritional needs of their children. Commercial pressures have compounded the problems in recent years as a growing number of women in poor communities have abandoned breast- feeding, unaware of the hazards to their babies' health from contaminated feeds in unsterilised feeding-bottles. [39]

THE REMEDIES

From the broad range of social, political and economic factors underlying ill-health in poor countries, it must be readily apparent that medicines *alone* cannot solve the problems. Disease that is rooted in poverty can only be prevented by an onslaught on poverty and inequality. In the words of the Tanzanian Food and Nutrition Council, a "society that is perpetuating malnutrition cannot be treated with medicine. It has to develop and be restructured in such a way that all its members are ascertained all their basic human needs". [40]

Most illness is in fact self-limiting through the body's own defence mechanisms. This makes good nutrition crucial in fighting disease. Dr. Klouda observes from Tanzania: "If the nutritional status of the nation improved, that, at one blow, would do more for the health of the population than any other measure. The health services have only a limited role to play in this." [41]

The ICSSR and ICMR report confirms that ill-health has to be tackled with political and economic measures. "... there are millions of individuals whose illness arises basically from malnutrition. No 'pills' can help them; and the only way to prevent their morbidity and mortality is to make a direct attack on poverty itself through such programmes as guaranteed employment at reasonable wages." [42]

This prescription for better health is borne out by the experience of developed countries such as Britain. The diagrams overleaf trace the rapid fall in infant mortality rates over the last century. Diagram 1 shows that deaths of babies in their first year of life had already fallen dramatically before the advent of modern life-saving drugs which, with the exception of small-pox vaccine, were not generally available until the 1930s. [43] In fact, as Diagram 2 demonstrates, the major impetus to better health in Britain from the mid-nineteenth century can be directly attributed to public health measures and social legislation which improved the living standards of working people. [44] Higher wages and welfare benefits made it possible for the poor to eat properly. Public health measures radically improved conditions in the densely-populated urban areas, particularly with the provision of clean water supplies, sanitation, sewerage and new housing. Finally, improved health care contributed to the prevention of early deaths. Infant mortality fell sharply at the turn of the century, when the Midwives Act (1902) came into force.

The fact that medicines can be seen to have played a relatively minor role in the trend to better health in countries like Britain is of course no argument against their potential value in developing countries today. Most deaths in the Third World are caused by infectious diseases that can now be treated with drugs.

It is also clear that when the first modern drug treatments became available their impact was soon felt in speeding up recovery and preventing deaths. TB was once a major killer in Britain. From the end of the nineteenth century public health measures, better diet and improved housing contributed to a dramatic fall in TB deaths. By the 1940s the TB death rate was still declining, by about 3% a year. But when the first modern antituberculous drugs became generally available in the early 1950s, the fall in TB deaths increased to 15% a year. [45]

Over the past thirty years drugs have made a tremendous impact in controlling some specific diseases. One of the most obvious successes is the eradication of smallpox with smallpox vaccine. There are numerous examples of drugs which have made major contributions to the relief of human suffering. These include

Diagram 1.

INFANT MORTALITY IN ENGLAND AND WALES

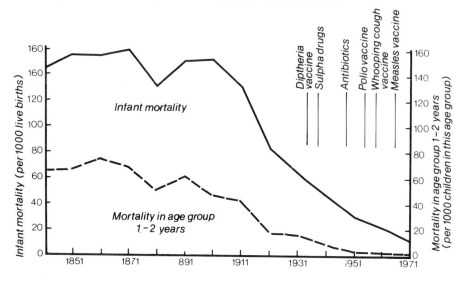

Diagram 2.

INFANT MORTALITY IN ENGLAND AND WALES

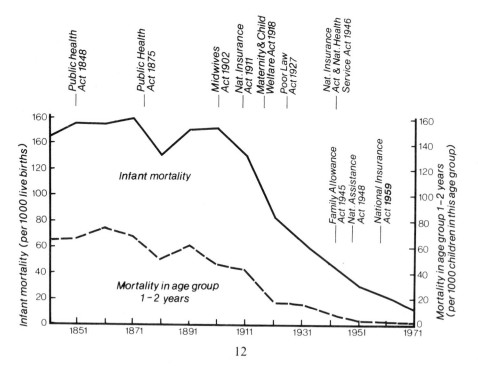

drugs to alleviate painful symptoms, but most vital are those that provide cures for killing diseases. An outstanding example is the development of antibiotics targeted to attack life-threatening infections without the patient suffering ill effects. Antibacterial drugs have made it possible to save lives on a massive scale. Their success has created what Dr. John Yudkin describes as the "antibiotic mentality", the belief in "a pill for all ills". [46]

The fact remains that medicines cannot tackle the social roots of ill-health. With a few notable exceptions, such as vaccines and antimalarials, they cannot prevent disease. But to make any major onslaught on disease, prevention is essential. The inevitable limitations of medicines are put clearly by a research and development director of Wellcome, one major British drug manufacturer. He points out that "drugs are not synonymous with health, ... there are many forces for the promotion of health, including nutrition, education and hygiene. In some parts of the world, these take priority before more sophisticated medicines are brought into play." [47]

Even vaccines which can be used selectively to protect young children from tetanus, diphtheria, whooping cough, polio, measles and TB may not all be entirely effective let alone cost-effective. [48] For example there is evidence to indicate that the anti-TB BCG vaccine is of unpredictable effectiveness . [49] It has been suggested that this may be related to the nutritional status of the recipient. In any case, no drug can be a substitute for food. Dr. Klouda highlights how vaccines may be an unrealistic option in terms of cost. "A good health budget will provide about £3 a head in a developing country [per year] . The cost for just measles vaccine for every child in Tanzania, including transport and other costs, came to about £1.50 in 1977. How can they even think of £1.50 a head for vaccines, which are not dealing with the major health problems?" [50]

Moreover, drugs are powerless to break the cycle of disease in an unhealthy environment. This is illustrated by the treatment, as against the prevention, of hookworm anaemia, a disease which is very common in poor communities that have no basic sanitation. Hookworm larvae thrive in moist soil where they have been deposited in human waste. The larvae break through the skin of people walking barefoot and work their way into the small intestine. Lodged in the intestine, the hookworm parasite leeches blood. A heavy worm infestation can cause severe iron-deficiency anaemia. If left untreated, an infected person gets steadily weaker and can die from heart failure. [51]

Hookworm anaemia can be treated effectively with modern drug therapy - worm pills in conjunction with iron tablets. But so long as the community remains ignorant of how the disease is transmitted, they will go on using the moist ground instead of latrines and keep on getting hookworm anaemia. The only long-term solution is to build latrines. Finding an appropriate method to dispose of human waste can be both technically difficult and expensive. But people could protect themselves from the disease if they knew how it is transmitted. For instance, many could buy cheap plastic sandals as a simple preventive measure. [52] Encouraging the poor to go on buying drugs without doing anything to stop diseases from recurring makes as much sense as continuously wallpapering a damp wall and failing to do anything to treat the damp. It is expensive, wasteful and ultimately doomed to failure.

So to improve health in poor countries disease has to be attacked simultaneously on a number of fronts. Amongst them clean water, sanitation and other public health measures are vital. The difficulty is that these require a great deal of capital investment. For example, it has been calculated that the basic cost of providing clean water supplies for the rural population of India by the year 2000 would require an investment of at least £277 million a year. This estimate excludes all the time-consuming and expensive business of coping with the technological and maintenance problems that would have to be overcome. [53] This sum is roughly equivalent to the £250 million calculated to have been invested in the Indian drug industry in 1977. [54] But whereas there are immediate returns to be made on medicine sales, there are clearly few attractions for private investors in providing poor communities with clean water.

However, lack of money to carry out preventive health projects need not be an insurmountable obstacle to better health. This is illustrated by the experience of Kerala, one of the most economically underdeveloped States in India. Kerala spends less on health per person that all but one of the 14 remaining states, but it has by far the best health statistics, even by comparison with the most affluent Indian States such as the Punjab. The death rate in Kerala is 7.2 per thousand, compared to 19.2 per thousand in the State of Uttar Pradesh. The significantly better health status of people in Kerala has been linked to its greater social and educational development. Women have relatively better status. The society is less rigidly segregated on caste lines. Literacy rates are high and women, in particular, are now benefiting from widespread adult literacy campaigns and elementary education. [55]

The experience of Kerala, that greater awareness can generate better health, is confirmed by OXFAM's experience of community development projects throughout the Third World. The poor only take an active interest in preventive health measures, such as devising basic sanitation, if they participate in making decisions. For this to happen, poor communities need to go through a process of social education, to gain the will and the confidence to organise to improve things. [56]

We have seen that the main health problems of the poor are rooted in their poverty and powerlessness, and that no single prescription for better health is likely to succeed. Improved living standards, more equal distribution of land, job opportunities, clean water, control of disease vectors and other public health measures are all essential elements, as are education and preventive and curative health care. All depend on the political will of governments to give priority to the needs of the poor. Consequently lack of political will and of money to implement changes remain the major stumbling blocks to meeting these needs.

14

ESSENTIAL DRUGS FOR PRIMARY HEALTH CARE

Over the past five years governments of all complexions have been expressing their commitment to extending health services to cover their entire population. The new emphasis on the universal right to health care dates back to the joint World Health Organisation (WHO) and United Nations International Children's Emergency Fund (UNICEF) international conference on Primary Health Care held in Alma-Ata in 1978. This set the ambitious target of "the attainment by all peoples of the world by the year 2000 of a level of health that will permit them to lead a socially and economically productive life". [57] Of course, the rhetoric obscures the reality in developing countries, but aims for politically neutral ground to galvanise governments into action.

The Alma-Ata Declaration defines primary health care as "essential health care .... made universally accessible to individuals and families in the community .... through their full participation and at a cost that the community and country can afford ...." [58] It is within the framework of these primary health care services that medicines could be used most effectively as part of a wider preventive strategy. In the words of WHO, "While medicinal products *alone* are not sufficient to provide adequate health care, they do play an important role in protecting, maintaining and restoring the health of the people". [59](WHO's emphasis)

The crucial issue for poor countries is that, whereas a limited number of drugs are vital to health needs, not *all* drugs are essential, let alone useful. Of the thousands of different drugs sold, WHO has identified a selection of approximately 200 which experts consider "essential", in other words "basic, indispensable and necessary to any nation's health needs". [60] The drugs included in the WHO *Selection of essential drugs* (Appendix 1) have mostly been in use for many years and are known to be relatively safe and cost-effective. WHO also urges individual countries to make a much more limited selection of drugs for their priority needs in primary health care. [61] Whilst different experts hold different views on exactly which drugs should be considered 'essential' for primary health care, many agree that as few as a dozen or so vital drugs are sufficient to cater for the most pressing needs of poor communities. [62]

In this chapter we have focussed on the relatively limited role of medicines in terms of the Third World's *overall* health strategy. But modern drugs are nonetheless, in the words of one United Nations (UN) report, "a marginal albeit essential technology". [63] As WHO stresses, drugs are "essential tools for health care and for the improvement of the quality of life". [64] Some key medicines could be used to save millions of the world's poor from unnecessary suffering and premature death.

Bearing in mind that the poor need a small number of essential drugs, in the next chapters we shall concentrate on the reality in the Third World today and examine the drug market and its relevance to the needs of the poor.

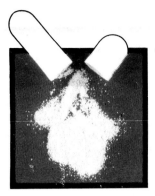

CHAPTER 2

UNEQUAL DISTRIBUTION

"The public health services of the 67 poorest developing countries, excluding China, spend less in total than the rich countries spend on tranquilizers." (Dr. Halfdan Mahler, Director General, World Health Organisation, *World Health Forum,* 2(1), 1981.)

CHOR ASHARIDAHA is an island in the middle of the Ganges, just inside Bangladesh, on the border with India. The island is really no more than a mud-flat thrown up by the river, but, because land is desperately short in Bangladesh, it has become the home of about 12,000 people. They are dynamic and industrious. Everyone is up before dawn and working: the men labouring in the paddy fields, the women straining over the monotonous task of husking paddy and the children tending the animals.

The island is at the mercy of the river. Every year, at the time of the monsoon, it runs the risk of serious flooding. As the water-level rises dramatically there is nothing to stop the water breaking across the island, washing away the crops and mud houses in its path. September 1980 brought a massive flood. Many people lost their homes and, as the year's main rice crop was destroyed, most lost their livelihood.

When this happens the poor landless labourers cannot find work, so they have no means of feeding their families. The powerful in the community who have their own land, suffer from the loss of their crops. But they have reserves to tide them over, and by selling their rice at inflated prices they can even amass more wealth at the expense of the poor. The landowners have little difficulty obtaining credit to buy seeds for the next crop. But the landless have nothing to fall back on. They are trapped in the day-to-day struggle to secure food and shelter.

For several days at a time the poorest go without even a bowl of rice. Amongst the worst off are young 'widows' and their children, abandoned by husbands who have left because there is no work. The health of the poor is seriously threatened by both lack of food and the insanitary conditions in the villages. There are no latrines or basic sanitation on the island and much of the water supply is contaminated.

As the flood water recedes, hookworm and roundworm thrive in the moist soil where people must squat to defecate. The skies are beginning to clear as the monsoon is nearly over. But every so often a sudden downpour leaves the villagers soaked to the skin as they work on, rebuilding the mud walls of their homes.

Adults and children look thin and weak from intestinal parasites and repeated bouts of diarrhoea. Many of the youngest children have pot bellies from the combined effects of malnutrition and heavy worm infestations. The eyes of those worst affected are dull and dry-looking. At night they stumble in the dark, showing the first obvious signs of nutritional blindness. Those who survive may have their eyesight damaged for life. Respiratory illnesses are common, and there are serious pneumonia and TB cases.

What both children and adults obviously need is more food and a healthy environment. The prospects of any far-reaching changes are remote. Even with the necessary resources and the political will, the process of improving health will take time. But the islanders could benefit from preventive health measures and a few key drugs could make the difference between life and death for some. Antibacterial and antituberculous drugs, deworming pills and some vaccines could all make an immediate impact on the islanders' health.

There are four government-paid health workers on the island. But people see little point in going to find them. They have no drugs. There is also a small drug dispensary, but its annual drugs allocation, worth Taka 5,000 (about £138), is hopelessly inadequate to cater for the needs of 12,000 people. Not only is the allocation meagre at little more than 1p a head, but supplies are so erratic that the dispensary only has stocks for a few months of the year. Most of the time its shelves are empty and the doors locked.

The island has no private pharmacy, but some traders do sell high-priced drugs to those who can spare the cash to buy them. Medicines are an impossible luxury for the poorest families, who spend about three-quarters of their income on food.[1] Across the water, there is a government health centre where medicines are distributed free. But the poor have neither the time nor the money to pay for the crossing and then make the 6-mile trek to the centre. They might queue for hours only to find that the dispensary has run out of the drug they require. So the poor are forced to treat illness as a fact of life and carry on regardless. They may not go for help until the problem is serious. All too often, by the time they go for treatment, it is too late.

The situation of the islanders is not unique. Throughout Asia, Africa and Latin America, millions of the world's poor have no means of obtaining medicines to help relieve suffering, or cure illness. [2] This is because the world distribution of medicines is like that of most commodities. It is dependent on purchasing power, not need. The rich take a disproportionate slice of the pharmaceutical cake, leaving the poor with the crumbs.

Nineteen of the world's richest industrialised countries (with a combined population of 684 millions) consumed 58% of drugs on the world market in 1976.

In the same year, thirty-four of the poorest nations, with almost double that population (1,317 millions) consumed just 3%. [3] The Third World as a whole has three-quarters of the world's population, but today accounts for little more than 20% of world drug sales, and nearer 15%, when China is excluded. [4]

Drug expenditure each year in the poorest countries averages less than 50p a head. In some industrialised nations it exceeds £35. [5] These figures underline the lack of purchasing power of the Third World poor. Essentially, they reveal more about wealth than health. It is, for example, highly debatable whether the level of drug consumption in much of the rich world represents a particularly 'healthy' state of affairs. But one conclusion is inescapable: whereas rich countries can afford to be extravagant with medicines without risking acute social consequences, poor people and their governments cannot. Because they have so little money, it is crucial that it is spent only on essential drugs.

In most countries drugs are distributed both through organised health services, either government or voluntary, and by private pharmacies and retailers. Patients in industrialised countries can usually obtain treatment through government-subsidised services or health insurance schemes. For example, in Britain anyone in need of medicine is entitled to a prescription subsidised by the National Health Service. In many developing countries medicines are also, in theory, available free of charge through the health services. In practice, only a privileged minority has easy access to treatment, mostly because they can afford to pay for drugs prescribed by private doctors, rather than relying on the desperately inadequate health services.

Drug distribution cannot be looked at in isolation from health care systems. The stark fact is that throughout most of the Third World almost three-quarters of the population has no access to basic health services. [6] This lack of a primary health care infrastructure to meet the needs of the majority is the single major obstacle to the safe and effective distribution of drugs in poor countries.

But the Third World poor face a double deprivation. In the absence of organised health services, they are particularly vulnerable to pressures from the expanding commercial drug market which is subject to a minimum of controls. There are of course exceptions. A few developing countries have succeeded in providing basic health services for the majority of their people and have introduced controls on private drug distribution to safeguard health. [7] However, in this chapter we concentrate on the problems of public and private drug distribution common to many very different developing countries.

LIMITED HEALTH BUDGETS

Much of the problem of people not getting health care or drugs is straight economics. Governments of poor countries lack resources not just to buy medicines, but to balance all the conflicting demands generated by underdevelopment. The deficiencies of the health infrastructure are, after all, just one problem area. Food production, transport and other sectors may present more

Diagram 3.

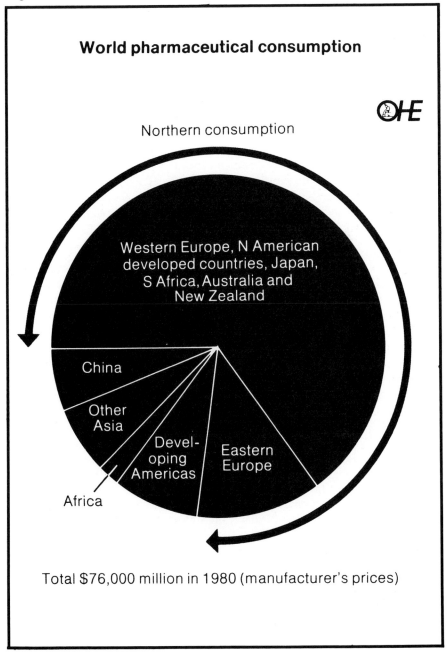

World pharmaceutical consumption

Northern consumption

Western Europe, N American developed countries, Japan, S Africa, Australia and New Zealand

China

Other Asia

Africa

Developing Americas

Eastern Europe

Total $76,000 million in 1980 (manufacturer's prices)

Source: **Taylor,** *Medicines, Health and the Poor World,* **OHE, London 1982.**

immediate problems. Many governments appear to rate 'health' as a low priority alongside more strategic sectors such as defence. For example, the Government of North Yemen spends 44% of its budget, and Bangladesh 20%, on the armed forces, compared with 3.5% which each Government allocates to health. [8]

Even governments whose policies commit them to achieving a greater degree of social justice will not necessarily allocate a lot of funds to their health budget. After all, health services play only a limited role in improving health. Governments may decide they can do more to improve health by investing more in agriculture, industry or education. [9]

Similarly, other sectors of government spending have some bearing on a government's ability to distribute medicines to the people. For example, funds allocated to setting up basic industries may be used to increase self- sufficiency in essential drugs, and good transport and communications are vital to an efficient drug distribution system.

Almost invariably the health budgets of poor countries are very limited. In 1978/9 the British National Health Service spent over 900 times more money providing services to 54 million people in Britain than the Bangladesh Health Ministry spent on health care for its 85 million people. [10] This lack of resources is of course a major stumbling block to making health care available to the mass of the people. But the difficulties have been greatly exacerbated by the fact that most Third World countries have modelled their health systems on the expensive curative services that form the basis of health care in rich industrialised countries. Even in these countries the bias towards high-technology curative care as opposed to more emphasis on disease prevention is increasingly questioned.

HOSPITALS OR HEALTH POSTS?

The escalating costs of health services are beginning to tax the governments of rich countries. But to poor countries the high recurrent costs of these Western-style curative services are crippling. Money is syphoned off to pay for costly medical equipment and keep hospital dispensaries stocked with all the latest drugs. The cost of extending this level of services to the mass of the people is unthinkable. So millions of the poor remain outside the system, denied the most basic health care. Part of the problem is that it is of course much easier to spend the health budget providing services for a compact urban population than on people dispersed in the rural areas.

The tremendous drain of paying for hospital services is illustrated by the situation in Tanzania, where the Government's 1979 *Evaluation of the Health Sector* reveals that the hospitals alone are eating up 60% of the entire health budget. Yet the same study shows how little of the population actually benefits from hospital services. Over half of all hospital in-patients and three-quarters of out-patients live within 5 to 10 kms of the hospital and almost all the hospitals are in the towns.

This means that most of the health budget is only benefiting people in the urban areas - little more than 14% of the population.

Recurrent expenditure on each Tanzanian hospital (seeing 137,000 out-patients a year) costs as much as it does to run 53 dispensaries (which, together, see 1,060,000 out-patients a year). The true cost of running the hospitals is clear from the fact that two out of three villages are left with no health facility at all. [11]

Dr. Klouda, OXFAM's medical adviser in Tanzania, reports that after paying for the hospitals, "Only a little [of the health budget] is left to keep the country's dispensaries and health centres going, as well as provide a tiny budget for preventive services. The amount left for the dispensaries and health centres covers salaries and a few drugs and other necessities. Little is provided for transport, repairs, maintenance, spare parts or equipment. But even the drug allowance does not cover the basic needs of a dispensary. This means that dispensary staff provide inadequate treatment, are very rarely supervised, very rarely visit the four or so villages they should cover, and are often demoralised." [12] Yet Tanzania is a country which has given a higher priority than many to the equitable spread of health care. [13]

The distortion between where money is actually spent on health care and where it is needed recurs throughout the Third World, and indeed elsewhere. For example, in Bangladesh, three-quarters of the money spent on curative health services is channelled through health facilities in the towns, where only 8% of the people live. There are specialised orthopaedic, cardiovascular and eye institutions already, and plans to set up more of each, in addition to a new cancer research institute. [14] Cancer and heart disease do not rank among the country's priority health problems, but they are an increasing concern for the urban elite.

Meanwhile, in rural Bangladesh most people have no access even to the most rudimentary health post. The 1977 official *Health Profile* states: "The seven million urban population is relatively well covered by Government and private health facilities but a major proportion of the 76 million rural population do not have health care of any sort." [15]

A factor that contributes to the misallocation of funds away from real health needs is that Third World governments and aid donors alike are keen on 'visible' projects. Brand new health posts in the north-east of Brazil have been kitted out with electric sterilisers where there is no electricity. Some of the buildings remain unused except by the occasional visiting dignitary. [16] These gleaming white elephants demonstrate the good intentions of planners frustrated by the shortage of money for running costs and, above all, the absence of trained personnel where they are most needed.

INAPPROPRIATE TRAINING

The chronic lack of trained health workers is one of the major obstacles to providing basic health care to the majority of the rural poor. Most governments recognise the urgent need to train paramedics and to develop referral systems to support them. But in most cases demand far outstrips the number of health workers successfully trained.

Meanwhile, large sums of money continue to be poured into training doctors who emerge from medical schools with no intention of working in the rural areas. Moreover, many of the skills the doctors acquire are not relevant to their country's most pressing health needs. Dr. Mahler, Director General of the World Health Organisation, underlines the deficiencies of conventional medical training: "Most of the world's medical schools prepare doctors not to care for the health of the people but to engage in a medical practice that is blind to anything but disease and the technology for dealing with it." [17]

Doctors' training is very expensive. It rarely opens the students' eyes to their country's major health problems or to an awareness of the social and economic roots of ill-health. In Bangladesh medical students spend far longer than their British counterparts studying subjects such as anatomy, at the expense of gaining an understanding of disease prevention and common health problems. They are encouraged to depend on medicines. For example, throughout five years' training, not a single lecture is devoted to appropriate non-drug treatments for diarrhoea, although diarrhoeal diseases account for over half the country's illness. [18] It is hardly surprising that these doctors prescribe expensive anti-diarrhoeal drugs and rarely encourage oral rehydration, which would enable people to take advantage of a safe and inexpensive means of saving lives.

Most Third World medical students come from wealthier families and many are totally ignorant about the reality of life for the mass of the poor. Neither their background nor their training motivate them to work in the rural areas where conditions are primitive and health facilities very basic. Many opt for private practice and specialised medicine. A Brazilian doctor sees the trend as so well-established that the first question invariably put to newly trained doctors is what they plan to specialise in. He comments that "Specialisation is getting so far-fetched that there will be specialists in the retina of the eye and the right hand". [19]

It is hardly surprising that Third World doctors congregate in the urban areas. In the towns of Bangladesh there is one doctor for every 1,200 inhabitants. But in the rural areas, where over 90% of the population lives, there is one doctor for every 31,300 people. [20] Similarly, in North Yemen, the hospitals in the country's three largest towns, catering for only 7% of the population, employ more than half the doctors in the country and 60% of all trained nurses. [21]

Often Third World countries lose out on the expensive investment they make in medical training as doctors migrate to richer countries for better pay and access to advanced technology that poorer countries cannot afford. Britain is just one of the rich nations benefiting from this drain on Third World resources. [22] The

Bangladesh Government is particularly concerned by the exodus of doctors to the Middle East "for better monetary gains". [23]

Most developing countries also suffer from a chronic shortage of trained pharmacists, who obviously have an essential part to play in the safe and efficient distribution of drugs. Like the doctors, many are creamed off by the private sector. A British professor of pharmacology writes: "Of the pharmacists who qualify either locally or overseas, very few enter government service. Most enter commercial pharmacy practice in the larger urban areas. Thus, although many students may train in pharmacy (at their country's expense), very few actually become available to deal with the basic pharmaceutical problems of their developing country." [24]

PUBLIC DRUG DISTRIBUTION

Different countries break down their health expenditure in different ways so it is difficult to make accurate comparisons of spending on drugs as opposed to other health inputs. For example, expenditure on drugs for hospitals may be shown under the hospitals budget, or under the national drug budget. Moreover, country-by-country comparisons are distorted by the fact that salaries are very much lower in most developing countries. However, WHO calculates that, whereas most developed countries allocate 10-20% of their health budgets for drug purchases, some developing countries are spending over 40% of their health budget on drugs. [25]

There is little doubt that out of total health expenditure, poor countries allocate proportionately more for drugs than many rich nations. However, in terms of meeting actual needs, the funds allocated for drug purchases are often hopelessly inadequate. For example, in Bangladesh the drugs budget in 1979 was equivalent to £4.6 million, an expenditure of about 5p a head. [26]

Furthermore, the distribution of drugs, like that of health facilities, is highly uneven. The situation in Tanzania is representative of other poor countries. The Tanzanian Government's 1979 *Evaluation of the Health Sector* shows that the main hospital in the capital is allocated 14% of the nation's drug budget. By contrast, all the government dispensaries put together only receive 15%. Thus, it is hardly surprising that little more than a third of the rural dispensaries were found to have an adequate supply of medicines. [27]

Shortage of key drugs is a problem common to dispensaries throughout the Third World, particularly in remote areas. But in some countries even the central medical stores are known to run out of essential supplies. For example, the central government stores in the capital of North Yemen sometimes exhausts stocks of penicillin and folic acid. By contrast, large quantities of less useful medicines, such as hormones, are freely available, and from time to time there is a glut of a particular drug which is farmed out to the dispensaries because the expiry date is close. [28]

Many Third World countries lack administrators with the technical skills needed to operate an efficient drug distribution system. To avoid wastage, officials responsible for drug supply need to be in a position both to assess actual drug requirements for the whole country, and to operate tight controls. In practice, they are seldom in a position to do either. The extremes of climate in many poor countries make the shelf-life of drugs a crucial factor. Bureaucratic inefficiency and lack of understanding that medicines cannot be treated as ordinary goods often means that drugs are left lying around in docks and airports, where the ambient temperature may be 100 degrees fahrenheit. Lack of refrigeration facilities and difficult transport compound the problems, so that the quality and potency of some drugs may be seriously impaired long before they reach the shelves of the rural health posts. For instance, this is often the case with polio vaccines transported over long distances in unrefrigerated vans. A physiotherapist in Nigeria finds that a number of the young polio victims she has to treat have cards showing that they were "immunised". [29]

A recent study of medicine distribution through the public sector in south Cameroon indicates the extent of wastage through inefficient record-keeping, ordering, storage and transport. The Dutch anthropologist who carried out the research calculates that because of the inefficiency of the central drug agency, only about 65% of the medicines they should receive actually reach the health centres. [30]

In some countries, because administrative controls are weak, drugs are stolen from hospital and clinic dispensaries and given to relatives or sold on the black market. In the capital of Bangladesh government hospital employees are known to be selling medicines from the hospital stores to traders in the well- supplied Mitford market. [31] In Zambia, in 1980, President Kaunda exposed a racket in which government doctors and nurses were known to be selling drugs from government clinics to private doctors who then sold them to their patients for three times the price originally paid by the Government. [32]

A detailed study of drug availability in three primary health care units in rural India relates the scarcity of useful drugs to wasteful drug purchases. The authors of the study found that "most of the drugs purchased were by trade names which were several times costlier than the equivalent drugs with generic names". An uneconomic assortment of different brands of almost identical drugs were stocked and "valuable resources were wasted in the purchase of drugs with doubtful or limited therapeutic effectiveness, namely enzymes and vitamins". [33] By contrast many of the most useful drugs were in very short supply. Consequently, on average over 40% of patients were sent away to buy drugs not in stock. "Since there were no chemists' shops at any of the primary health centre villages, the villagers had to obtain them either from the city market or go without them." [34]

Clearly, lack of money is only one cause of the serious shortages of drugs for primary health care. Problems of mismanagement, wasteful purchases and overprescribing have to be tackled to avoid even greater wastage as drug budgets are increased. The most obvious consequence of rural dispensaries running out of drugs is that people stop going to them. Meanwhile governments have to go on paying for health facilities that are under-used, and paramedics find it doubly hard gaining acceptance as health educators when they cannot deliver basic drugs.

PRIVATE DRUG DISTRIBUTION

The shortcomings of the public health sector and the relative and growing affluence of a small sector of the population have encouraged the rapid growth of private medicine in most developing countries. In Third World cities, in particular, where those with the greatest purchasing power live, there is a concentration of private doctors and retail pharmacies, mostly run by non-pharmacists. In most Third World countries private drug sellers have also made significant inroads into the rural areas and a largely haphazard, uncontrolled system of drug distribution has evolved. A major problem in the rapid expansion of the private drug market is that, whereas drug manufacturers and retailers have been quick to develop the potential market in the rural areas, they have shown insufficient interest in contributing either capital or technical expertise to developing the necessary infrastructure for medicines to be distributed safely and efficiently. Consequently, transport and communication facilities remain bad and drugs are frequently dispensed by untrained salesmen and unlicensed traders. [35]

Private drug sales have boomed and dwarfed distribution by the public sector. In some developing countries the value of drugs distributed through the private sector is over 90% of the total. This is the case in Bangladesh, Nepal and North Yemen. [36]

Few Third World governments have succeeded in imposing any meaningful controls on private drug sales. Consequently, medicines that can only be obtained on a doctor's prescription in developed countries are freely available over the counter or from street traders in poor countries. Whereas less than a quarter of drugs sold in Britain are products that do not require a prescription, it is estimated that in some developing countries up to 75% of medicines are bought without prescriptions. [37]

Drug control agencies in developing countries are generally very poorly funded and understaffed, so they are in no position to carry out regular inspections of drug stores or crack down on illegal sales. Some Third World governments are also reluctant to regulate the sale of drugs too strictly, on the grounds that medicine sellers may be providing the only source of treatment available especially to the poor. A 1979 official report explains that in Bangladesh: "Restrictions regarding prescriptions are not strictly enforced, particulary because of the small number of qualified physicians in the country and the low level of medical coverage." [38]

There are potential benefits to be weighed against the risks in allowing some drugs to be sold without a prescription. For example, in Bangladesh the contraceptive pill is sold in pharmacies, general stores, even on market food stalls by people with absolutely no medical training. One month's cycle costs about 1p. A relatively

25

small number of women will suffer adverse, even dangerous, side-effects from taking the pill without medical supervision. But if the pill were only available on a doctor's prescription, as in developed countries, many poor women would have to go without it, because there are so few doctors and they are expensive to consult. Consequently, they would be deprived of a relatively safe and reliable contraceptive, when the risks of pregnancy and childbirth are much greater in poor communities.

Nevertheless the uncontrolled distribution of drugs on the private market presents major problems, particularly for the Third World poor. The situation in Bangladesh, described in a Government report, is in no way atypical of other developing countries: ''Almost all the retail drug shops are owned and run by non-pharmacists and/or untrained persons. Drugs and medicines, including dangerous drugs, are often sold as ordinary articles of commerce ... leading to misuse and waste.'' [39] Drug sellers are not in business to recommend cost-effective treatments. They are out to earn a living.

It is sometimes argued that controls and rationalisation of commercial drug distribution will be of little benefit to the poor since the main drug consumers are the rich. There is no doubt that the wealthy in developing countries spend more on drugs than the poor, but the differential can be surprisingly small. For example, a study of drug use in a town in southern Brazil revealed that families in the richest neighbourhood spent only two-and-a-half times more a month on medicines than poor families from the shanty towns. [40]

But the weight of evidence suggests that it is the poor who stand to gain most from controls on private drug sales. In the absence of adequate health services, the poor turn to drug sellers for treatment and advice. An anthropologist has made a detailed study of where people in a small town in El Salvador go for treatment when they fall ill. She has found that the commercial drug sellers are an important source of treatment for rich and poor alike. But it is the *poorest* who rely on them most. They cannot afford to consult a doctor as well as buy medicines, so they go straight to the drug stores. [41] There, they may be victims of pressurised sales tactics as ''clerks and owners consistently recommended more expensive medications and more medications to their customers seeking health care advice''. [42]

In most developing countries, neither the public nor the private drug distribution system caters for the needs of the poor. As the Dutch anthropologist who studied the government and commercial distribution in south Cameroon concludes, ''The present inefficiency favours exactly those who are least in need of medical help and, moreover, are most able to pay for it. In other words, the current inefficient medicine distribution perpetuates and aggravates existing inequalities both in economic and health conditions.'' [43]

The poor are at the mercy of the drug sellers and the dictates of the market. In the next chapters we look at the implications of this dependence and examine the conflict between what the poor need and the rich choose to sell.

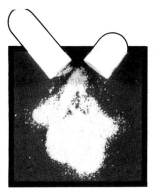

CHAPTER 3

PRODUCERS' MARKET

IN MOST countries, rich and poor alike, drugs are produced and sold by private business. So even life-saving medicines are subject to normal market forces. In developing countries the mass of the poor lack purchasing power, so they have little impact on the dynamics of the drug market. Consequently, the type of drugs marketed may bear no relation to a poor country's most pressing disease problems.

An Indian doctor puts the problem forcefully: "The drug industry, like any other industry, produces only to the extent that drugs can be sold at a reasonable profit in the market, irrespective of the needs of the people. The majority of our population is very poor. It is precisely this poor section that requires more medical attention and hence larger quantities of drugs. But since these people do not have money to buy the drugs, the industry ... neglects this section of the populace ... This happens because the logic of present day society is such that production is geared to the demand in the market, irrespective of the needs of the people." [1]

Scientists and managers within the industry are acutely aware that poor people are deprived of vital drugs. Poverty is the main constraint and drug producers are in no position to end poverty. The pharmaceutical industry acknowledges, however, that it has "special" obligations "arising from its involvement in public health". [2] In practice actual marketing policies are inevitably determined by the demands of running a viable and profitable commercial operation. Companies have workers to pay and shareholders that want a return on their investment.

A spokesman for the British drug industry did not mince words in explaining the constraints on manufacturers: "You must understand that the reason multi-national companies try to grab back as much profit as possible out of the less developed countries is frankly because they are suspicious of the future stability of their operations there." "I would just be talking rubbish if I were to say that the multinational companies were operating in the less developed countries primarily for the welfare of those countries... They are not bishops, they are businessmen." [3]

Bearing in mind that there are business constraints, in this chapter we examine how far the drugs marketed in poor countries are relevant to public health needs - ultimately whether the drug market is contributing more to alleviate or to perpetuate poverty.

RICH WORLD CONTROL

We have seen the extent to which the world distribution of drugs is skewed in favour of the rich. There is a similar imbalance in drug production. About 70% of world drug production (by value) corresponds to drugs manufactured in Western industrialised countries. A further 19% of total production is located in Eastern European and other centrally planned economies. As little as 11% of pharmaceutical production takes place in the Third World as a whole. [4]

The imbalance is even greater in the control of world trade in pharmaceuticals. The US, France, West Germany, Britain, Switzerland and other rich industrialised nations dominate 90% of drug shipments. About two-thirds of these are controlled by just 50 European and US-based transnational companies. [5]

Production has remained largely concentrated in the major industrialised countries because some (but not all) stages in the manufacturing process require sophisticated and costly technology. The image of monolithic difficulties in all areas of drug production is false. It serves to reinforce the poor world's dependence on the rich. No country can be entirely self-sufficient in drug production without a fine chemicals industry to provide *chemical intermediates* which are the starting point for producing most modern drugs. But a chemical industry is not essential. Switzerland, one of the world's leading drug producing nations, does not produce its own intermediates, but imports them for processing into *bulk drugs*. [6]

The technology needed to produce some bulk drugs from imported chemical intermediates is relatively straightforward, with the necessary technical know-how and resources. [7] But some bulk drugs production can be particularly difficult. For example, the fermentation plants needed to produce antibiotics are expensive and uneconomic without large-scale production. There are also varying degrees of difficulty in the third stage of processing the bulk drugs into *formulations* or finished dosage forms (i.e. the actual tablets). For example, it is complicated to manufacture ampoules for injections because sterile conditions are essential, but relatively simple to produce tablets and capsules. The final stage of *packaging* or repackaging finished drugs is easy and requires minimal equipment. This cost-saving processing is well within the technical capacity of even the least developed countries. [8]

But most Third World countries either have no manufacturing facilities at all, or local manufacture consists of little more than repacking and simple formulation of some bulk drugs. Forty-five of the world's smallest and poorest nations are totally dependent on imports of finished drugs. They are mostly in Africa which accounts for only 0.5% of world production (compared with 5.61% of world production in Asia and a further 5.26% in Latin America in 1977). [9]

In countries with local production, there is a wide variation in how much each country continues to rely on imports of finished drugs. For example, Kenya and Nigeria respectively import about 75% and 90% of finished drugs consumed locally, whereas Bangladesh imports under 20% and Colombia only 5%. But all these countries share a heavy dependence on foreign suppliers for large quantities of drugs and some intermediates. [10]

Little more than a handful of developing countries have an advanced drug industry. Between them, India, Egypt, Brazil, Argentina, Mexico and South Korea account for two-thirds of all Third World production. With the exception of Korea, these countries all have a chemical industry capable of producing most drug intermediates, and the technical expertise to carry out research and development into drugs and manufacturing processes. Indian state-owned and private companies now export not only drugs but also their own technology to other developing countries. [11]

Despite the sophistication of local production, even India, Brazil, Mexico and other industrialised countries still rely on foreign manufacturers for some bulk drugs, chemical intermediates, and advanced production technology. For example, in 1978/9 India was still importing over 40% of its bulk drug requirements and a recent study on foreign technology in the Indian pharmaceutical industry highlights the fact that the local industry is held back because it lacks advanced technology developed by foreign manufacturers. [12]

The continuing dominance of foreign firms in the Third World drug market is confirmed by a 1981 report from the United Nations Centre for Transnational Corporations (UNCTC), which includes case studies on developing countries with varying degrees of local production. [13] With the exception of Egypt, where the large public sector caters for 70% of the country's drug requirements and leaves foreign companies only a 14% share of the market, in all the countries studied foreign companies take the lion's share of the market: 59% in Argentina (1978), 70% in India (1977), 82% in Costa Rica (1977), 88% in Brazil (1979), 90% in Kenya and Colombia (1978) and 95% in Sierra Leone (1976). [14]

There are more than 10,000 companies producing drugs around the world, but 90% of pharmaceutical trade is dominated by little more than 100 manufacturers.[15] The top twenty-five European and US-controlled transnationals controlled 44% of world drug sales in 1978. [16] They are shown in the diagram overleaf which also shows that the market leaders each account for only 2-4% of world sales. This low degree of concentration in overall sales is misleading because the drug market is fragmented into about a dozen sub-markets (such as antibiotics, antihistamines, tranquilizers and other specific types of drugs). In each of these sub-markets sales concentration is very high with individual manufacturers controlling from a quarter to over half of total sales. [17]

According to UNCTC, "At the level of bulk drug production, the evidence for concentration is even more striking". [18] 650 bulk drugs were produced in the United States in 1975, and of these only four were made by more than four manufacturers and nearly 500 were produced by a monopoly supplier. [19]

The market power of these major producers accounts for the rich industrialised countries' strong trade surplus in pharmaceuticals. [20] By contrast the poor world had a negative trade balance in pharmaceuticals with the rich world amounting to around 4,000 million dollars in 1980. [21]

Diagram 4. THE MAJOR PHARMACEUTICAL COMPANIES OF THE WORLD, 1978–1979

1978 Rank	Name	Pharmaceutical Sales $M 1978	$M 1979	As % Total Sales in 1979	As % World Total 1978	1979 R&D Expenditure $M	As % Drug Sales	Origin
1	Hoechst	2 200	2 300	16	3.8	200	9	German
2	Bayer	1 890	1 850	13	3.2	300		German
3	Hoffmann La Roche	1 380		44	2.4	300		Swiss
4	Merck	1 355	2 004	84	2.4	180	9	American
5	Ciba-Geigy	1 355	1 595	28	2.4	190	12	Swiss
6	American Home Products	1 279	1 448	43	2.2	90	6	American
7	Sandoz	1 242	1 289	48	2.2	170	13	Swiss
8	Pfizer	1 193	1 430	52	2.1	120	8	American
9	Lilly	1 063	1 003	45	1.9	150	15	American
10	Takeda	1 062	1 092	59	1.9	80	7	Japanese
11	Boehringer-Ingelheim	1 027	1 092	77	1.8	120	11	German
12	Warner-Lambert	971	1 045	32	1.7	80	8	American
13	Rhône-Poulenc	907	1 242	16	1.6	100	8	French
14	Upjohn	859	956	63	1.5	120	13	American
15	Bristol-Myers	745	946	34	1.3	100	11	American
16	Squibb	723	900		1.3	60	7	American
17	Schering-Plough	690	757	53	1.2	70	9	American
18	Abbott	683	830	49	1.2	70	8	American
19	Smith Kline	671	862	64	1.2	90	10	American
20	Glaxo	670	955	68	1.2	75	8	British
21	Sterling-Winthrop	661	768	58	1.2	50	7	American
22	Schering AG	640	635	42	1.1	90	14	German
23	Beecham	635	711	31	1.1	70	11	British
24	Johnson and Johnson	608	760		1.1	80	10	American
25	ICI	599	697	6	1.1	65	9	British

Figures from company reports and from information from Interpharma; *Scrip*, various issues; Aries, *op. cit.*; *European Chemical News*, various issues. R&D expenditures are approximate and should be used with caution. They have however been considered as realistic estimates by industrial experts consulted.
Table A.2., page 243 of the English original study.

In recent years Third World countries have been doubling their expenditure on medicines every four years, whereas their GNP has been doubling only every sixteen years. [22] Pharmaceutical imports average only about 2% of the value of all commodity imports to developing countries, but according to WHO, "For developing countries importation of pharmaceuticals is one of the fastest growing drains on hard foreign currency..." [23]

Spiralling drug costs present an acute problem for most developing countries because of their dependence on imports. The Health Minister of Zimbabwe drew attention to this when he addressed a regional meeting of African pharmacists in April 1982. "We are all aware that this country like practically every Third World country, is experiencing the ill-effects of inflation, falling commodity prices, rising prices of imports leading to unfavourable terms of trade. Foreign exchange allocations which were adequate for the import of 'essential' medicines a year or two ago now fall far short of the mark. This is due to the increase in the rates levied by the traditional manufacturers or agents outside Zimbabwe." [24]

This dependence can have both social and economic costs. In the words of WHO: "In developing countries the pharmaceutical sector is a captive market which has an effect on the health care system, and especially on the *cost* and *type* of drugs supplied." [25] (our emphasis) We shall concentrate in this chapter on the *type* of drugs marketed in the Third World and look at the question of cost in the next.

PLACEBOS IN WASTEFUL ABUNDANCE

To recap: developing countries need large quantities of a small number of essential drugs, above all those that can prevent and treat disease. These include antibacterials and antimalarials; drugs that are needed for specific conditions (such as insulin for diabetics), and some key medicines to provide effective relief from painful symptoms. The terms 'essential' and 'non- essential' are obviously very loose. Any attempt to evaluate the usefulness of specific drugs is likely to produce as many views as experts - depending on the criteria behind the selection and where the drugs are to be used. A clear illustration of the difficulties is that the same combination of two anti-tuberculous drugs which was defined as extremely useful by one WHO working group on tuberculosis was rejected by the expert committee that drew up the WHO Selection of Essential Drugs. [26]

But there is a clear consensus of independent expert opinion on some types of drugs that are either wasteful or unnecessary or both - and therefore harmful to the needs of the Third World poor. These have been expressly excluded from the WHO list. [27] The obvious categories include most combination drugs (particuarly irrational mixtures such as antibiotics and vitamins); the latest and most expensive formulations of drugs like antidepressants, and the mass of multivitamin and mineral tonics, and cough and cold preparations which have little value except as placebos. [28]

The 'ideal' of what the poor need clashes with the reality of the drug market. In the words of two senior pharmacologists: "Unfortunately a good proportion of

31

the drugs available are of little importance in terms of essential health care and they are marketed mainly because they can be sold and not because they benefit the health of the population." [29]

Throughout the Third World there is evidence that drug consumption habits have been indiscriminately transferred from rich nations to poor. The causes have been pinpointed by WHO. "In recent years many medicinal products have been marketed with little concern for the differing health needs and priorities of different countries. Promotion activities of the drug manufacturers have created a demand greater than the actual needs." [30]

There are countless illustrations of distorted priorities in the type of drugs manufactured and imported into developing countries. The value of vitamins and tonics imported into North Yemen in 1980 was 17.8% of total pharmaceutical imports. But only 1.3% of the total was spent on importing drugs to treat three of the country's most widespread diseases - malaria, bilharzia and TB - affecting an estimated 800,000 people. [31] On one estimate, at least 65% of all imports are for non-essential drugs, both placebos and symptomatic treatments for self-limiting conditions. [32]

The WHO Essential Drug List includes one cough suppressant: codeine. On the drug market in the Philippines there are 162 different brands of cough suppressants, and under a dozen are based on codeine. Spending on these cough preparations represented 12% of total drug expenditure in the Philippines in 1980. [33]

A 1977 report on local production in Sri Lanka by the Chairman of the State Pharmaceutical Corporation underlines the distortion between what will sell and what is needed in a market with 97% of local production controlled by just seven manufacturers, five of them subsidiaries of leading transnationals. "Vitamin preparations, soluble aspirin and cough remedies accounted for over 50% of production. They were elegantly presented, heavily promoted and used by the affluent. For example, the two largest firms made 18 different combinations of vitamins with or without iron, which were swallowed by the well-nourished who did not need them. The undernourished could not afford to buy them." [34]

MULTIVITAMIN TONICS

The quantity of multivitamin tonics marketed is just one illustration of the wider problem of wasteful products that swamp the market in even the poorest countries. In Nepal a 1980 study found that out of 2,000 different products on the drug market, 733 - more than one third - were 'tonics'. Anaemia and malnutrition are major health problems in Nepal, but as the report concluded, "Those who need iron and vitamins can seldom afford to buy these expensive proprietary preparations... A few inexpensive preparations of iron and vitamins could effectively and easily replace the 733 formulations, and enormous savings could be made as a result." [35]

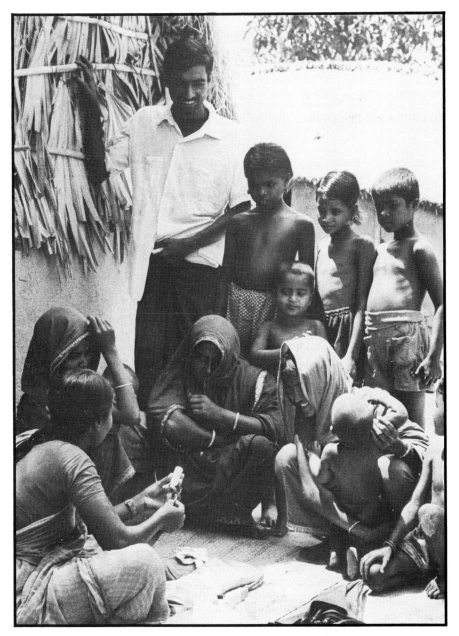

Primary health care brings appropriate treatment to the rural poor. Health workers are trained to dispense a limited range of the most effective drugs where they are really necessary.

One of the most glaring examples of demand being wastefully stimulated in poor countries is for preparations containing vitamin B12. This essential drug is prescribed in Britain only for pernicious anaemia and other vitamin B12 deficiency states. In contrast to developed countries, pernicious anaemia is relatively rare in the Third World. Of course many poor people suffer from dietary deficiencies, but these are far more commonly due to lack of folate or iron, than to vitamin B12 deficiency. [36] But vitamin B12 is amongst the most widely sold drugs in many Third World countries. There were no less than 126 formulations containing B12 on the Indian market and 160 on sale in Brazil in 1978, compared with 16 listed in the *British National Formulary*. [37] Many of the formulations containing vitamin B12 are multivitamins. This is highly wasteful according to the *British National Formulary:* "There is *no* justification for prescribing multiple-ingredient vitamin preparations containing these substances". [38] (original emphasis) Moreover, many are tablets or liquids, but since most cases of B12 deficiency are caused by a problem of malabsorption from the stomach, taking B12 by mouth is "futile" according to the experts. [39]

Doctors in Brazil have also expressed concern that some of the injectable preparations of vitamin B12 are sold in highly wasteful dosages. Of the products marketed in Brazil, 106 ranged from dosages of 5,000 to 30,000 micrograms per millilitre. They included two formulations sold under the brand name Retar B12 by the British manufacturers, Glaxo. This, despite the fact that in Britain the highest dosage form recommended or sold by Glaxo for B12 injectables is 1,000 micrograms per millilitre. [40] According to the *British National Formulary* : "There is no evidence that larger doses provide any additional benefit in vitamin B12 neuropathy." [41]

ESSENTIAL DRUGS IN SHORT SUPPLY

In most developing countries private importers and chemists stock a wide range of expensive - mainly foreign - brands of all sorts of different products. But basic drugs like penicillin are invariably in short supply and rarely available at all outside the health service dispensaries. Their low cost makes them a particularly unattractive proposition for private importers, especially when they are held to fixed price mark-ups. The situation in Mozambique before independence closely resembles the reality in other non-drug-producing countries today. Penicillin could only be bought in fancy film-coated capsules. These were sold in small packs at several times the prices of ordinary penicillin tablets used in British hospitals at the time. Only one distributor had even bothered to import oral penicillin. It would have been against the company's interests to shop around for a good price, so they chose an expensive brand that guaranteed them a good profit margin on sales. [42]

Attempts to control profit margins on drug sales in the free market have also acted as a disincentive on local production of low cost essential drugs. As a result, even India - a major drug producing nation - experiences shortages of supplies of essential drugs due to the skewed pattern of drug production. This was highlighted

34

in a recent joint report by the Indian Council of Social Science Research (ICSSR) and Indian Council of Medical Research (ICMR) which describes the situation as one where "the drugs required by the poor are not produced on the main ground that there is no profitable market and adequate demand for them, while the country continues to be flooded by a plethora of costly and wasteful drugs meant for the minor illnesses of the rich and well-to-do." [43]

The ICSSR and ICMR explain that out of total drug production in India in 1976, "25 per cent is taken away by vitamins, tonics, health restoratives and enzyme digestants mostly consumed by the relatively well-fed urban population. Twenty per cent is covered by antibiotics, only 1.3 per cent by sulphonamides (a very cheap and useful anti-infective) and 1.4 per cent by antituberculous drugs" ... "Dapsone, the basic drug for leprosy costing only Rupees 5 [under 30 pence] a year's treatment, is always in short supply." [44] Yet India has a third of the world's leprosy sufferers (about 4 million people) and an estimated 8 million active TB cases - the equivalent of the entire population of London. [45]

India has literally thousands of drug manufacturers, ranging from very small local units to about 100 large-scale manufacturers under varying degrees of Indian and foreign control. All must share responsibility for producing and creating demand for non-essential drugs. In terms of the total *numbers* of these products, many more are marketed by local than foreign producers. A United Nations Conference on Trade and Development (UNCTAD) study quotes figures for 1972 showing that foreign companies accounted for 15% of all the different brands of vitamins and tonics, 21% of antacids, 14% of digestive enzymes and 13% of cough and cold preparations. [46] But the UNCTAD study also revealed that up to one-third of all the drug formulations marketed by foreign- controlled companies in 1972 consisted of vitamins and tonics, cough syrups, tranquilisers, sedatives and painkillers. [47]

A number of studies have concluded that the way in which local production in India started up as an 'off-shoot' of the rich world drug industry is to a large extent responsible for its failure to cater for the needs of the mass of people. [48] For example, according to the Hathi Committee on the drugs industry which reported to the Government in 1975, "In India, in spite of efforts to plan socio-economic growth, the drugs and pharmaceuticals industry ... operates on the principle of free market economics. The drugs industry is dominated by the foreign units which set the pattern in this industry. The drug needs of any country are characteristic of the climatic conditions, social behaviour and economic conditions in each society. The foreign units which evolve their policies for the rich countries in temperate climates, with radically different socio-economic conditions, operating in free-market systems, promote the same systems in India, which are adversely detrimental to our national interests." [49]

Controls introduced in India to try to limit production of non-essential drugs have failed to break the mould. Ironically in some instances they have backfired and actually held back increased production of essential drugs. [50] For example, we have already singled out the shortages of dapsone - for treating leprosy. The Indian

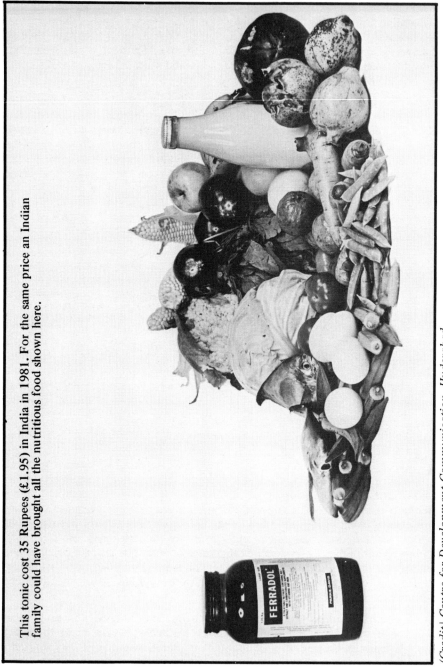

This tonic cost 35 Rupees (£1.95) in India in 1981. For the same price an Indian family could have brought all the nutritious food shown here.

(Credit) Centre for Development Communication, Hyderabad.

subsidiary of Wellcome which produces the drug confirm that "Dapsone is not commercially an attractive proposition for us to manufacture". [51] But they point out that Wellcome has been producing 12-14 tons of dapsone a year, when it was officially only licensed to produce 10.8 tons. By contrast, they say that the only other dapsone producer in India, a public sector company, has been unable to produce more than 5-6 tons, despite their licensed capacity of 15 tons. In 1978 Wellcome attempted to get permission to more than double their dapsone production capacity but this was not forthcoming for two-and-a-half years. [52]

The complex situation of drug production in India, added to what one analyst has described as its "labyrinthine regulatory statutes", [53] illustrate the obvious fact that it would be simplistic to ascribe all blame to manufacturers for shortages of essential drugs. Nonetheless, subsidiaries of European and US manufacturers are aggravating the problems for developing countries by producing marginally useful drugs - and in some cases even drugs that they would not be authorised to sell on the home market. We can best illustrate the problems by taking a closer look at drug production in Bangladesh which, in contrast to India, is more typical of the situation in developing countries as a whole.

BANGLADESH: A CASE STUDY
In 1982 there are 166 licensed drug producers in Bangladesh. But the local market is dominated by just eight foreign-controlled manufacturers - mostly subsidiaries of European and US transnationals - which account for three- quarters of local production. [54] Besides taking the lion's share of sales turnover on the private market, these companies have been near monopoly suppliers of drugs for the public health services, controlling about 80% of total government purchases. [55]

According to Drug Administration officials, by comparison with other sectors of manufacturing industry the drug producers are to be congratulated for the dramatic rise in production they have achieved. In the decade after independence, production capacity has more than trebled. [56] The drug market has also been growing rapidly - by about 20% a year at the end of the 1970s/early 1980s. Total sales turnover will have more than doubled in just four years from 1978 to 1982. [57]

Over 80% of drugs on the market are now locally produced. But all this means is that they are formulated and packaged in Bangladesh. No more than a handful of bulk drugs are actually produced there. The majority have to be imported and paid for in foreign exchange, and they are costing the country about Taka 600 million a year - a sum equivalent to 1.7 times the 1979/80 health budget. [58] This drain on foreign exchange, but above all the fact that about three-quarters of the population still has no regular access to vital drugs, makes it crucial that local production cater for priority needs. [59]

Faced with the needs of the poor, the reality of drug production in recent years jars. Market estimates for 1978 produced by the local branch of one foreign company reveal the skewed pattern of production: vitamins, iron tonics, cough and cold preparations, 'tonics and restoratives', 'volume restorers', enzymes and digestants, antacids and psychotropic drugs make up 33% of the market. By contrast, on these estimates, antibiotics, antiparasitic drugs and skin preparations for treating some of the country's major public health problems together account for under 23% of the market. [60] Market estimates drawn up for the previous year by another foreign company set the share of the market for vitamins and tonics alone at 30%, with a further 8% for tranquilisers, anti-depressants and sedatives. [61]

An expert committee reviewing the Bangladesh drug market in May 1982 concluded that of total drug expenditure in the country, "Nearly one third .... was spent on unnecessary and useless medicines such as vitamin mixtures, tonics, alkalisers, cough mixtures, digestive enzymes, palliatives, gripe water and hundreds of other similar products". [62]

NON-ESSENTIAL AND NOT SOLD IN BRITAIN

An analysis of products marketed by the subsidiaries of two leading British manufacturers with factories in Bangladesh reveals a product range top-heavy with drugs that are not relevant to priority needs. Full details of products listed in the 1981 price lists of the Bangladesh subsidiaries of Glaxo and Fisons appear as Appendices II and III. Only a quarter (14 out of 56) products marketed by Glaxo (Bangladesh) Limited and as few as 4 of the 31 products of Fisons (Bangladesh) Limited are formulations included in the WHO Selection of Essential Drugs. [63]

No less than 22 of Glaxo's range of 56 pharmaceutical products listed in the 1981 product list are vitamins and tonics. Only 3 of these are brands marketed in Britain and only 2 are basic formulations of vitamin A and vitamin B-complex. Most of the 19 extra vitamin products they have chosen to market in Bangladesh are "fruit-flavoured" and "sugar-coated" multivitamins and mixtures of multivitamins and minerals. Vitamin B12 which is an essential drug has been promoted by Glaxo in Bangladesh for non-essential uses as a general tonic. [64]

Of Fisons' 31 products listed as available in Bangladesh in 1981, less than a dozen are formulations marketed in Britain. Over half are vitamin, calcium and mineral preparations, only 2 of them single-ingredient preparations of folic acid and iron dextran that are considered essential by WHO. There are two antacids; one brand of aspirin and one of paracetamol; two cough preparations and two inappropriate antidiarrhoeals - one containing clioquinol - a drug that can have serious toxic side-effects crippling to the nervous system. [65]

Framycort ointment and Framygen Eye and Ear Drops marketed by Fisons in Bangladesh include neomycin sulphate. But in Britain the formulation of these products is different, as they contain framycetin sulphate instead of neomycin sulphate. [66] Some experts have expressed the view that "the rare but potentially serious adverse effects of *neomycin* in skin products makes it unacceptable, particularly because it has not been proven effective in such products". [67] (our emphasis)

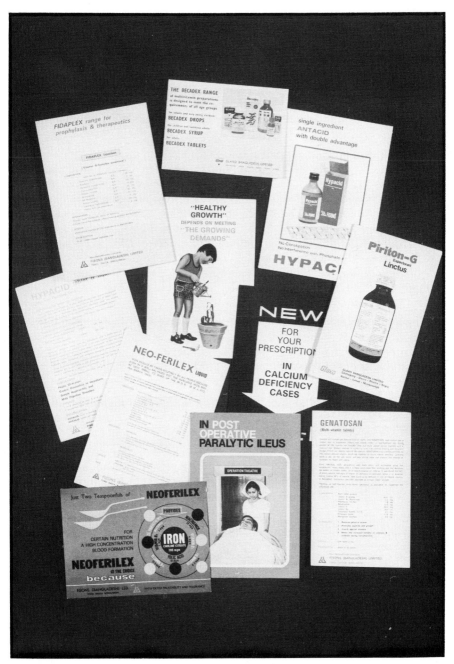

Glaxo and Fisons promotion material.

A number of multivitamin preparations can be highly wasteful because they contain amounts of vitamin far in excess of what the body can absorb. Commenting on one multi-ingredient "geriatric preparation" that Fisons has marketed in Bangladesh, a British Professor of Clinical Pharmacology (who is also a member of the Committee on Safety of Medicines - the British Drug Regulatory Agency) expressed the view that it is "inconceivable that Decatone would receive a Product Licence for sale in Britain". [68] We understand that Fisons (UK) have said that this product was withdrawn from sale in Bangladesh in 1979, although this has not been confirmed to us. [69]

Another Fisons' product that is not marketed in Britain, but has been widely sold in Bangladesh, is Digeplex - a liquid preparation of two digestive enzymes and some vitamin B-complex. The advertisement reproduced here claims that: "Its vitamin B-complex content will correct the underlying deficiencies which are the basic cause of digestive disorders. Digeplex gradually helps the patient in building up the natural emzymes." In the opinion of a British doctor this is a ludicrous claim with no scientific basis. [70] Another British doctor, Dr. Schweiger, who has worked in rural Bangladesh, is concerned about the widespread use of Digeplex for any abdominal complaint. He points out that "Gastric ulcers are already very common in Bangladesh... do you really want to put pepsin into such an ulcer? It will only make it worse." [71]

Commenting on the range of products manufactured in Bangladesh by Glaxo and Fisons, Dr. Schweiger concludes: "Bangladesh is a poor country and can ill afford to spend foreign exchange on non-essential items. The nutritional problems of the poor will not be solved by expensively packaged multivitamins which will only divert limited resources from other more relevant purchases." [72]

The comments received to date from Glaxo and Fisons on their product range appear at note 73. However, in our view, these do not provide a full answer to our criticisms.

Of course, the two British companies, whose product range we have studied in some detail, are not alone in marketing non-essential medicines in Bangladesh. Both the locally-owned companies and other foreign manufacturers are selling products of little relevance to the country's needs.

In terms of sheer *numbers* of different brands of cough syrups, tonics and other over-the-counter products, most are marketed by the national companies. [74] But by value the products that sell best are those of the transnationals. Amongst the top-selling tonics are Squibb's Verdivitone Elixir and Hoechst's Polytamin Tonic, the latter described in the May 1982 Expert Committee Report as a "combination vitamin tonic including vitamin B12 and alcohol; one of the most abused drugs on the market". [75] Hoechst argue in support of Polytamin that "Bangladesh is in a chronic state of malnourishment, the vital supply of polyvitamins is essential in countries where a balanced diet is not available"; and that "The ready-for-use liquid formulation is essential for those countries where safe drinking water supply is not available". [76]

DIGEPLEX

Digeplex relieves all symptoms which are due to improper digestion of protein and starch.

Digeplex offers more than just temporary relief of symptoms. Because its Vitamin B-Complex content will correct the underlying deficiencies which are the basic causes of digestive disorders. Digeplex gradually helps the patient in building up the natural enzymes.

COMPOSITION

Each 4 ml. (approximately one teaspoonful) contains :

Diastase	1:2000	(in tablet form)	...	12.5	mg.
Pepsin		...	...	...	10	mg.
Thiamine Mononitrate	U.S.P.	...	...	4	mg.
Riboflavine	B.P.	...	...	0.5	mg.
Pyridoxine Hydrochloride	B.P.	...	...	0.5	mg.
Cyanocobalamin	B.P.	...	...	2	mcg.
Nicotinamide	B.P.	...	...	10	mg.
dl -Panthenol		...	...	...	2	mg.

With adjuvants, flavouring and vehicle.

Digeplex is stabilised at a PH of 5 to 5.2 to ensure the stability of Diastase in presence of Hydrochloric acid secretion of the stomach.

DOSAGE

Adults : 1 to 2 teaspoonfuls immediately after meals.
Children : 1 teaspoonful after meals.

PRESENTATION

Bottles of 100 ml. & 170 ml.

 FISONS (BANGLADESH) LIMITED.
DACCA.

But the reality is that people in Bangladesh without safe water supplies and in a "chronic state of malnourishment" are in no position to buy multivitamin tonics costing more than a poor family's entire daily income. There are much cheaper sources of nutrients in local foods. Indeed, the chairman of ICI's local subsidiary explained to us that although doctors and drug sellers in Bangladesh add multivitamin preparations to almost any prescription, he considered that these products could not represent value for money in a country where spinach, limes and other fruit and vegetables are readily available. [77]

The growing dependence on vitamin and mineral tonics can have a damaging impact on the nutrition of the poor. This is the case when they spend money on tonics instead of food, but it can even present problems when they do not have to buy them. Dr. Schweiger who worked in rural Bangladesh explains: "Malnutrition is not treatable at all by drugs and it is the biggest single problem - malnutrition is treated with food. People will die from lack of calories long before they die from lack of a particular vitamin. I wonder very much about the patients I treated with my previous organisation. We gave a lot of multivitamin tablets there for children with malnutrition and I saw a lot of those children go slowly downhill because obviously the teaching message of more food requirement was not really accepted by the parents. If we gave tablets then the feeling may very well be, well we can't remember all the junk the health workers have told us, but these tablets 3 times a day is all we need...." [78]

When we spoke to local company managers in Bangladesh and queried the relevance of many of their products to the country's needs, most expressed their sensitivity to the sufferings of millions of their fellow citizens. None tried to suggest that the major health problems were anything other than malnutrition and infectious disease. Most argued that, so long as they were not in a position to help the poor, what harm could there be in catering for the needs of the affluent minority?

The Marketing Manager of Fisons (Bangladesh) Ltd expresses a view shared by others which he gives "as a citizen of Bangladesh", "not as a vitamins seller". He puts the question: "Why, on one hand, as a government, or as a policymaker of my country, do you allow me to buy and drive foreign cars, enjoy foreign colour television, put on expensive foreign clothes and smoke expensive foreign cigarettes and on the other, forbid me to take locally produced (under foreign collaboration) quality vitamins at locally competitive prices, specially when I think, or my doctors think that I need to take them! ... Please consider the country's situation in its entirety and if you cannot provide even sub-standard vitamins to everybody in the country who needs vitamins, at least do not put a bar on those who can afford to buy quality vitamins at lesser cost than the sub-standard vitamins". [79]

Critically, the argument hinges on how far medicines can be bracketed with cars, televisions and clothes, if this means that placebos intended for the well-to-do are produced *at the expense* of vital drugs needed by everyone, but particularly by the poor. The distortions in production in Bangladesh and other developing countries appear all the more acute when industry has set itself the "obligation" of producing drugs that "have full regard to the needs of public health". [80] Dr. Mahler, Director General of the World Health Organisation, is one of a growing number of people to have reached the clear conclusion that "We can no longer treat these vital components of people's health as normal commodities in the market-place. They have to be taken out of the market-place, and other ways may have to be found to produce these essential drugs." [81]

But apart from the difficulties of treating medicines as any other commodity, more holes can be knocked in the argument that the production and marketing of non-essential drugs does not really hurt the poor. As the ICSS and ICMR point out, it is misleading to suggest that only the well-off consume these unnecessary drugs. "They have a demonstration effect which misleads the poor also and becomes an additional channel for their exploitation." [82]

The poor are encouraged to buy multivitamin tonics and other non-essential products. These are routinely prescribed by doctors and chemists and are often bought at the expense of useful treatments. Some of the hard-hitting facts are revealed by a study of precriptions given to a sample of 90 women patients at an Indian hospital. This showed that when these women returned for treatment, only 26 had been able to buy all the medicines prescribed on their first visit; 27 had not had enough money to buy more than the first two items on the prescription, which were almost invariably a tonic and vitamin B-complex; 37 had been too poor to buy any of the drugs prescribed. [83]

Of those who had bought all the drugs prescribed, four had had to borrow money; some even used the cash they had been paid for being sterilised; one found the money by economising on what she bought with her son's daily wage of 4 rupees (about 20 pence). She had been prescribed two tonics and vitamin B-complex capsules. Almost all the prescriptions were identical; with tonics, vitamins and aspirin at the top of the list, and the important treatment often appeared in only about fifth position. Most of the drugs prescribed were well known brands. [84]

Turning back to our review of the product range of leading foreign manufacturers in Bangladesh, we discussed the wastage of a poor country's resources on non-essential drugs with the Association of British Pharmaceutical Industries. They advanced the argument that manufacturers in Bangladesh are merely catering to demand, and not actively creating the market for non-essential products. [85] This is not a view shared by Dr. Hye, the former Director of Drug Administration in Bangladesh, who states categorically: "Manufacturers are responsible for creating the demand for non-essential drugs in the first place and they are stimulating it with promotion sometimes even with forced sales." [86]

An insight into how demand can be created is given by the "Merck in Bangladesh Marketing Plan 1980(-1982)" of the local branch of the West German manufacturers, E. Merck. This reveals that they at any rate have little doubts about the effectiveness of promotion in creating demand. Merck's biggest selling product on the local market in 1979/80 was Neurobion, (containing vitamins B1, B6 and B12). [87] According to the Marketing Plan, Neurobion alone accounts for over

68% of the total market in neurotropic preparations. The marketing strategy outlined in the Plan states: "Our objective will be to achieve at least 75% market share by intensifying more promotional effort ..." and that "remarkable results can be achieved by motivating field force". The Marketing Plan also reveals that the "major threat" to business "is that the government may ban import of one or more of our fast moving items". Thus a key strategy will be "to maintain very good relations with government officials in Health and Commerce Ministry to guarantee importability for our products". [88]

Merck's promotional strategy has obviously paid off. According to Dr. Hye, the popularity of Neurobion (in its injectable form) is demonstrated by the fact that in 1980 £77,777 worth of the product was imported. [89] This was equivalent to 1.94% of total imports of all finished drugs in 1980. [90]

Poor countries like Bangladesh have enough problem with the adverse balance of trade without having to foot the bill for imports of non-essential finished drugs. [91] But the unnecessary drain on foreign exchange is not confined to drugs in final dosage form. The value of imported raw materials in 1980 was 38 times greater than that of finished drugs. [92] To take the raw materials imports of one company alone, commenting on the situation in 1980/81 Dr. Hye writes: "Almost 40% of the foreign exchange allocation to Fisons (Bangladesh) Ltd for the import of pharmaceutical raw materials is used up for making non-essential, practically useless preparations." [93]

But the non-essential medicines produced with these raw materials are not only draining valuable foreign exchange, they are also taking up limited production capacity that could be used to produce the drugs the country really needs. In the words of the Expert Committee reporting to the Bangladesh Government on drug policy in May 1982: "Though the multinationals have all the technologies and know-how to produce sophisticated essential drugs and basic pharmaceutical raw materials, in Bangladesh these companies are engaged mostly in formulation of simple drugs including many useless products such as vitamin mixtures, tonics, gripe water etc." [94] As a result 90 of the 182 essential drugs needed for the public health services are not produced at all in Bangladesh. [95]

* * * * *

The situation in Bangladesh is not unique. Other detailed case-studies in very different developing countries have shown up similar problems in production and wide-scale promotion of drugs which are far removed from priority needs. An illustration of this comes from the research carried out by a French pharmacist into the products marketed in Mexico by the three Swiss pharmaceutical giants. Of 165 products marketed in Mexico in 1978 by Roche, Ciba-Geigy and Sandoz, only 36 were drugs included in Mexico's selection of 426 drugs essential for public health care. Of these 16 were formulations on the WHO Essential Drug List. [96]

But some of their top-selling products were hardly 'essential'. [97] For example as much as 62% of Roche's sales turnover in Mexico in 1978 was made up of just 5 products. [98] One of these was Cal-C-Tose (a chocolate-flavoured mixture of vitamins and minerals) popular amongst the well-to-do in Mexico. [99] A second of Roche's best-selling products was Redoxon. This, despite the fact that Dr. Brudon - who carried out the research - calculated that Mexicans could have obtained their necessary vitamin C intake by buying oranges - at one tenth of the cost of Redoxon. [100]

* * * * *

In the next chapter we focus on the critical area of prices. But to sum up the equally important question of the *type* of drugs that major manufacturers choose to market in developing countries: lip service is increasingly being paid to the need for a limited selection of essential drugs for developing countries. But in most cases the need to stick to priorities to benefit the majority is applied only to the public requirements of the public health services. Attempts to reduce private sales of non-essential drugs have often been fiercely resisted. [101]

A 1980 report "based on the opinions of individuals in the industry", with the title "Opportunities for Pharmaceuticals in the Developing World over the next twenty years", is - to say the least - not encouraging. It states: "The most important requirements for drugs by the developing countries will continue to be for antibiotics, cough and cold preparations, vitamins, analgesics, hormones and tonics, but demand for other types will increase in line with the extent of greater urbanisation and industrialisation." [102]

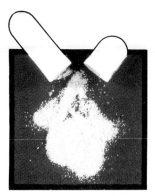

CHAPTER 4

POOR VALUE
FOR THE POOR?
Drug prices

"It has now become common knowledge that international trade - and specifically North-South trade in pharmaceuticals - bears hardly any relation to the objective costs faced by suppliers, but is rather one of the most striking manifestations of unequal exchange which has the ultimate effect of creating and sustaining the underdevelopment of the Third World." (Dr. Rainford, Deputy Secretary General of the Secretariat of the Caribbean Community (CARICOM), 1980.) [1]

TO POOR PEOPLE throughout the Third World drug prices are astronomically high both in relation to wages and to the cost of basic necessities. In Mexico the best-selling brand of the antibacterial drug cotrimoxazole is Roche's Bactrim. Just 20 tablets - enough for a short course of treatment - cost Pesos 138.60 (over £3) in 1978. A peasant family lucky enough to have a few hens would have had to sell 110 eggs to buy those 20 tablets of Bactrim. For the same amount of money a family of four could have bought enough black beans to provide their basic diet for two weeks, or 33 kilos of tortillas, equivalent to bread in Europe or chapatis in India. [2]

The same drug, cotrimoxazole, is available locally from other manufacturers at less than half the price. But Mexicans buy over a million packs of Bactrim each year. The products of the 'big name' manufacturers are usually the most expensive. Promotion ensures that they are also the market leaders. Out of about 9,900 different pharmaceutical products on the Mexican market in 1978, just 80 cornered a third of the total market. Without exception, these top-selling drugs are brand-name products of the major US and European research-based companies. Only six were developed within the last 2-6 years. The remainder are well-established and many are now off patent. They could be bought far more cheaply from non-research-based manufacturers. [3]

The situation in Mexico is in no way unique. Throughout the Third World poor people pay high prices for expensive brands when far cheaper alternatives exist. In this chapter we explore the huge variations in drug prices and the problems created by an obvious conflict of interests. On the one hand, poor people and governments need to obtain reliable drugs at the lowest possible prices. On the other, the leading companies claim they need to charge high prices in relation to other manufacturers to pay for their costly research establishments.

There are striking differences in drug prices from one market to another, between different manufacturers and in the prices that the same producers charge different buyers. Pricing is a complex issue, not least because of all the external factors that influence prices, including the size of the market, the degree of competition between similar products, the extent of government controls, taxes and the margins added by wholesalers and retailers.

Recent cooperation between Caribbean countries on drug policies has unearthed some major discrepancies in the prices of identical drugs. One supplier sold methyldopa tablets (for high blood pressure) to Trinidad at six times the price quoted in Barbados for the same quantity, and roughly three times the prices charged in Guyana and Jamaica. Meanwhile the small island of St Kitts obtained the same drug from another manufacturer under a group purchasing scheme for about a ninth of the price paid by Trinidad. These and similar price differentials cannot be explained away by different market size, or variations in freight and insurance costs. [4]

An important factor underlying different prices between both developed and developing countries is the degree of government price control. A recent UNCTAD report reveals that in the Philippines, where the Government exercises few controls on the market, prices are generally much higher than elsewhere. For example, the least expensive tetracycline capsule cost over 8 times more than the cheapest available in the USA and four-and-a-half times more than in neighbouring Malaysia. Similarly in the Philippines Roche's products Librium and Valium were priced 8 times and 14 times higher than in Britain. [5]

£14 FOR 100 ASPIRIN

Contrary to some popular misconceptions actual drug prices are not always higher in developing countries. On a straightforward currency conversion, actual prices are often much lower than prices in developed countries, even in manufacturers' own home markets. For example out of 24 identical products marketed in Bangladesh and Britain in 1980/81 by seven transnational companies, with two exceptions, prices were all lower in Bangladesh. [6]

But direct price comparisons can be misleading because they ignore vast differences in purchasing power, in this case between the majority of people in Bangladesh and in Britain. In terms of purchasing power the real cost of these products is much higher in Bangladesh. One 60 ml bottle of Beecham's ampicillin syrup, sold under the brand-name Penbritin, costs a poor family in rural Bangladesh about 66p - or 6% of their total monthly income. If a British family with a net income of £7,000 a year had to spend the same percentage of their monthly income on the drug, one bottle would cost them about £35. Similarly, the cost of 20 capsules of ICI's oxytetracycline, Imperacin, represents 5.3% of the Bangladeshi family's monthly income. So proportionately, this short course of antibiotics would eat

47

up about £31 of the British family's budget. One hundred aspirins sold under Fisons' brand name, Genaspirin, have a maximum retail price of 82p in Britain. In Bangladesh their actual cost is 27p or 2.5% of the poor family's income - equivalent to £14.57 for the British family. [7]

A French pharmacist, Dr. Pascale Brudon, has used the United Nations purchasing power parity system to calculate the true cost of identical products in a number of different countries. Her analysis reveals that, particularly in the least developed countries, the real cost of drugs is very much higher than in the major drug producing nations. For example, Ciba-Geigy's antidiarrhoeal, Mexaform, costs one-and-a-half times more in Mexico than Switzerland, 6 times more in Indonesia, 13 times more in Niger and 20 times more in Upper Volta. [8]

"WHAT THE MARKET WILL BEAR"

There is every indication that drug prices are determined as much by market factors as the actual costs of production and supply. [9] Some of the most compelling evidence is the way that manufacturers have dropped their prices massively in competing for orders for the public sector, as opposed to acting as monopoly suppliers to private importers. [10]

The extent to which prices are influenced by competition on the local market is indicated by the following extract of E. Merck's "Bangladesh Marketing Plan 1980 (-1982)". This refers to the company's product, Neurobion, which accounts for most of local sales turnover. "The movement of both tablet and ampoules are very fast and *being the leader* overshadowed other neurotropic vitamins. The reasonably good turnover of Neurobion has drawn the attention of our competitors and some of them are seriously thinking to produce identical product locally. Although *the high price is acceptable by the market,* but becoming burden to the consumers and it's constant complaint from the doctors". [11](our emphasis)

Our research supports the conclusion reached by earlier studies that manufacturers appear to charge what the market "will bear". [12] But external market forces alone do not account for all the price discrepancies. The stucture within the industry makes it inevitable that identical drugs are sold at very different prices. There are exceptions, but as a rule the research-based companies charge one set of prices, and the non-research-based producers another.

IT'S ALL IN THE NAME ...

Perhaps surpirsingly, the easiest way to focus on the reasons underlying manufacturers' very different price strategies is by looking at the *name* under which a drug is marketed. Initially, the research chemists who develop a new drug will refer to it by its chemical name, as for example, '7-chloro-I, 3- dihydro-I-methyl-5-phenyl-2H-I, 4 benzodiazepine-2-one'. The active ingredient or drug is then patented and - fortunately for non-scientists - it is given its *generic* or *non-proprietary* name. The *generic* name, 'diazepam' in this case, means the drug can be easily recognised internationally. When the drug is ready to be launched on the market, its manufacturers give it an exclusive *proprietary* or *brand* name.

48

Promotion ensures that most of us will recognise the drug by its brand name -in this case 'Valium'.

A company that develops a new drug is granted monopoly rights over its production, import and sale in countries that recognise patents - in many for up to 20 years. The effective life of patents may in fact be only half as long by the time a new drug is fully tested and ready for sale. But while manufacturers enjoy this monopoly their new products can sell at high prices. Once the patent expires (or before that in countries that do not recognise patents) the drug can be copied by anyone with the technical know-how to produce it. So non-research-based companies can step in and market the drug either under its generic name or their own brand.

Keeping to the example of diazepam, this is now off patent and sold in Britain both under its generic name and half a dozen brand names, including Valium, the trademark of its originators, Roche. [13] Two characteristics distinguish the brand name product from the generic. Valium is well known, diazepam less so, and the trade price of Valium to the National Health Service is over twice the price of the generic. [14] The differences can be greater. A comparison of prices of thirteen top-selling brands and their generic equivalents on the British market in 1979 revealed that the generics cost only two-thirds to one- tenth of the price of the brand-name products. [15]

The situation in the Third World is similar. For example, in Bangladesh Valium costs approximately four-and-a-half times more than diazepam from a local generics factory. [16] According to UNCTAD, in the Philippines the retail price of Smith, Kline & French's Isona 500 tablets was over 22 times more than the generic equivalent (isoniazid) from the generics producer Rhea-Pilusa. [17]

THE COMPETITIVE RACE

Price competition is crucial in the generics market, with obvious advantages for the Third World poor. [18] Generics producers have nothing like the overheads of the research-based manufacturers, so they can sell drugs profitably for slightly more than their actual manufacturing costs. As the Director of Operations of Beecham explains: "Imitators will always be able to charge less than originators because they have no research and development costs of to recover." [19]

The research-based companies have rarely tried to compete with the low prices of the generics producers. An industry document points out that "innovators hardly ever reduce their prices when their products are copied". [20] Broadly speaking price-cutting is against the interests of research-based companies that need to maximise their prices and profits to cover their large overheads. [21] The market leaders compete by bringing out new products that can sell at high prices while they are covered by patents. Each aims to increase its share in about half a dozen different sub-markets. Glaxo, for example, specialises in antibiotics and drugs for asthma, rheumatism, ulcers, skin complaints and heart conditions. [22]

Dr. von Grebmer of Ciba-Geigy exlains the position of the market leaders: "The innovator is compelled to develop new innovations if he is not to fall behind in the competitive race. Theoretically, the research-based company could defend its market share, even after expiry of the patent, by effecting price reductions. Such a strategy, however, involves the danger of its tying down a growing proportion of its resources as a company to this generics market and thus weakening its capacity for research and development." [23]

BRAND PROLIFERATION

The results of this "race" are that the world market is flooded with what Senator Edward Kennedy has described as "a myriad of competing drug products". [24] There are about 1,000 different active ingredients or drugs but of these little more than 200 are considered as essential to priority needs by WHO. Moreover, these active ingredients are sold under thousands more trademarks and dosage forms. In Britain alone there are an estimated 17,000 different drugs on the market, including all brands and formulations, but excluding homeopathic and herbal medicines. [25] In India there are about 15,000 products on the market, and a similar number in Brazil. In Nepal alone there are 67 different brands of chloramphenicol, 79 antacids, 63 cough syrups, 63 brands of phenobarbitone and 42 of aspirin. [26]

Although there are only seven combination drugs on the WHO Selection of Essential Drugs, there are over 10,000 in the Mexican prescribing guide. Many are more expensive than single-ingredient drugs. Arguably they have more to offer manufacturers in securing new patents than in any clear therapeutic advantages to doctors. [27] The proliferation of different brands of similar, if not identical, drugs, all on sale at different prices, can easily present headaches for doctors. For prescribers in developing countries the choice of the most cost-effective treatment is even more fraught with difficulty than it is for their counterparts in developed countries. The Third World doctor rarely receives any objective drug information from any non-company source.

The inevitable consequence of this variety of competing brands is that manufacturers must spend large sums of money on promotion to convince doctors that their products are superior to their competitors'. These marketing costs can add up to as much as 20% of sales turnover. [28]

Inevitably the costs of innovation and advertising have to be paid for in higher drug prices. As a result actual production costs can account for as little as 20-30% of the research-based companies' prices. Dr. von Grebmer explains that "Between 70% and 80% of the sales figure goes towards general costs and profit". [29] The Third World's heavy reliance on the market leaders means that the poor are helping to foot the hefty bill for research and promotion. According to Dr. von Grebmer: "Owing to the special nature of the costs structure in the research-based pharmaceutical industry, the only economically reasonable accounting procedure to adopt is to calculate for each product a so-called 'contribution margin' (= price minus directly chargeable costs) which includes an extra percentage to cover general costs." [50] However, the price discrepancies we have described make it clear that this 'contribution margin' cannot be distributed evenly. [31]

This system of adding a premium to the actual production cost of *all* drugs has the advantage that a few of the best-selling drugs effectively subsidise the cost of drugs for rarer diseases. (Commonly 50% of a company's sales are made up by only about 5% of their product range.) [32]

Third World patients do of course benefit, because rich world purchasers are helping to pay for drugs for tropical diseases that might otherwise be even more prohibitively expensive as their sales volume is low.

But drugs for specifically 'tropical' diseases are only one aspect of a poor country's needs. Most of the medicines urgently needed by the Third World poor are for common infections and are decades old. Hardly 5% of the WHO selection of essential drugs are covered by valid patents, so they could be obtained as generics at competitive prices. [33] Furthermore, as the British industry-funded Office of Health Economics points out, the research and development costs for these drugs "have largely been paid for". [34]

SHOULD THE POOR SUBSIDISE NEW DRUGS FOR THE RICH?

Without doubt, new drug research is vital. It offers the only hope to many suffering from incurable diseases. Research and development is, of course, a high-risk and costly business. This is beyond dispute. The question is, should the Third World poor have to help pay for it and how relevant is the research to their needs? [35]

On average it takes about a decade and costs around £35 million to develop a new drug. It can cost as much as £50 million. [36] When a company makes a major breakthrough its huge investment in time and money is usually amply rewarded, although not of course immediately. It was reported that Smith Kline & French's record-breaking new drug Tagamet, for gastric ulcers, should bring in £2,000 million in sales over ten years on an investment of about £17 million. After its launch the company reported a 45% rise in turnover and a 90% rise in profit. [37] It has recently been forecast that the British company Glaxo, which spent about £45 million on research and development in 1980/81 may make profits of between £30 and £40 million a year averaged out over the next five years from the launch of its rival anti-ulcer drug, Zantac. [38]

But these major breakthroughs are obviously relatively few and far between. Profitability depends on bringing out *new* products, irrespective of whether they offer any major advantage over existing drugs. A 1981 report by the British licensing authorities reveals that of the 604 new product licences approved in 1980, only 23 were for new chemical entities as opposed to new formulations of existing molecules and active compounds. Over the period from September 1971 to 1980 less than 6% of licences granted in Britain were for new chemical entities. [39]

Some new formulations of existing compounds are of course extremely valuable. But figures from the United States Food and Drugs Administration (FDA) reveal that only a minority of new products licensed offer any *major* therapeutic advance. Out of a total of 484 new drug applications approved over a five year period, 112 were new chemical entities, 106 new formulations and combinations and 253 replicas of existing formulations. According to the FDA, of these 31 represented an important therapeutic gain, 62 a modest gain and 391 a minimal or non-existent gain. [40]

The majority of these new drugs may therefore do little more than add to the cost of treatment, which can only be harmful to the poor. The British licensing authorities concluded from their study of new drugs that innovation is "directed towards commercial returns rather than therapeutic need". Most new drugs are not directly relevant to the needs of the Third World poor, but are for "conditions which are common, largely chronic and occur principally in the affluent western society". [41]

Of course the poor could potentially benefit from research into heart disease, cancers and other chronic and viral diseases common to both developed and developing countries. Because of this industry commentators argue that "it is misleading to split off pharmaceutical research oriented towards the health problems of countries like Britain from that for poor nations". [42] A second argument advanced is that all research is relevant to the poor because a breakthrough, for example on immunology techniques for rheumatoid arthritis, may turn out to be helpful in preventing parasitic diseases. [43]

But there is a wide gap between theoretical benefits and concrete advantages to the poor. The Third World poor are still not benefiting from essential drug technology developed in the 1950s and 60s. Since they are expected to contribute to the cost of this research (in paying higher prices for brand-name drugs) it is essential to question how far the research actually sets out to benefit people in developing countries.

In 1976 WHO estimated that total world expenditure on research and development for tropical diseases amounted to about £17 million a year - a sum equivalent to 2% of the money spent each year on cancer research alone. [44]

An article that appeared in the Roche staff journal in 1978 stated: "It has unfortunately become apparent that in recent years a number of university institutes and pharmaceutical companies have reduced or even ceased their research activities in the difficult field of chemotherapy of tropical diseases." [45]

The explanation given is that research costs have increased because of stricter clinical trials now needed before a drug can be marketed. This makes it unlikely that profits from sales of tropical medicines will be sufficient to cover the initial research outlay, given the lack of purchasing power of people in the Third World. Roche also suggests that with the severing of colonial ties the British and French now give less priority to tropical medicine. [46]

According to Roche: "It is today mainly pharmaceutical companies in Switzerland (Roche, Ciba-Geigy), Germany (Hoechst, Bayer), France (Rhone-Poulenc) and, to a lesser extent, in Great Britain (Wellcome) which are engaged in the development of new drugs against tropical diseases. In the US it is mainly the Walter Reed Army Institute of Research which is involved in research in this field." [47]

Amongst the latest and most useful medicines developed for Third World needs are rifampicin for the treatment of TB and leprosy (the product of collaboration betweeen Ciba-Geigy and Lepetit); Roche's new antimalarial Fansidar, which is effective against chloroquine-resistant strains of malaria, and Bayer's new schistosomicide Praziquantel, which is less toxic than early drugs. [48] Wellcome's commitment to research into tropical diseases dates back to the turn of the century. It has since brought out a range of drugs including treatments for malaria, intestinal parasites and a vaccine to cater for the needs of a minority threatened by Pig-bel, a disease which claimed a few thousand lives each year in Papua New Guinea. Research is currently being undertaken by Wellcome into the six major tropical diseases, which are also under investigation by scientists of other manufacturers, including Roche and Ciba-Geigy. [49]

Other companies such as ICI and May & Baker have produced useful antimalarials and Janssen, Bayer and Merck Sharp & Dohme have contributed anthelmintics, relevant to Third World needs. These are just some examples, but by no means a comprehensive list of manufacturers' valuable contributions to tropical medicine. At least a dozen of the major research-based companies are actively cooperating with WHO's Special Programme for Research and Training into Tropical Diseases. [50] The amount of these companies' research budgets specifically directed towards the needs of developing countries is comparatively small. [51] But the majority of manufacturers spend nothing on research into Third World diseases. [52]

In fact, out of total research and development expenditure of around $5,000 million (£2,100 million) in 1980, according to an industry analyst, "The international pharmaceutical industry spent over $50 million [£21 million] on specifically 'third world' drug research". [53] In other words, in 1980 the international industry overall allocated just 1% of research and development spending to poor world diseases - or about half as much as it costs to develop just one new drug.

The extent to which the specific needs of the Third World are neglected is pinpointed by Andras November of the Geneva Institute of Development Studies. He identifies 87 diseases specific to poor countries. Of these, there are vaccinations for ten, and satisfactory drug treatment available for a further 23. But there are no drugs to treat 32 diseases and the remaining 22 can only be treated with very unsatisfactory drugs, with toxic side effects. [54]

REVOLUTION WITHOUT THE POOR

Meanwhile leading manufacturers continue to increase their research expenditure. Pfizer for example is committed to a 20% a year increase for each of the next five years. [55] The industry has high expectations of exciting new technological advances in bio-engineering and other fields. In September 1982 the British industry held a conference on the expected "Second Pharmacological Revolution". But the "revolution" is apparently mainly of interest to the rich. George Teeling-Smith of the Office of Health Economics explains: "... we took a fundamental planning decision that this meeting should be concerned only with pharmaceutical innovation relevant to the advanced world. We are always conscious of the risk of trying to cover too wide a front on any one occasion and felt that we could not do justice to the very important Third World issues if we simply tried to tack them on to a meeting dealing with very high technology '21 Century' innovation." [56] The implication seems to be that "21 Century innovation" is not relevant to the needs of two-thirds of the world's population. A further symposium is planned for later to look at the "equally important problems of health care for the world's poor". [57]

There is no straightforward answer to the intractable problem of who can afford to pay for research into new drugs for tropical diseases. Both industry and international agencies see the best hope for the future in joint collaboration. By contrast the Third World's need for low-cost generics is clear-cut. Some years ago WHO officials estimated that if world drug consumption reached $42,533 million (£18,254 million) by 1980, the poor world would be paying the rich a contribution of over $800 million (£343 million) towards research and development costs. [58] World consumption has more than doubled that figure and the poor continue to shoulder the bill. [59]

AN IRREVERSIBLE TREND TO GENERICS

Poor countries are not forced to buy brand name drugs at uncompetitive prices from the research-based companies. There are alternatives. Working in the Third World's favour is the fact that there is a growing demand for generics. A Ciba-Geigy policy document explains: "The amount of products no longer enjoying patent protection is becoming more and more important, giving way to increased competition, specially with regard to prices, and thus encouraging the production of the so-called generics." [60]

Much of the impetus is coming from within rich countries, as governments and health insurance funds attempt to curb spiralling drug bills. For these reasons Ciba-Geigy sees the trend towards generics as "an irreversible course of action, which the pharmaceutical industry will not be able to keep at bay". [61] In the US, generic prescriptions now represent about 14% of all new prescriptions written and some forecasts suggest that, by 1989, generics will account for nearly half of the total US market. Not surprisingly, 15 out of 20 major research-based companies in the US are now involved to some extent in generics production. [62] Clearly their strategy, as outlined by Ciba, is to hold on to the market: "Our main aim remains innovation through research. Where generics have *already* captured a very large share of the market and represent a threat to our traditional business or in cases where *additional* markets can be opened up by means of generics, we are prepared to enter into the business of generics." [63] (our emphasis)

As this suggests, research-based manufacturers are not going out of their way to push generics at the expense of their brand name products. In 1980, the value of the world generics market was only 4-6% of the total drug market and brand name products accounted for an estimated 90% of total UK drug exports. [64] A publication of the British industry-funded Office of Health Economics (*Brand Names in Prescribing*) indicates that many research-based companies see no role for themselves in responding to the growing demand for inexpensive generics. It states: "Older unbranded medicines which are by now long- established in the various national formularies can usually be adequately and cheaply manufactured in even the less developed local world markets. International trade in these unbranded products is consequently negligible." [65]

This statement obscures the very real difficulties that developing countries face in setting up local production. To start with they must obtain the necessary technology and technical know-how. These may be available from other developing countries that have already set up local production. But rapid technological refinements in the rich world can leave local production vulnerable to price undercutting. Third World producers also remain heavily dependent on rich world producers for supplies of bulk drugs and chemical intermediates. [66]

Not all countries are in a position to set up local production. Those attempting to break the monopoly of traditional suppliers by buying bulk drugs on competitive tender, have other problems to overcome. Many Third World countries lack both skilled administrators and the necessary market intelligence to operate an efficient purchasing system. In some cases patent laws may debar them from buying from cheaper generic suppliers or obtaining technology to produce the drugs themselves. It is open to patent-holders to attempt to enforce their monopoly rights, even when they have no intention of producing a drug locally themselves. [67]

A further major obstacle is the high cost of quality control facilities essential to test drugs produced locally or imported from unknown suppliers. Lack of quality control can enforce dependence on the market leaders especially if promotion exacerbates fears about the reliability of products from generic imitators. Some countries with chronic foreign exchange shortages may be forced to go on buying from the leading companies, and paying high prices, because cheaper suppliers cannot give them credit. [68]

But manufacturers cannot be expected to want to relinquish their existing markets. Even research-based companies that have diversified into generics production like Ciba will of course not wish to threaten the market power of their brand name products. They wait for governments to make the first move. A Ciba document explains the strategy: "This policy of ours is deliberately of a reactive type, which explains why we refrain from entering into the generic business in markets where such products are still of no great significance." [69]

The research-based companies attach considerable importance to their exclusive trademarks as a source of market success. This is borne out by the results of a survey conducted by the Office of Health Economics. Twenty-eight companies were asked to rate various factors in an order of priority in deciding whether they would enter a Third World market. Not surprisingly, the main consideration chosen was "confidence in the future of the market". But, significantly, the second factor they singled out was "pressures for generic prescribing and attack on brand names". By contrast, "strictness of price control" rated fifth in order of importance. [70]

OPPOSITION TO GENERICS

Any moves to generic prescribing are resisted. A common reaction is for major manufacturers and producers' associations to stimulate concern amongst doctors and the general public that the quality of drugs may suffer without the guarantee of brand names. Doctors are also encouraged to resist any curtailment of their 'freedom' of choice. [71] National companies that have managed to establish their own brands will also oppose a generics policy. As UNCTAD points out: "They may fear a generic policy more than the transnational firms do because, owing to their higher costs, they may be less well equipped to face competition in the market for generics." [72]

In 1980 the Indian Government made a significant step to encourage generic prescribing by abolishing brand names on five commonly prescribed drugs. [73] Soon afterwards a spate of industry-funded advertising appeared in the Indian press in an apparent attempt to discredit the new generics policy. [74] An example of this propaganda is the advertisement reproduced on the opposite page: *"Would you rather have your doctor choose a medicine for you - or somebody else?"*

The issues the advertisement raises are crucial to people's acceptance of generic prescribing and consequently to cutting drug costs in poor countries, so we shall take a closer look at the arguments advanced.

> "The move to abolish brand names is motivated by the
> erroneous belief that if there are no brands, drugs will
> become cheaper."

We have seen that brand names *do* disguise big price differentials. For instance, Limbitrol Forte, a tranquiliser promoted by Roche in Lesotho, contains amitriptyline and chlordiazepoxide. This combination product was in 1980 five times as expensive as the two single ingredients. [75] WHO is in no doubt that "There is great pressure to use brand names rather than generic names for pharmaceutical products. Use of the latter could facilitate the availability of alternative, cheaper drugs that are still satisfactory from the medical point of view." [76] Hence WHO's recommendation: "To ensure standardisation and *reduction in price,* generic names should be utilised in drug procurement in developing countries." [77] (our emphasis) Many doctors concur including the President of the Indian Medical Association: "Of course generic drugs will become cheaper for the consumer and so far our experience with the drugs that are required to be manufactured under their generic name has not been unhappy." [78]

Would you rather have your doctor choose a medicine for you-or somebody else?

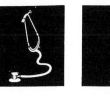

Somebody other than a doctor may choose a medicine for you if brand names for drugs are abolished and doctors are compelled to prescribe by generic name only.

A generic name is the common name of a drug — usually a long chemical name. When this drug is made by several firms, each one gives it an easy-to-remember brand name, which is usually simpler than the generic name.

Simplicity or Confusion ?

"Bromodiphenhydramine Hydrochloride" is a generic name. It is marketed by companies under their own brand names. "Ambrodryl", for example, is a brand name for this drug. Similarly, "Dihydro-ergotamine Methanesulphonate" is the generic name of a drug marketed as "Dihydergot", a brand name. "Otrivin" is a brand name of a drug generically named "Xylometazoline Hydrochloride".

Brand names usually have no similarity in spelling or pronunciation. Hence the chances of wrong dispensing of a drug prescribed by a brand name are negligible.

In contrast, several generic names are similar in spelling and pronunciation, although the drugs concerned may be quite different in their therapeutic action. Example: Quinidine Sulphate is a cardiac drug, while similar-sounding Quinine Sulphate is an anti-malarial.

If doctors are forced to prescribe drugs by generic names, the chances of wrong dispensing by chemists can be very high, especially if prescriptions are illegibly written as they often are.

Layman's View

Laymen think that all products with the same chemical composition have the same degree of

effectiveness. But chemical equivalence is not the same as therapeutic equivalence, as every good doctor knows.

This is because drug quality and effectiveness are not simply a matter of how a medicine is named or marketed, but how and by whom it is made. Several critical factors, which differ from company to company, vitally affect the effectiveness of a drug in patients.

These differences can, and often do, result in variations in the degree and speed of therapeutic response –how much of the drug is absorbed, where in the body and how rapidly it is assimilated, allergic reactions or other side-effects, tolerance by the patient in specific condition, etc.

Doctor Knows Best

This being so, the doctor, who knows the patient's condition better than anybody else and has previously observed the action of different brands of the medicine, chooses a brand he knows to be effective and is best for the patient.

If brand names are abolished, the doctor will have to prescribe by generic name. When you take the prescription to the drug store, the chemist will decide which com-

pany's product should be given to the patient.

And the chemist, unlike the doctor, has no knowledge of the patient's condition, nor has he any experience of the therapeutic effects of products made by different companies.

Ensuring Quality

When a company markets a product under a brand name, it stakes its reputation on the brand. This is a less expensive way of ensuring quality than administrative controls.

The Soviet Union has retained the brand system. When Pakistan abolished brands, spurious and substandard drugs took over. The country has gone back to brands.

It is obvious that the abolition of brand names will jeopardise the interests of the consumer without any corresponding benefit like lower prices. There is no justification for taking this risk in such a vital field as medical care.

> "Somebody other than a doctor may choose a medicine
> for you if brand names are abolished and doctors are
> compelled to prescribe by generic name only."

This is a bogus argument as it implies that doctors are invariably well- informed about the special properties and possible side-effects of drugs, or that there is necessarily any significant difference between generics and brand name drugs. It also ignores the fact that in India the great majority of drugs are not sold on prescription.

> "Simplicity or confusion?" Generic names are long and
> complicated. Some are similar and could be confused.

The suggestion that generic names are more easily confused than brand names is once again a non-argument. Whereas similar generic names like digoxin and digitoxin or chlorpromazine and chlorpropamide can cause confusion, it is very easy to compile an equally lengthy list of confusing brand names, like Aramine and Avomine, Daritran and Dartalan or Jadit and Jonit.

In fact, generic names are often more helpful in giving clues about the nature of a drug. For instance, the generic names ampi*cillin,* cloaxa*cillin* and carbeni-*cillin* indicate that all three are penicillins, whereas no clues are given by their corresponding brand names Penbritin, Orbenin and Pyopen. [79] Brand names decidedly do not make life any easier for a doctor. A Bangladeshi doctor wanting to prescribe oxytetracycline, is confronted with the choice of Aldacycline Forte, Clinmycin, Edrucycline, Imperacin, Kedoxyline, Oxaline or Terramycin. [80]

> "Laymen think that all products with the same chemical
> composition have the same degree of effectiveness. But
> chemical equivalence is not the same as therapeutic
> equivalence as any good doctor knows ... Several critical
> factors, which differ from company to company vitally
> affect the effectiveness of a drug in patients. These
> differences can, and often do, result in variations in the
> degree and speed of the therapeutic response - how much
> of the drug is absorbed, where in the body and how rapidly
> it is assimilated...."

What the argument boils down to is: whereas a generic drug may well be *chemically* identical to a brand name drug, it will not necessarily be as *effective.* The implication is that a generic is usually less effective.

One key determinant of therapeutic effectiveness is bioavailability: the rate and amount at which the active ingredient of a drug is absorbed into the blood stream. This is a significant problem with a relatively small number of drugs. In the case of one, digoxin, differences between brands that could prove fatal have been found. A US Congressional investigation concluded that the vast majority (85% to 90%) of chemically equivalent drugs can be used interchangeably because their therapeutic equivalence is not a problem. [81] A British pharmacist, writing to the *Daily Telegraph* to counter arguments against generic prescribing, confirms that "the variation in bio-availability in different brands has been shown to have a negligible effect involving less than 0.5% of patients." [82] The problem of bioavailability is not sufficiently widespread to justify its blanket use against all generics.

> "When a company markets a product under a brand name, it stakes its reputation on the brand. This is a less expensive way of ensuring quality than administrative controls."

But brand names are no guarantee of quality. According to UNCTAD, "The US Food and Drug Administration has shown that branded and generic producers can have substandard products with about equal frequency. A non-branded product from a reliable firm is just as likely to be effective as a branded product." [83]

Substandard drugs can present very real problems in developing countries. One estimate puts the incidence in India as high as 20%. Foreign firms and large national producers have excellent records on quality. The problems arise with the mass of small firms. [84] Nonetheless, the fact that substandard generics are produced is no argument for reliance on brand names, only for the crucial importance of adequate quality control facilities to test *all* drugs.

WHO is similarly dismissive of the claim that a brand name ensures quality: "The image of drug quality is often linked with the brand name and the name of the producer ... However, exaggerated claims of high quality may not be related to better therapeutic performance of the product but may be used to justify higher prices and to increase market power." [85]

Dr. Hye, formerly Director of Drug Administration in Bangladesh, explains: "One common practice of multinationals is to set the quality specifications of their branded products a little higher or above the specifications laid down in the official Pharmacopoeia, involving additional refining or processing. This is unnecessary so far as the efficacy or usefulness of the drug is concerned, but very useful for the company to justify branding of the product and for claiming that it is a superior product to other similar products. It also helps to justify higher prices." [86]

Another factor that makes a nonsense of the claim that brand name drugs are intrinsically superior to generics is that brand name producers sometimes buy drugs in final dosage form from identical sources to generics producers. For example, in US Senate Committee hearings it was revealed that one generics manufacturer was producing capsules of chloral hydrate for seventeen companies. The identical drug was then marketed both by generics producers and research—based companies. The only difference being that under the exclusive Merck Sharp & Dohme, and Squibb trademarks, the drug cost three times more. [87] It was also reported in 1979 to be standard practice for small British generic producers to manufacture brand name products under contract to the big-name manufacturers. "The extraordinary situation arises in which the same drug is made in two guises in the same factory for sale at two different prices, the branded price often being at least twice the unbranded." [88]

OVERPRICED RAW MATERIALS

The need to assure high quality is often used by local subsidiaries of manufacturers formulating drugs in the Third World as a justification for importing high-priced raw materials, sometimes exclusively from their parent companies. Similarly, locally-owned companies producing drugs under license may be forced to buy raw materials from the licensors in developed countries and pay inflated prices.[89]

A Third World country can operate strict price controls on finished drugs, and still find itself paying exceptionally high prices if the cost of imported raw materials is ignored. A WHO document explains: "The most difficult components in determining the prices of drugs are the costs of production of raw materials and especially the cost of active ingredients, which are generally known only to the producer. Such costs are the most important in determining the prices of drugs by cost calculation because the pricing system is generally based on a percentage mark-up of raw materials costs ... As drugs are moving internationally, many transnational companies decide on the transfer of prices according to their own interests." [90]

An industry analyst confirms that the transfer prices of raw materials bear very little relation to actual production costs. Prices carry a premium for research and development and "centrally incurred costs". It is very hard for anyone outside the company to quantify these costs, so in the words of the same analyst it is possible for "appreciable profits to be transmitted from the local affiliate to the parent company." [91]

This mechanism of transfer pricing is commonly used by transnational corporations to shift capital around the world, avoiding government controls and minimising taxes. [92] Transnational companies, by their very nature are in a position to set their own rules and get by unchallenged by purely national price controls. Probably the most notorious instance of transfer pricing came to light in 1973, in Britain, with the publication of the Monopolies Commission Report on the supply of chlordiazapoxide and diazepam. Roche had been charging its British subsidiary £370 and £922 per kilo for the active ingredients used to formulate Librium and Valium in Britain. The Commission found that these active ingredients were available from Italian manufacturers at £9 and £20 a kilo. Thus they estimated that although Roche had been declaring profits generally below 5% on capital employed, its real profits were over 70% between 1966 and 1972. [93]

When developed countries like Britain, with sophisticated market intelligence sources to hand, are hard put to monitor transfer pricing, it is hardly surprising that developing countries end up paying high drug prices because raw materials are overpriced.

HIGH TRANSFER PRICES TO BANGLADESH

The difficuties for developing countries as a whole are illustrated by the situation in Bangladesh. Figures for imports during 1979/80 show that local subsidiaries and licensees of major manufacturers paid their parent companies inflated prices for imported raw materials. A number of manufacturers - such as Glaxo - operate an enlightened policy by allowing their Bangladeshi subsidiaries to buy all raw materials on the open market from the cheapest reliable sources. [94]

The US-based manufacturer, Squibb, buys only 12 of the 195 materials used locally from Squibb sources. But it has imported raw materials at considerably higher prices than other local manufacturers. For example, it paid almost twice as much as Pfizer and over three times more than the locally-owned company K.D.H. to import tetracycline. [95] The manager of Squibb Bangladesh explains: "We buy them from our affiliates because we are guaranteed the materials will conform in every particular to the exacting Squibb standards. It is strict adherence to these quality standards and therefore product efficacy, that has made Squibb trusted by the medical profession throughout the world and nowhere more than in Bangladesh where we cannot risk wasting precious foreign exchange import licenses on critical materials from outside vendors that may prove to be sub-standard and therefore unusable." [96]

The Wellcome Foundation also cites the "stamp of Wellcome's quality control" in explanation of the fact that trimethoprim was imported into Bangladesh on its behalf at five times the price paid for this drug by the local manufacturer, Square Pharmaceuticals. [97] Trimethoprim is one of the ingredients formulated into Wellcome's brand name product Septrin in the factory of ICI Bangladesh, where it takes up a sizeable part of production capacity. The high import price of the raw material influenced the local Drug Administration's decision to hold down the price of Septrin when a representative of Wellcome visited Bangladesh to try to negotiate a price rise from Taka 2 to Taka 3.50 a tablet. [98]

Similarly, ICI's local subsidiary paid five times more for a consignment of levamisole than another local manufacturer and over twice the price Janssen of Belgium (that originally invented and patented the drug) charged its local licensee, Square. [99] The Chairman of ICI's Pharmaceuticals Division comments that the price of Taka 5,400 per kilo CIF "referred to a single shipment of special grade material manufactured exclusively to meet the special requirements of ICI Bangladesh Manufacturers Ltd. (ICI BM). Since then we have been able to modify the formulation of 'Ketrax' syrup and tablets so that ICI BM could use a simpler starting material, and from February 1980 all supplies have been shipped at prices in the range Taka 2,070 - Taka 3,130 depending principally on the exchange rate applicable at the time." [100] ICI's Pharmaceuticals Chairman also points out that "the question of fair pricing is examined by the office of the Drug Controller". [101] Indeed, according to the Director of Drug Administration at the time, a written warning was sent to ICI telling them that the import price of levamisole must be reduced. After some argument ICI agreed to drop the price. [102]

BPI, the joint-venture company managed under contract by May & Baker UK, buys raw materials on the open market, but because of the conditons of a UK Government tied-aid grant some raw materials have had to be bought at uncompetitive prices through the Crown Agents in London. [103] BPI has imported metronidazole at 5 times the price paid by other local manufacturers. [104] Some

61

locally-owned manufacturers have found themselves paying high prices for raw materials when they are bound by licensing agreements. The local manufacturer, Therapeutics, a licensee of American Cyanamid, paid Cyanamid over 2½ times more for its initial consignment of dimethyl carbamazine citrate than the price paid by BPI for the same raw material. After Government pressure the price was reduced. [105]

According to Dr. Hye, then Director of Drug Administration in Bangladesh, "One reason for high prices of drugs is due to practices of price transfer by the multinational companies through procurement of raw materials from chosen single sources."[106] A 1979 report on the viability of local production, commissioned by the World Bank, confirmed that local manufacturers were charging strikingly high prices for some finished drugs, compared with the cost at which they could be produced. [107]

The study team compared actual finished drug prices with their assessments of production costs (on a no profit, no loss basis) using raw materials purchased from the cheapest reliable sources. On this basis they calculated that tetracycline capsules could be produced for only one-fifth of the average commercial prices. Prices charged locally for penicillin tablets were estimated to be three-and-a-half times higher, for chloroquine phosphate one-and-a-half times more, and for vitamin C over ten times more than their production costs. On the study team's calculations, all but one of the 31 essential drugs selected for primary health care could have been imported at much lower cost than the local manufacturers' prices. Furthermore, the team came to the conclusion that local production of 23 of the 31 drugs would be even more economical than importing them from the cheapest reliable sources.[108]

CHOICES CONFINED TO THE RICH?

In rich developed countries there is growing concern about the escalating cost of drugs to the health services. Just over 90% of drugs prescribed by GPs in Britain are brand-name products. The British Government has considered the possibility of cutting costs by reducing consumption of expensive brand-name products, through generic substitution. [109] This is already happening in some developed countries. In the view of the British industry-funded Office of Health Economics, rich countries have a choice to make. "Europe faces an important economic question. It has an option of a cheap drug policy to keep health service costs low ..." But, if Europe opts for generics "it will at the same time drive out its innovative pharmaceutical industry. The alternative is to pay the price of the new wave of innovation ... by supporting a research-based pharmaceutical industry through paying relatively higher prices for medicines ..." [110] The promised rewards are new drugs for Europe's problem diseases and, of course, a flourishing drug industry improving the trade balance.

What choice can there be for the Third World poor? As long as unnecessarily high prices are paid, many of the poor must go without vital medicines.

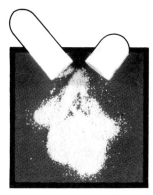

CHAPTER 5

INFORMATION OR MISINFORMATION?
Drug Promotion

"Medical representatives must be adequately trained and possess sufficient medical and technical knowledge to present information on the company's products in an accurate and responsible manner." (Association of the British Pharmaceutical Industry Code of Practice.) [1]

THE QUEUE of patients stretched out into the dark corridor and down the stairs. Inside the doctor's consulting room a row of chairs was filled with still more patients. Some would obviously have a very long wait. The dingy walls were brightened with glossy calendars from big-name drug manufacturers. An eye-catching display of tins of artificial baby milk stood on a shelf above the window. The advertisers' images of healthy babies beaming from the tins made a poignant contrast to the very sick children waiting to be seen. Harassed parents tried to stop them crying.

Looking decidedly unperturbed, the doctor was inspecting a patient's injured knee. Then he saw us in the doorway. Immediately he abandoned his patient and came to greet us. His warm welcome was mainly directed at the familiar face of the drug salesman whom we were accompanying on his rounds. We had stopped off here to deliver a stack of prescription pads specially printed with the doctor's name. This was part of the 'special service' to doctors, we were told, besides providing a means of keeping tabs on their prescribing habits. (Later the salesman could go to the pharmacy and check just which products the doctor had prescribed.)

Outside in the heat and the dust, horns blared as cars, people and animals negotiated their way through the narrow streets. Fully veiled women hurried along silently. This was Sana'a, capital of the Yemen Arab Republic (North Yemen) one late afternoon in August 1980. The salesman's car was parked alongside the doctor's Mercedes, its boot crammed with more prescription pads and an assortment of free samples.

Somewhat bizarrely, our first encounter with the salesman had taken place in the offices of the Supreme Board of Drug Control - the government agency responsible for controlling drug marketing. The salesman was employed there in the mornings as an administrator. But in the afternoons, to supplement his meagre government pay, he worked for the Mohdar Corporation, agents and wholesalers for a number of leading drug manufacturers. [2]

When we had expressed interest in his work the salesman enthusiastically offered to take us on his rounds. Evidently *he* saw no conflict of interests in regulating drugs in the mornings and promoting them in the afternoons. He described his job as handing out free samples and lavishing praise on whatever drugs he was asked to promote. He had had some training as a salesman, none in medicine or pharmacology. He candidly admitted that his understanding of medicines was minimal. [3]

* * * * *

In this chapter we look into promotional practices in the Third World and their impact on the poor. One analyst has commented that, on the logic of the free market system, industry is "condemned" to promote its products. [4] The Association of the British Pharmaceutical Industry explains: "It is necessary ... for the manufacturer, operating as he does in a keenly competitive industry and serving professions for which freedom of choice is essential, to draw attention to the existence and nature of a particular product; for example by appropriate promotional measures and the dissemination of further knowledge and experience gained in widespread use." [5]

THE COSTS

From the perspective of the poor, the logic of the market is costly. Promotion adds to manufacturers' costs, so these have to be passed on to the patient in higher prices. The United Nations Centre for Transnational Corporations states that "The amount of money spent on promotional competition in the pharmaceutical industry is extraordinary. Approximately 20% of all drugs sales at the manufacturer's level goes for promotion". [6] It is estimated that in Colombia the money spent each year by foreign companies on marketing their drugs adds up to more than half the country's national health budget. [7]

Promotion aims first and foremost to encourage sales. But it can be very helpful to prescribers, as two senior pharmacologists point out: "The pharmaceutical industry plays a very important role in providing information on drugs to the medical profession and doctors have come to rely heavily on such information in the choice of a drug." [8] Consequently, promotion can determine what doctors prescribe. This is illustrated by research carried out in Switzerland which found a close relationship between drugs that are heavily promoted and drugs that are heavily prescribed. The study concluded that prescribing 'freedom' is something of a myth because although they prefer not to admit it, doctors are clearly swayed by promotional pressures. [9]

According to these two pharmacologists, the evidence suggests that "heavy promotion has to a great extent been responsible for excessive and irrational prescribing" - problems that are all the more acute in the Third World. [10] After all, no one could expect a salesman to point out to doctors that a rival product to the one he is promoting, costing far less, is likely to be equally effective. Nor is it realistic to expect salesmen to discourage doctors from reaching for the prescription pad. One company executive says candidly: "All salesmen are biased in that they talk about the virtues of the drug they are selling and cannot be expected to extol the virtues of somebody else's product." [11] In recognition of these difficulties, the British industry's code of practice recommends to member companies that information must be "accurate, balanced and must not mislead either directly or by implication". [12]

In Britain manufacturers operate a system of self-policing within the guidelines of their voluntary code, which one industry source has described as "virtually monastic in its strictures". [13] But the Government also monitors advertising standards and has the legal powers to take action against offending companies. [14] It also keeps doctors supplied with more objective drug information, particularly on cost-effective prescribing - an element frequently played down by sales promotion.

Very few Third World governments are in a position to control promotional activities, much less foot the bill for providing objective drug information. The problems created by this information vacuum are set out graphically by an Indian pharmacologist and WHO consultant. "Once our doctors pass out of medical college and set up practice, they are cut off from the world of pharmacology. Only those who are interested enough and find the time will keep themselves abreast of the latest developments in medical therapeutics - and these form a very small minority. The others are thus .... vulnerable to glib medical representatives ... This situation is quite different from that in developed countries like the US and UK, where there are well organised services rendering a constant flow of information about drugs to prescribing doctors. Thus we have a gaping lacuna in our country and most firms take full advantgage of it." [15]

Companies employ a variety of sales promotion tactics, including sponsorship of medical meetings, advertising in journals and prescribing guides, and direct advertising to the public. Among the key target groups in ensuring market success are doctors, drug retailers and government officials. The "Marketing Plan 1980 (– 1982)" of E. Merck in Bangladesh includes all three as central to its marketing strategies. Its authors propose "To maintain very good relation with Government officials in Health and Commerce Ministry to guarantee importability of our products". [16] Chemists are an important target group because according to the marketing plan 80% of Merck's products are distributed through wholesalers and retailers, and over-the-counter sales without a doctor's prescription make up a large percentage of total sales. Strategies proposed to distribute Merck products include: "To take sales goods during up-country trips and make direct sale to chemist on cash base." [17]

Merck's sales force apparently already covers a quarter of the country's doctors. But the Marketing Plan includes as a strategy: "To create more demand of our products by the way of effective promotion through *better doctor selection*." [18] (our emphasis) The Marketing Plan also indicates that in 1978 the company's "average sales proceeds per man per year" were 22 times greater than his average cost to the company. [19]

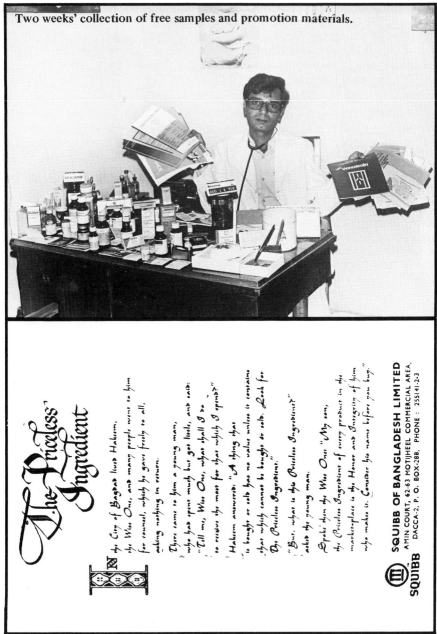

Two weeks' collection of free samples and promotion materials.

Details of manufacturers' spending on promotion in the Third World are not made public. But Dr. John Yudkin, who studied the Tanzanian market, estimated that the amount which "the companies spend each year on 'educating' doctors about which drugs to use is more than the annual budget of the Faculty of Medicine, which is used to educate doctors in every other sphere including how to use drugs properly". [20]

The figures suggest that there is a much greater concentration of sales representatives to doctors in the Third World than in developed countries. Whereas in Britain there is approximately one for every 18 doctors, in Bangladesh the ratio is estimated to be 1:7; in Tanzania 1:4; and as high as 1:3 in Nepal, Brazil and several Central American countries. [21]

Sales promotion can take up a considerable amount of a doctor's time. A 1975 report gives the example of a Brazilian senator (and doctor) who decided to test out just how much sales activity was directed at doctors. "For 21 working days he kept track of salesmen's visits to his clinic. He was visited on 18 of the 21 days by a total of 69 salesmen. He was given 452 free samples of drugs (after refusing extra quantities so as not to distort the counting); he received 25 gifts including coffeepots, notebooks, etc." [22] The photograph opposite shows the promotional handouts and drug samples accumulated by one general practitioner in Secunderabad, India, over just *two weeks*. [23]

Promotion is directed at both private and health service doctors. In North Yemen sales representatives have been banned from visiting government clinics during the mornings, because they were found to be taking up too much of the doctors' valuable time. But the main prices paid for uncontrolled promotion are that it encourages both overprescribing and a demand for unnecessarily expensive drugs.

BRAND LOYALTY

Promotion is often designed less to point out the merits of a specific drug than to create 'brand loyalty' to the manufacturer's range of products. The emotionally-charged advertisement "The Priceless Ingredient" reproduced opposite from a prominent position in the Bangladesh Prescriber's Guide 79 aims to impress upon doctors the superiority of *Squibb* products and, by implication, the notion that doctors would be unwise to prescribe anything but drugs marketed by a big name manufacturer.

The Indian Hathi Committee which reported on the drug industry in 1975 identified pressurised promotion of brand image as central to the foreign companies' consolidation of market power: "Attractively got-up medical literature and international brand names of drugs appearing in advertisements in foreign medical journals with which top consultants in the medical profession were acquainted, played their part in popularising the drugs of the foreign companies. Large sums of money were spent by foreign companies in systematically training their 'medical detailers' [sales representatives] and the general tone of detailing resorted to was that their products contained 'something plus' over products with identical

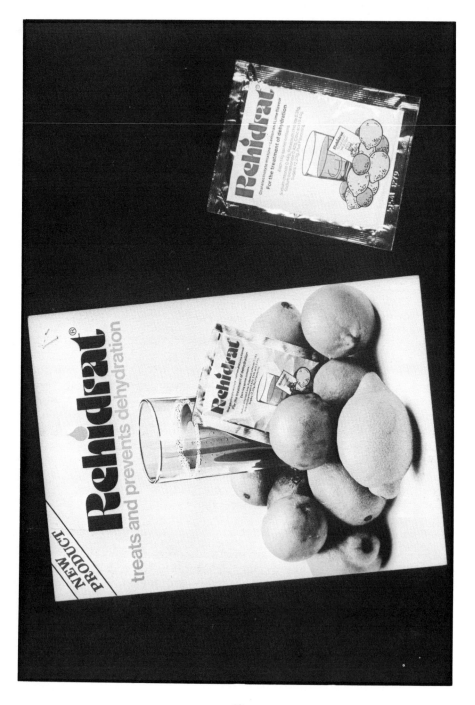

composition marketed by Indian units and that the edge in their quality was the outcome of their superior expertise and international standing." [24]

This promotion stressing the intrinsic superiority of the big name producers continues to threaten the viability of small local producers attempting to market inexpensive generics. It also confirms the prejudices of many medical students who leave college with a glowing respect for *new* drugs. This predilection is easily reinforced by sales promotion to the point that, as a British pharmacist found in Nigeria, "Doctors are sceptical of my comments in favour of cheap, well-established, unbranded drugs and against new, fancy, inadequately documented and expensive drugs". [25]

COST IS SECONDARY?

One example of a 'new' product which was promoted to doctors in Sierra Leone in 1980 is Searle's Rehidrat. As the name suggests, Rehidrat is a rehydration salts preparation. Rehydration saves lives, particularly when children become severely dehyrated through diarrhoea. Rehidrat comes in individual sachets and contains a "special granule" to preserve its "lemon-lime flavour", as explained by the eye-catching promotional leaflet, with its refreshing-looking lemons and limes. But this obviously useful new product has its price. The medical volunteer who sent us the leaflet explains: "This has made the physician specialist here furious because the cost of a sachet to make up 250 mls of solution is 80 cents. I've found that by buying sodium bicarbonate, sodium chloride and glucose at the local supermarket in small quantities, but using potassium chloride from England, the cost is just under 10 cents. Moreover, the formula which the rep said followed the WHO recommendation for oral rehydration fluid is in fact quite different, with more than twice as much glucose, half as much sodium chloride and also includes citric acid. To make up the same volume of the WHO solution would in fact cost about 5 cents" (one-sixteenth of the manufacturer's price). [26]

Searle's Director of European Clinical Research stresses Rehidrat is quite deliberately different from the WHO recommended product. Children, he explains, may be put off by the taste of the WHO solution and some experts argue that its sodium content is too high. [27] He comments: "Rehidrat is made in Norway, packaged in England, and exported and distributed throughout Africa and Asia. It contains micro-encapsulated flavouring and is stable. When properly reconstituted, and in contrast to the WHO soluton - it provides a palatable source of fluid, glucose and electrolytes for the oral treatment of dehydrated infants. *It is necesarily more expensive.* In context, it costs slightly more than a bottle of Coca Cola in such countries as Kenya, Nigeria and Zambia." [28] (our emphasis)

But in Sierra Leone the cost of just one sachet to mix a ¼ of a litre of Rehidrat is about equal to the daily wage of a poor labourer. A dehydrated child weighing 10 kilos will need about 8 times that amount of fluid in just 24 hours. [29] Cost is crucial because rehydration saves lives. Poor families could easily improve the taste of a basic cheaper solution by flavouring it with local fruits. [30] Advertising is designed to catch the doctor's interest and imagination. A salesman for Merck

If <u>your</u> child was suffering from a bacterial infection

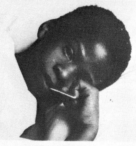

wouldn't you prescribe Septrin?

Septrin*

The original trimethoprim and sulphamethoxazole antibacterial specially formulated as a pleasant tasting suspension which children find easy to take.

Septrin's broad spectrum 'double blockade' action ensures decisive results against a wide range of pathogens and its excellent absorption also ensures rapid clinical results. Septrin is ideal in many kinds of children's bacterial infections, gastrointestinal and urinary tract infections.

Without doubt, Septrin is the most acceptable and proven antibacterial in the world today.

Paediatric Suspension

Wellcome

*Trade Mark

in rural Bangladesh stressed to us that Iliadin drops, a nasal decongestant, were taken by Neil Armstrong, the first man to walk on the moon. [31] Similarly a promotional leaflet for Wellcome's Septrin makes a direct appeal to the doctor's emotions: "If *your* child was suffering from a bacterial infection wouldn't you prescribe Septrin?" This type of advertising is breakfast reading for doctors the world over. But in the Third World there can be acute social consequences when doctors are encouraged to overlook the relative cost of treatment between brand name products and generic equivalents or between patented products and older medicines .

A doctor who has worked in both rich and poor countries sums up the pressures against cost-effective treatment: "Therapeutics is largely taught in isolation from questions of cost. Once a student has graduated he is usually granted freedom to prescribe any drug he wishes, and the medical establishment in most countries fight strenuously to protect the right. For the rest of his professional life the doctor is subjected to advertising pressure to prescribe the latest types of expensive proprietary preparations. Most of this advertising is aimed primarily at the doctor's emotions, appealing to his sympathy for patients, his professional self-esteem, etc. Such advertising is undoubtedly very effective." [32]

The most serious consequence of doctors' fighting for freedom to prescribe *any* drug is that many in the Third World actively oppose even the suggestion that they should be restricted to a limited selection of drugs. But it is precisely this limited selection which, both WHO and industry agree, now offers the best hope of catering for the needs of the Third World poor. The International Federation of Pharmaceutical Manufacturers Associations (IFPMA), for example, has stated that they "especially appreciate the problems that arise in those countries which have few physicians, trained para-medical staff, hospitals or diagnostic facilities and where distribution arrangements, particularly in rural areas, are lacking ... In these circumstances, there is an obvious necessity to provide health-workers with a limited number of drugs which they can prescribe with reasonable safety." [33] But here, in contrast to WHO, the IFPMA is not saying that *doctors* should be limited in the drugs they prescribe - only health-workers.

"ACCURATE, FAIR AND OBJECTIVE"

According to the 1981 IFPMA voluntary code of marketing practices, one of industry's obligations is that "Information on pharmaceutical products should be accurate, fair and objective, and presented in such a way as to conform not only to legal requirements, but also to ethical standards and to standards of good taste." [34] But in the Third World, the information imparted both by sales representatives and promotional literature is not always as "accurate" and "objective" as it might be. The Director General of WHO has focused attention on the problem that sales representatives "often have inadequate medical and scientific training, insufficient knowledge of the actions of the products they promote and of the comparative safety and efficacy of competitive products" [35]

The evidence suggests that the sales promotion of the big foreign companies maintains higher standards than that of some of the smaller local companies. For instance, in the experience of a pharmacist working at a Nigerian hospital: "The multinational company reps come 4 to 6 times a year. They bring the usual gimmicks and loads of samples. They try to persuade me to buy branded products, not the cheaper, alternative brands and they push new drugs... The multinational reps tend to be intelligent and well-informed, and are often pharmacists or trained nurses. The smaller firms often use less intelligent reps who sound like tape recordings. One even showed me his 'script' to emphasize the point. It read something like this: 'Doctor I'm sure you'd be interested in a drug even more effective than ..... (old, well-established drug like chloroquine) ... (wait for doctor to agree) ... Well ..... (their new product) has been shown to be ......''[36]

There are also problems with sales promotion by European and US-based companies. In a small drug store in the Bangladesh town of Rajshahi in September 1980 we encountered a Senior Field Organiser promoting the products of the West German company E. Merck. As soon as we expressed interest in his work, the Senior Field Organiser started reeling off the merits of Merck's products: Neurobion, Encephabol, Iliadin drops and Pasuma Strong. He told us that the last product (containing hormones, strychnine and other ingredients) for 'male sexual potency', was not officially available, but added reassuringly that it was quite easy to get hold of it in Dacca. We interrupted him, to ask what he saw as his main duties. He replied quite simply: "to convince doctors to prescribe Merck products". We then asked how important he saw it to *inform* prescribers of problems with drug use. Would he, for example, advise them of any products being withdrawn from the market in West Germany. He answered, with some surprise, "No, I don't do that." [37]

Officials of E. Merck in West Germany advise us that "It is, of course, problematic to draw conclusions on the activities of a pharmaceutical manufacturer by interviewing a member of its field force. Regardless of the country in which he practices his profession, no responsible doctor will prescribe a product without being thoroughly informed on its indications, properties and side-effects, and also without being convinced about the benefits of the particular product for his patients. Your question as to whether he would advise prescribers when a product was withdrawn in Gemany, which caused surprise to a member of our field force in Bangladesh, is also surprising to us as none of the products marketed by us in Bangladesh has been withdrawn in Germany." [38] They also comment that Pasuma has never been registered or marketed by Merck in Bangladesh and that any packs on the market must have been smuggled into the country through channels outside their control.

Turning now to the "Merck in Bangladesh Marketing Plan 1980(-1982)", there is decidedly less emphasis on the need to keep doctors "thoroughly informed" than on other aspects of promotion. For example, a seven point strategy is listed for increasing sales of one product, Neurobion. These include: "1. Promotion of Neurobion throughout the year. 2. Presentation of attractive literature with adequate samples. 3. Presentation of prescription pads. 4. Distribution of stickers and gift articles. 5. Fair distribution of stocks in rural markets. 6. Motivation of field force with clinical reports. 7. Promotion to the fresh graduates and quack doctors in rural markets." [39] The seven point plan for marketing another Merck product, Syptobion, includes as point 6: "Promotion to fresh graduates and potential quacks." [40] It is only in the strategy for promoting Encephabol that any specific mention is made of "Providing field force with sufficient scientific information and clinical support". [41]

A British professor of pharmacology comments that "The marketing plan's 'strategy' plumbs the depths when it urges its Sales Force to undertake 'promotion to the fresh graduates and quack doctors' ". [42] E. Merck in West Germany have expressed surprise at our queries about their marketing strategies and assure us that "In Bangladesh, all our pharmaceutical products are promoted only to doctors and we always take care that our field force is provided with full information on their properties and use". [43]

PARTIAL INFORMATION
Some manufacturers are not always consistent in the standards they operate from country to country in the critical area of drug information. In the next chapter we focus on potentially dangerous double standards in the promotion of drugs like anabolic steroids and antibiotics in poor countries. First we shall consider why Third World doctors need to be sceptical about some of the claims made in promotional literature, particularly when these are not balanced with precautions on use or warnings of unpleasant and serious side-effects.

A number of studies have documented the widespread problem of substandard drug information in the Third World. For instance, a report by Dr. Milton Silverman of the University of California published in 1976, showed that only 2 out of 23 manufacturers were consistent in what they told US and Latin American customers about their products. In the US most product literature consisted of a relatively short list of recommended uses for a drug, balanced with an extensive list of precautions and possible side-effects. But in Latin America identical products were recommended for many more uses, and warnings were conspicuous by their absence. [44]

The explanations advanced by manufacturers at the time included the fact that legal requirements are different in different countries so there is nothing 'illegal' about not disclosing all warnings that must be given on the home market. [45] Some manufacturers explained that they had accumulated "a wealth of convincing evidence to show that our product is safe and effective for the conditions we claim. Unfortunately, the evidence is not convincing to the FDA [US Food and Drugs Administration] . What we have ... therefore is a dispute between honest scientists." [46] And a Latin American "drug promotion expert" saw the discrepancies as part of normal business practice: "... if your competitor claims five indications for his product, you claim at least six. And if he discloses three adverse reactions, you are senseless if you disclose more than two." [47]

Thai and British versions of package inserts. Note the paucity of information available to the Thais.

But blatant discrepancies in drug information are not just past aberrations. Dr. Silverman concludes from his more recent research that whilst "some companies have changed their policies in Latin America ... the situation remains bad there and probably worse in Africa and Asia". [48] The offenders include Western research-based companies, Eastern bloc producers and nationally-owned companies. [49]

Our own research has brought to light many examples of apparent double standards. Two package inserts for the Roche products, Valium and Mogadon, forwarded from Thailand in 1980 and reproduced opposite, illustrate the problems. Like the English versions of these leaflets, the Thai translations include information on 'composition', 'properties', 'indications', 'dosage' and 'packings'. But the Thai versions expressly exclude the information given to English readers on 'tolerance' and 'precautions'.

Roche advise us that these leaflets "dated from 1974 and are no longer being supplied. Subsequently, the Thai regulations have changed." [50] The Thai product information leaflets now contain "warning" boxes. Roche comments: "We should stress that in general Roche are not in favour of variations in product information leaflets in different parts of the world." Moreover, "It is a policy of Roche Basle to review, from time to time, the leaflets being used by Roche companies in other countries and to examine the differences which exist. Such a review is currently taking place." [51]

In Bangladesh Glaxo's local subsidiary has distributed promotional leaflets for corticosteroids omitting warnings on possible side-effects, precautions and 'contra-indications' (i.e. information on when not to use the drugs) which Glaxo makes available to British doctors. The promotional leaflet for Betnovate-N (see page 76) stresses that the product is "unequalled in effectiveness" and that it "swiftly suppresses dermatoses". But it does not warn that prolonged use should be avoided, particularly in infants, children and pregnant women. Glaxo advise us that the data sheet currently in use in Bangladesh for Betnovate-N contains a very full statement of contra-indications, precautions and side-effects, including 4 separate statements warning doctors of possible adverse results of prolonged treatment. [52]

Similarly, the promotional leaflet for Glaxo's Betnelan oral corticosteroid tablets specifically draws attention to their effectiveness in rheumatoid arthritis. But it does not include specific warnings given in Britain that they should use "the lowest dosage that will produce an acceptable result", or that the dosage should be reduced in stages. The recommended dose for rheumatoid arthritis given in Britain is 0.5 -2mg daily. The Bangladesh leaflet, reproduced on p 77 gives the recommended initial dose as 3 mg, reducing to 0.75 mg. [53]

A tendency to keep any 'negative' information to a minimum is also evident in advertising to the general public. The 'rosy' picture given is particularly striking in advertisements for the high-oestrogen oral contraceptive pill, Maya, that appeared in Bangladeshi newspapers during 1980. The distribution of Maya is

BETNOVATE-N

Trade Mark

SWIFTLY SUPPRESSES SEVERE DERMATOSES

Dramatic and impressive results have been obtained with Betnovate-N (0.1% betamethasone 17-valerate with 0.5% neomycin sulphate) in the treatment of severe inflammatory and allergic dermatoses. Extensive clinical usage has confirmed that Betnovate-N is unequalled in effectiveness in the field of topical corticosteroids.

Doctors have particularly noted the speed and intensity of its action and its ability to obtain a response in conditions that have proved resistant to treatment with other preparations.

INDICATIONS

Psoriasis

Atopic dermatitis : infantile eczema, food eczema, allergic eczema, neurodermatitis

Contact dermatitis : including the eczematous type ; patchy eczematous dermatitis

Seborrhoeic dermatitis

Stasis dermatitis

Chronic dermatitis of the hands and feet

Otitis externa

Ano-genital and senile pruritus

Lichen simplex chronicus

Hypertrophic lichen planus

PRESENTATION

BETNOVATE-N Cream, Ointment
(0.1% betamethasone 17-valerate with 0.5% neomycin sulphate)

Creams and Ointments are available in 5 gram tubes.

Glaxo **Glaxo Bangladesh Ltd.**
Chittagong   Dacca   Khulna   Bogra
Sylhet   Barisal   Mymensingh

- Betnelan is a corticosteroid and is about 8 to 10 times as potent as prednisolone on a weight-for-weight basis.

- Betnelan is virtually free from risk of causing oedema and hypertension.

- Betnelan has a negligible effect on potassium balance.

- Betnelan is indicated when corticosteroid therapy is required in a variety of conditions, including acute asthma, intractable hay fever and some inflammatory skin diseases. Other indications include rheumatoid arthritis, the nephrotic syndrome and various blood dyscrasias.

Betnelan Tablet contains 0.5 mg betamethasone. The value of Betnelan in allergic conditions such as eczema, urticaria, asthma and food and drug eruptions is already known and acknowledged. Usefulness of Betnelan in rheumatic inflammatory disorder such as bursitis, tenosynovitis, epicondylitis and synovitis is fully established. In majority of these cases, though rheumatic pain is relieved with analgesic, but the mobility of the patient remains impaired due to inflammation. In these cases Betnelan can be of great help. A short and safe course of 21 tablets given over 6 days reduces the inflammatory condition and enables the patient to move more freely. This extremely small dosage is effective and safe.

Recommended dosage for short-term therapy of Betnelan:

To start (a) 2 tablets 3 times a day for first 2 days
Followed by (b) 1 tablet 3 times a day for next 2 days
"   "   (c) ½ tablet 3 times a day for last 2 days

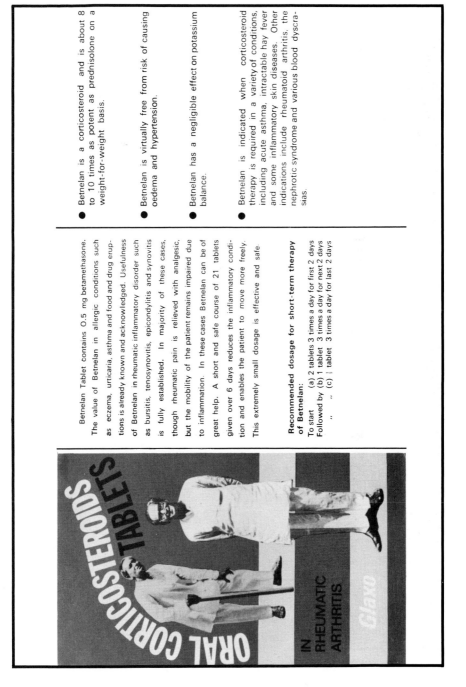

ORAL CORTICOSTEROIDS TABLETS

IN RHEUMATIC ARTHRITIS

Glaxo

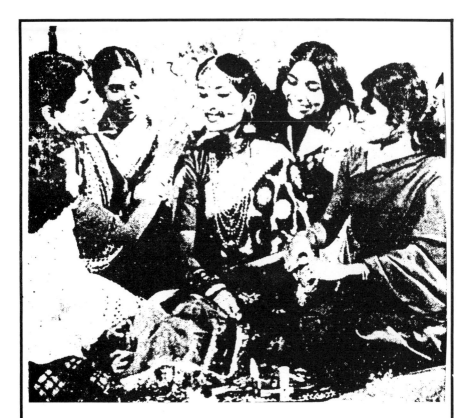

From dreams to reality.....

A reality that could remain as sweet as dreams once you make Maya part of your way of life. Maya the highly reliable imported birth control pill will help keep the woman in you alive and young.

Maya also ensures menstrual regularity, relieves you from cramps and discomforts and improves your complexion.

MAYA — the choice of millions

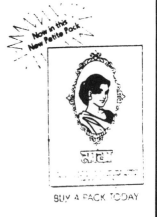

Bangladesh newspaper advertisement

"HOW EFFECTIVE IS MY METHOD OF BIRTH CONTROL?"

As a physician, you may be asked this question by your patients concerning numerous contraceptive techniques.

"The Pill", a daily dose of medicine has achieved an almost perfect record of preventing pregnancy.

The Pill had to await the discovery of 'hormones' regulating human fertility. A woman who takes the pill is adding a small daily dose of estrogen and progesterone in synthetic form to her body's own production of hormones, the effect of which is to prevent conception.

M A Y A

— a presentation of Population Services International — is a 28 day low-dosage 'Pill' that provides a continuous oral contraceptive regimen for females of Bangladesh. MAYA consists of 21 **white pills** and 7 **brown pills**. MAYA is available in a consumer pack of 2 monthly cycles.

HOW TO TAKE MAYA ?

The course should be initiated on the first day of well established menstruation or on the subsequent menstrual day with the first white pill with this ——→ arrow mark and then to be followed until 21 **white pills** have been fully taken. After finishing the 21 white pills, the **brown pills** should be taken from the 22nd day through to the 28th day. Next menstruation will usually start while taking these brown pills.

A new pack should be started on the day after the last brown pill is taken. It is vitally improtant that MAYA should be taken every day without fail. If however a pill is missed on any one day, it should be taken the next day as soon as it is remembered, along with the normal regimen of that day. The pills should be taken with food or drink preferably at bed time.

WHAT IS THERE IN MAYA ?

Each **white pill** contains : Norethindrone 1mg. with mestranol 0.05mg. Norethindrone is a potent progestational agent with chemical name 17 a- ethinyl - 17 hydrooxy - 4 estren.

Mestranol is an estrogen with the chemical name ethinyl estradiol 3 - methyl ether.

Each **brown pill** contains : Ferrous Fumerate 75mg.

Ferrous Fumerate is a well-tolerated Iron salt having 33% elemental iron and indicated in Iron deficiency anaemia.

WHO IS OFFERING YOU MAYA ?

MAYA is offered by

PSI POPULATION SERVICES INTERNATIONAL
House No : 51, Road No : 2, Dhanmondi Residential Area, Dacca-5.

 FISONS (BANGLADESH) LIMITED
is the Sole Distributor of MAYA in Bangladesh.

subsidised by Population Services International and the local subsidiary of Fisons has been involved in repackaging and distributing it locally. The advertisement reproduced on p. 78 ,"From dreams to reality",which appeared in the *Bangladesh Times*, fails even to hint at the possibility of side-effects from the use of the high-oestrogen pill. But even more disturbing is the fact that a promotional leaflet was circulated to the medical profession bearing the name of Fisons (Bangladesh) omitting any warnings of possible side-effects or precautions for use. [54]

CURE-ALLS

In Britain each 'indication' (or recommended use) of a drug has to be approved separately. This is not the case in developing countries, such as Bangladesh. [55] Manufacturers appear on occasion to have taken advantage of these loose controls, and the fact that few doctors have easy access to independent drug evaluations, to claim indications for their products that are not accepted on the home market.

For example, in Britain the only uses Glaxo recommends for its vitamin B12 preparation, Cytamen, are "pernicious anaemia" and the "prophylaxis and treatment of other macrocytic anaemias associated with vitamin B12 deficiency". [56] But the promotional leaflet from Bangladesh, reproduced opposite, recommends its use for a wide variety of problems, includng "poor appetite", "poor growth" and "sterility". We understand from Glaxo that the data sheet in use in Bangladesh since March 1980 does not include any of these indications, which would make the advertisement out of date.

At the time of going to press we have no comments from Glaxo on why these extra indications were ever included. But Glaxo did respond to an earlier query we raised about their promotion of Calci-Ostelin syrup as a general tonic in another developing country, when not only does Glaxo not do this in Britain, but the *British National Formulary* describes this use as having "no justification". [57] Glaxo's Senior Medical Adviser responded then by stressing that "different countries" have very "different concepts of medical practice". [58] If people in developing countries want to use vitamin B12 as a general tonic, why should we stand in their way? - was the gist of the argument. What it ignored was the manufacturer's role in creating this demand through its own promotion in the first place.

It may require some effort to sift through all the indications claimed for just one product. For example, E. Merck's top-selling product in Bangladesh - Neurobion (containing vitamins B1, B6 and B12) - is promoted for a wide range of uses, as illustrated by the advertisement on page 82 . A British professor of clinical pharmacology commenting on this variety of indications points out that the individual vitamins in Neurobion are certainly useful for some specific nerve disorders. For example, vitamin B1 is effective for treating the nutritional disorder beri-beri, which causes peripheral neuritis (nerve inflammation). One specific form of drug-induced neuropathy, caused by the anti-tuberculous drug isoniazid, does respond to vitamin B6. But it has no effect on many other types of drug-induced neuropathy. Vitamin B6 is also taken by women suffering from depression associated with oral contraceptives and Vitamin B12 is useful for neuropathy connected with pernicious anaemia. [59]

CYTAMEN

Pure crystalline Vitamin B_{12} Cytamen represents all known effects of liver extract and is painless on injection. For specific treatment or as a tonic in general debilities, Cytamen is an injection of value and has gone through the test of time.

Indications :

Tropical macrocytic anaemia
Macrocytic anaemia of pregnancy
Poor appetite
Poor growth
Sterility
Herpes zoster
Trigeminal neuralgia
partial haemeplegia
and other neuropathies

Mode of Issue :

250' 10 ml & '1000' 10 ml vials

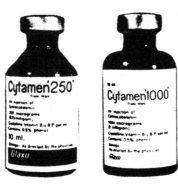

GLAXO BANGLADESH LIMITED
Chittagong Dacca Khulna Bogra
Barisal Sylhet Mymensingh

For disordered cell metabolism

Neurobion

means a quicker return to normal

Composition

Each 3 ml ampoule contains:
Vitamin B_1
(thiamine hydrochloride)   100 mg
Vitamin B_6
(pyridoxol hydrochloride)   100 mg
Vitamin B_{12}
(cyanocobalamin)   1000 µg

Each coated tablet contains:
Vitamin B_1
(thiamine disulfide)   100 mg
Vitamin B_6
(pyridoxol hydrochloride)   200 mg
Vitamin B_{12}
(cyanocobalamin)   200 µg

Indications

Neuritis and neuralgia, especially cervical syndrome, shoulder-arm syndrome, lumbalgia, sciatica, facial paresis. Alcoholic polyneuropathy. Diabetic neuropathy, including impotence due to autonomic neuropathy. Metabolic and neuropathic changes due to pregnancy and oral contraceptives. Drug-induced neuropathies. Supplemental therapy following major surgery or debilitating illness.

Dosage and Administration

For initial treatment 1 or 2 ampoules daily by deep intramuscular injection. After the acute symptoms have subsided and in less severe cases 2 or 3 ampoules per week. On days without injection and for follow-up and maintenance therapy 1 or 2 tablets 3 times daily.

Presentations

Neurobion ampoules:
Packs of 2 5 ampoules

Neurobion coated tablets:
Packs of 20 tablets

MERCK

Information for doctors.

Professor Rawlins concludes that the individual vitamins "are effective in alleviating certain specific forms of neuropàthy but their use in a blunderbuss fashion for the wide range of indications quoted... would be as inappropriate in Bangladesh as it would be in the United Kingdom". He also states that "The indications claimed by the company (including neuralgia, neuritis, diabetic neuropathy) would be appropriate in patients also suffering from coincidental malnutrition but in the vast majority of patients with these disorders Neurobion would be valueless. Moreover, adequate nutrition would be a much more appropirate method of treating such patients." [60]

E. Merck argue in defence of their claims that many patients have nerve disorders resulting from "a sub-optimal supply of vitamins", and that the "first clinical sign of this [vitamin deficiency] is often in the peripheral nervous system". [61] Both claims are undoubtedly true in specific cases such as beri-beri, but neither argument supports the use of Neurobion for the specific indications: neuralgia, neuritis or diabetic neuropathy. Merck also argue that a deficiency of a single B vitamin is rare and that "As the diagnosis of a specific vitamin deficiency is more expensive than a course of Neurobion ... it is again a reasonable therapeutic decision to cover the patient by administering a combination of B vitamins". [62] A single vitamin deficiency is indeed rare in Bangladesh where malnourished people suffer from lack of *food*, not lack of vitamins. Consequently, it makes more sense to 'prescribe' food, especially when the cost of daily treatment with Neurobion adds up to more or less the entire daily income of a family in rural Bangladesh. [63]

SALES INDUCEMENTS

In both developed and developing countries, manufacturers offer gifts and inducements to doctors to prescribe their products. In Britain the industry's voluntary code limits these to gifts that are "inexpensive and relevant to the practice of medicine or pharmacy". [64] But in most Third World countries, the parameters of 'normal' promotional practices are very much wider. Not all countries even have manufacturers' associations to define and monitor ethical standards - let alone governments that enforce controls.

Promotion in the Philippines is on a noticeably lavish scale. One doctor explains that some "drug companies, in order to get the physicians' commitment to prescribe only their products, offer the following incentives - a car (Volkswagen), a refrigerator or other home appliances. A drug company has been known to get the bank account number of physicians with a promise that within the week a 4 digit cash deposit will be added to the physician's bank account, if and when the physician commits himself to prescribing their products." [65]

The sales inducements described by the Filipino doctor are a far cry from the ethical guidelines laid down by the ABPI code. He also reports that some "drug companies now employ beautiful women as drug representatives (or drug detail persons) to advertise their products to doctors". [66] "Doctors in remote areas are encouraged by the drug companies to sell drugs on a consignment basis. The doctors are given 20-30% discount (meaning prices that are 20-30% lower than the market value). The doctors are told they can sell them at any price as long as they pay the designated prices of the drugs.'' [67] In one specific case a doctor, on the island of Samar, was offered two Ford cars by a drug company to encourage him to set up a pharmacy selling exclusively their products. His store would have had a total monopoly on sales, as he was the town's only doctor and there were no pharmacies. [68]

From Indonesia a doctor reports that bonuses are paid to doctors and even government officials receive both impressive discounts and special gifts from drug companies. [69] In Bangladesh, as elsewhere, the transnational companies support doctors' travelling expenses to attend seminars and meetings abroad. ''These are disguised as neutral scientific gatherings,'' explains the former Director of Drug Administration, ''but are in fact meetings sponsored by big companies to promote their special products. This makes it possible for them to offer 'paid holidays abroad' as gifts to doctors who 'matter'.'' [70] In some cases influential doctors have a direct stake in a company's profitability. [71]

The evidence suggests that the big transnational companies are by no means the worst offenders in using over-zealous sales promotion tactics. An article in :i Business India magazine quotes a ''knowledgeable wholesaler based in Bombay's Princess Street'' as pointing out that ''It is mainly the Indian sector companies that give expensive gifts like cars and refrigerators to class A doctors who have what is known in the trade as a 'prescription following'. The multinational companies with their established brand names don't have to be so lavish.'' [72]

It is not of course only manufacturers that offer inducements to doctors to boost drug sales. For example, in North Yemen doctors are known to receive a 10% commission from drug retailers who dispense their prescriptions. [73] Throughout the Third World it is not only business interests - manufacturers, wholesalers and retailers - that profit from sales of prescription medicines. Doctors and sales assistants often have a direct stake in sales and an obvious incentive to overprescribe.

An OXFAM Field Director comments on the situation in Brazil: ''... pharmacy salesmen make commissions on over-the-counter sales to boost their meagre salaries. Hence, they try to push the most expensive drugs onto customers, which are often inappropriate. Doctors also receive commissions, sometimes from pharmacies, on the basis of patients and drugs turnover.'' [74]

At the receiving end, the poor end up paying for unnecessarily expensive treatments. An anthropologist who investigated the money spent by people buying medicines over the counter in a town in El Salvador, found that the companies' promotion and distribution methods were directly responsible for unnecessarily high spending on medicines. The poor were most dependent on over-the-counter sales from the drug stores. The most expensive treatments were those recommended at the town's two pharmacies which depended on travelling sales representatives for their supplies. Customers who asked for advice in these pharmacies ended up paying on average 260% more than those who consulted the sales staff in the town's two other pharmacies, supplied directly by wholesale pharmacies in the capital. [75]

This grassroots research into the economic consequences of company promotion highlights the fact that when salesmen depend on commissions, poor patients are more likely to end up paying unnecessarily high prices for treatment. The basic monthly pay of the travelling salesmen in El Salvador was very low. But they could earn 6 to 7 times more with sales commission. If pharmacies failed to place big orders for a wide range of products, the salesmen would no longer find it worth their while to include them on their sales trips. With their drug supplies at stake, the pharmacies were under pressure to stock a wide range of expensive products. As a result sales staff "used the opportunity presented by customers seeking advice to unload products which in many cases would not sell quickly because of their higher prices". [76] Compounded with this, when the sales staff behind the counter earn a percentage on sales, it is in their interests to sell higher-priced brands.

BY-PASSING THE SYSTEM

There are a number of reports of ways in which sales representatives have been able to get their products bought for the health services when these drugs are excluded from the national formulary. For example, Dr. Yudkin observed these pressurised sales tactics in action in Tanzania: "Doctors above a certain rank are allowed to prescribe non-scheduled drugs at their discretion, and representatives offer to help by taking local purchase orders to the Medical Stores to facilitate ordering. These orders are frequently of great cost but little use; one representative for A. H. Robins persuaded a doctor at a district hospital to order 300 bottles of Dimetane (a cough syrup), 300 of Robitussin (another cough mixture), and 120 of Donnagel (a mixture for treating diarrhoea) with the offer to take the local purchase order to the Medical Stores. *The cost of this order .... would supply a dispensary with enough drugs for three years.*" [77] (our emphasis)

SAMPLES ABUSE

A major element of sales promotion in the Third World is the lavish distribution of free samples. Whereas guidelines in developed countries stress the need to restrict the distribution of samples to a minimum, in poor countries large quantities are offered and snapped up by doctors who can sell them profitably. [78] For example, the Hathi Commission reported that in India, "Unfortunately, this practice of distributing samples has degenerated into a rat race among manufacturers, each trying to excel the other in the quantity of drug samples distributed to doctors. The scale of distribution of samples ... leads to malpractices. Reports have been received of physicians' samples being found on the premises of drug dealers." [79]

There is evidence of the wasteful and dangerous misuse of free samples from many developing countries. A nurse reports from Upper Volta that samples usually contain too little of a drug to provide a complete course of treatment. But this does not prevent them from being used indiscriminately - by people in need of drugs, but not because the free sample is what they actually need. For example, one man suffering from bilharzia was delighted to have been given six different free samples by a friend working in a hospital. He was taking all of them

85

concurrently. They included two different forms of injectable penicillin (neither sufficient for a full course), two eye ointments, a nasal decongestant and a drug for vertigo. Not one of these free samples was any use for treating bilharzia. [80]

In North Yemen research carried out in the remote mountainous region of Raymah unearthed 'free samples' stocked on the shelves of local drug sellers. [81] In the capital, the practice of taking advantage of free samples avilable from drug manufacturers has been institutionalised. Companies are required by law to hand over 20% of all samples imported into the country to the Ministry of Health. They are earmarked "for the stores of the General Office of Pharmaceuticals and Medical Supply in the Ministry of Health to support government drug services". [82]

From Tanzania, Dr. Yudkin reported that samples have been used by sales representatives as a means of creating demand for their products within the health services. In this way they have effectively by-passed centralised controls on drug purchases. "Along with the donation of a free sample to the doctor usually goes a box or bottle of the drug to the hospital pharmacy, and a message to the doctor that the drug is available in the pharmacy. This may happen whether or not the drug is approved by a Hospital Pharmacy Committee, or even if it is a non-scheduled drug (one which is not included in the Central Medical Stores List). When the doctor prescribes the drug, the pharmacist dispenses it, and will often order more when the doctor continues to prescribe and the free sample has been consumed." [83]

SLEDGE-HAMMER THERAPY

Overprescribing by doctors, health workers and drug sellers is a worldwide epidemic. But it hits the Third World hardest. There are many causes, including uncertainty over diagnosis, lack of training in alternatives to medicines, patient-demand and, as we have seen, the fact that prescribers often have a direct stake in selling more drugs. In each case advertising aggravates the underlying problems. We know of numerous specific cases of overprescribing from many very different developing countries.

A classic example from North Yemen is that of a patient referred to a doctor in the town of Hodeidah by a rural clinic with a note recommending that his nasal arteries should be cauterised to stop his nose bleeds. *He needed no medicines.* Two days later he returned to the rural health centre. He was still suffering from nose-bleeds. The straightforward cautery had not been performed. But, over the two days he had spent in the town, he was prescribed 12 different drugs by one qualified doctor. These included a total of 1,000 ml of intravenous fluid (both sodium chloride and dextrose); antibiotic injections (Pfizer's Terramycin); 3 different brands of vitamin injections and multivitamin tablets (15 of Bayer's injectable vitamin B-complex, Campovit; vitamins A and C; and Roche's Cal-C-Vita); two injectables to stimulate blood-clotting (vitamin K and Luitpold-Werk's Clauden); Otrivin nasal drops, and Hoechst's painkiller, Novalgin, in *both* tablet and injectable forms. This prescription was not the end of the story. The man returned with a bulging carrier bag full of drugs which also contained a further

86

four preparations of vitamin and antibiotic preparations, that were not included on the doctor's prescription, but had been sold to him nonetheless. [84]

The tragic consequences of this overprescribing are easily apparent in poor countries. In Upper Volta a typical prescription for a simple illness like a cough or cold will include a cough syrup, a decongestant, vitamin injections in case the patient is run down and sometimes even penicillin injections. Patients are generally prescribed medicines for a whole range of *symptoms,* rather than for the specific *cause* of their illness. An OXFAM researcher writes that "One can often see in the always crowded Ouagadougou pharmacies people forlornly clutching their prescriptions for a number of drugs. The assistant tells them how much each item costs, and then the would-be buyer must decide whether he can afford all the drugs. If not, he must choose amongst them, and generally unless well-informed, or with a friendly assistant, he will select the cheapest one or two." [85] So the poorest are most likely to end up with the multi-vitamins, rather than the vital antibiotic.

Meanwhile, manufacturers turn a blind eye to irrational and wasteful drug use. Some even appear to condone this tragic state of affairs. An example of this apparent endorsement of overprescribing is the advertisement reproduced on p. 88 : "Some patients treat prescriptions like menu cards: they pick and choose the medicines" ... "Give your doctor's prescription the importance it deserves. Have faith in it," from Roche, "World leaders in Vitamins". The manufacturer ignores the fact that the poor *are forced* to "pick and choose".

Roche comment that this advertisement placed in Indian papers during 1980 "was not aimed at doctors and, therefore, was not expected to have any effect on prescribing. The audience would be the literate and the better-off members of the community and the intention was to improve the understanding of, and confidence in, the practising physician by the patient ... Thus we do not think it reasonable (nor do doctors) to regard such an advertisement as an appeal either to over-prescribe or to over-consume." [86] Are doctors not "literate and better-off members" of Indian society? Can patients - above all poor patients - afford to have 'confidence' in doctors' multi-item prescriptions?

Professor Nurul Islam, head of the Dacca Institute of Post-Graduate Medicine and Research, stresses that virtually all doctors prescribe drugs unnecessarily and members of the medical establishment are often responsible for setting a bad example to medical students. Some routinely prescribe seven, eight or nine drugs. [87] For example one of Bangladesh's leading paediatricians is reported to have used this sledge-hammer approach in prescribing treatment for a 19-*day*-old baby, suffering from diarrhoea. The prescription included an anabolic steroid (Orabolin), a drug that is "specifically not recommended for children" in Britain. [88] The infant was also prescribed Flagyl (a powerful antimicrobial drug), and two antibiotics: Beecham's Ampiclox Drops and a tetracycline preparation (a drug not to be given to "children under 12" on the recommendation of the British National Formulary). [89] The baby's prescription was rounded off with the inevitable multivitamins *and* Polyvison, Mead-Johnson's baby vitamin drops. [90]

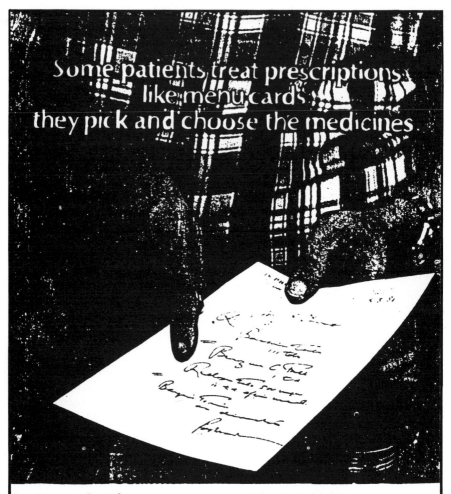

Some patients treat prescriptions like menu cards; they pick and choose the medicines.

Do you?
Do you take your prescription with a pinch of salt?
Do you drop some medicines because you believe too many medicines are bad?
Cut down doses at your whim and fancy?
Then you're not on your way to recovering very fast!
Your doctor's prescription is the most compatible and effective combination — of the right medicines in the right doses, to be administered at certain times daily for so many days. If you alter this combination in any way, you are reducing the efficacy of the treatment. And only delaying your recovery or intensifying the ailment.
Give your doctor's prescription the importance it deserves. Have faith in it. After all, you should be the last person to prevent him from getting you well.

World leaders in Vitamins ⟨ROCHE⟩

Advertisement from an Indian general readership magazine.

بسم الله الرحمن الرحيم

الدكتور

عبد الله حمــود الشيخ

بكالوريوس في الطب

Date ٨ ١ ٤ ٦ ٢ التاريخ

Name _____ محمد ____ الاسم

١. Procain penicillin 8 cap

أسبوع ايام لعلاج يوما سبرة بل
يوم ل ل

٢. Ilveco   Tab
          ٢ × ١

٣. Bronchorioa   syp ١ ج
          حبايتين ٢ / ١   ٥
                            ٥

٤. Calcivita   Tab   ١٢
          قرص يوم / ٢ فوار   ١٧
                            ٧
                            ٧

٥. Panadol   Tab   ٢٧
          قرص ٢ / ١

٦. Becomplex   Tab

          ٢ × ١   الموعد من ٤ – ٧ مساء

عبد المعاينة القادمة يستحسن احضار الرشده القديمة .

Prescription from the Yemen Arab Republic. Typical example of overprescribing.

89

CHALLENGING DRUG DEPENDENCE

The problems arising from promotional practices underline the need for controls on drug marketing practices. But these alone cannot succeed unless they are backed by concerted efforts to change the attitudes of medical students and practising doctors. This is one of the conclusions reached by the recent Indian Council of Social Science Research and Indian Medical Council's joint report. "One of the most distressing aspects of the present health situation in India is the habit of doctors to over-prescribe or to prescribe glamorous and costly drugs with limited medical potential. It is also unfortunate that the drug producers always try to push doctors into using their products by all means - fair or foul. These basic facts are more responsible for distortions in drug production and consumption than anything else. If the *medical profession could be made more discriminating in its prescribing habits, there would be no market for irrational and unnecessary medicines.*" [91] (our emphasis)

UNCTAD question whether the all-important area of providing doctors with drug information should be left to drug manufacturers: "It is debatable if the methods used at present are the correct ones. In fact many of the current malpractices in drug consumption are connected with this mode of drug promotion and high-pressure salesmanship, with their many exaggerated claims of the usefulness of the particular products and only a vague mention (if any) of possible side effects. *Ideally, this information should be provided only by professional bodies such as medical associations in collaboration with the drug control administration, absolutely independently of interested companies.*" [92] (our emphasis) This is of course an expensive task for Third World governments to take on.

However, as a doctor in North Yemen explains, commercial pressures from drug sellers remain a serious obstacle to rational drug use: "It takes a brave doctor to stand against the tide. He may refuse to see the sales representatives or be swayed by promotional literature. But the salesmen still promote their products to the pharmacies. They in turn put pressure on doctors to prescribe a large number and wide range of the products they stock. The pharmacies are, after all, in a position to destroy a private doctor's livelihood. Patients asking in the pharmacy for the name of a good doctor, could be told: 'Avoid Dr X. She's terrible' (ie she prescribes very few drugs). 'Dr Y, on the other hand, is excellent' (ie his prescriptions are usually for six drugs or more)". [93]

The attitudes of patients who expect or even demand to be prescribed drugs add to doctors' difficulties. Professor Nurul Islam in Bangladesh explains that doctors stake their professional reputation each time they decide not to prescribe any medicine. But no one doubts the judgement of the doctor who doles out multi-item prescriptions. [94] (Professor Islam himself often writes a prescription "No Medicine Required", to convince his patient that their condition does not need drug treatment.)

Next, we shall explore more of the hidden dangers of doctors always reaching for the prescription pad, and patients rushing to the market to buy medicines.

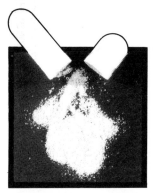

CHAPTER 6

BUYERS BEWARE
Uncontrolled Sales
and Problem Drugs

POOR PEOPLE make sacrifices to buy drugs. Rarely are these a solution to their problems. The story of one little Bangladeshi girl, struggling for life in a Children's Nutrition Unit in Dacca, is representative of the predicament of many of the world's poor.

She came from a village in Comilla, a district about 30 miles from Dacca. Her mother was poor, a widow, with five other children to feed. The little girl had fallen ill. She got progressively worse, so to get money for medicines and a doctor her mother sold some cooking pots and a few other possessions. She even sold their small piece of land so they could travel to the city. The doctors at the first hospital they tried said she would have to pay for the child to be admitted. So they went to Dacca Medical College. The doctors there examined the little girl and sent them away with a prescription for half a dozen drugs, mostly antibiotics and multivitamin tonics.

Her mother bought some but she could not afford all the drugs. The child was getting weaker so she turned to some relatives for help. But they had nothing to spare. Fortunately, when the mother was getting desperate, some neighbours told her about the Save the Children Fund Nutrition Unit where she would not have to pay. By the time the little girl was admitted, she weighed just over 5 kilos (about 11 pounds). At the age of 6, she was only a litle heavier than a newborn baby. The doctor diagnosed severe protein-energy malnutrition and anaemia. The child's life was in immediate danger because the haemaglobin level in her blood had dropped so low that her heart was in danger of stopping. That was not all. She had other complications, including a chest infection, a urinary tract infection and worms.

To stand any chance of surviving, the child needed intensive nutrition treatment. She would have to be fed milk through a nasal tube because she was nearly unconscious, and she also needed several blood transfusions.

But her mother had been sent away to buy expensive drugs. Even if she had found the money to pay for them, they could not have saved the little girl's life. The prescription would have meant money down the drain, because the underlying cause of the child's serious condition was lack of *food*. The tragic irony of this little girl's case is that to get her to the city, to see doctors and buy medicines, her mother had been forced to sell the best guarantee of her children's health. Without that piece of land, it was going to be even harder to stop the other children from getting more seriously undernourished. [1]

* * * * *

91

YOU GET SICK, YOU BUY MEDICINE

People everywhere share a need to believe in the healing powers of someone or something. Most of us will readily believe in the power of a drug and in this there is little difference between an educated Westerner and a poor, illiterate man or woman. All medicines, whether traditional herbal remedies or modern factory-produced drugs, have a special mystique.

In the eyes of the poor, modern medicines embody the power and status of the well-fed, Westernised people who are powerful in their societies. This encourages the poor to try to emulate the small minority who consume most of the medicines, in the same way as more and more poor people buy expensive factory goods like tinned foods and fizzy drinks.

Prevention may be better than cure. But prevention takes time. The poor need a quick solution to their health problems. Drugs hold out the promise of an instant cure. They tempt people with the illusion that there is a pill for every ill, provided you can afford to pay for it. In turning to local drug sellers for help, the poor may also be swayed by their status in the community. They may be literate and *seem* very knowledgeable. All these factors leave the poor and sick extremely vulnerable to sales pressures and to dangers from the actual drugs that neither they, nor the medicine sellers suspect.

A doctor working in North Yemen explains how people increasingly depend on buying medicines to solve ill-health problems: "Yemenis have come to want, indeed to feel they need what they perceive as Western medicine. This means for most of them Western *medicines,* simply because drugs, attractively packaged and efficiently marketed, are the only aspect of Western health care they have any experience of. With the emerging demand for medicines from the West, there has been no growing awareness of modern concepts of health and disease. The rudimentary principles of hygiene, nutrition and sanitation are practically unknown. The train of thought for both the patient and the practitioner is simply - you get sick, you see a doctor, nurse or pharmacist, he prescribes a medicine (or more often several medicines, at least one of which should be an injection) and you are made well again." [2]

The problem is not just the lack of organised health services. Health planners and doctors are responsible for encouraging dependence on medicines, as David Werner, author of *Where There is no Doctor,* explains: "In Latin America, many of the new programs under the Ministry of Health, Ministry of Education, and other agencies to deliver services and promote community health in rural and marginal areas have been designed by prestigious but poorly informed and out-of-date doctors and nurses. The result is that training and manuals for village health workers still tend to promote bottle feeding rather than breast feeding, restricting food to children with diarrhoea, and overuse and misuse of medication like Entero-Vioform, cough syrups, diarrhoeal plugs, etc." [3]

The widespread promotion of modern drugs has had a decidedly negative impact on some poor communities. An anthropologist, analysing the situation in Central

America, concludes: "The growing reliance on modern medicines has not only served to alter local health care traditions and means of coping with illness, but also to drain away resources without providing any long term improvements in health or living standards in the community. Dependence on these products and the agents and institutions which make them available, fosters the notion that the solution to illness resides in the purchase and consumption of medications rather than in improvements in living conditions." [4]

As we have seen, the poor will even put their health at risk by going without food to buy medicines. There has been little detailed research into just how much of their income goes on medicines. But a study in one town in Brazil found that poorer families were spending about 6% of their monthly income on medicines from the *farmacias*. [5] A survey in the Philippines revealed that another poor community spent more - about 10% of their income - on paying for treatment. This, despite the fact that the people defined their main health problems as diarrhoea and low wages which cannot be cured with drugs. [6]

The poor come under direct sales pressure from local traders whose livelihood can depend on selling as many medicines as possible. An anthropologist describes how in South-Cameroon petty traders selling drugs and other commodities are more in evidence at certain times of the year: "Particularly in the cocoa season, when the villagers have money, one meets these traders in large numbers, either on foot or on bicycle. Although the sale of medicines by ordinary traders is against the law, it is practised openly and is socially accepted." [7]

Advertising may also act as a powerful inducement encouraging people to see medicines as the key to health. For example, British doctors working in Nepal make a direct connection between advertising and overspending on drugs. They diagnose that overspending "arises from ignorance and the assumption that the more expensive the medicine the better it will be. This attitude either wholly or partly originates from the copious ... advertising carried out in the towns of Nepal's developed areas by Indian and multi-national drug companies. Likewise, partly in response to this market pressure there is a tendency to use sledge-hammer therapy." [8]

Growing numbers of the Third World poor, particularly migrants to the towns and cities, are now exposed to radio jingles and street hoardings advertising vitamin supplements, painkillers and antidiarrhoeals. Anne Ferguson, the anthropologist who studied attitudes to medicines in El Salvador, concluded that mass media advertising was reinforcing people's dependence on packaged drugs. "Although ... remedies made on the premises of the town pharmacies are still used in the community, reliance on pre-packaged medications is promoted on a national level through mass media commercial advertisements regarding their effectiveness. Prescription products are not advertised on radio or TV, but large companies ... indirectly promote the use of these medications by advertisements suggesting that the quality and efficacy of their products is superior to that of other companies, and that *the solution to illness resides in the purchase and consumption of modern pharmaceutical products.*" [9] (our emphasis)

Direct advertising is of course mainly targeted at the privileged minority in poor countries. But it has exerted a strong influence on the poor, such as in encouraging them to bottle-feed their babies and smoke expensive foreign cigarettes. The direct impact of drug advertising is more difficult to gauge. But advertising aimed exclusively at the educated minority clearly has a strong indirect impact on the poor. It conditions the attitudes and prescribing habits of doctors, who in turn influence the retailers who sell drugs to the poor.

There are few meaningful controls on advertising standards in developing countries. Some advertising appears to increase dependence on medicines by playing on fear and ignorance. The advertisment for Calcium-Sandoz, reproduced opposite, appeared in a magazine in India - a country that operates more controls on drug marketing than many. Its message is unambiguous. If you do not hurry to start your child on a calcium supplement, it may soon be "too late. No amount of calcium given later can repair the damage." By implication, *only* these calcium tablets can provide enough calcium for a growing child. This type of advertisement is clearly aimed at India's better- nourished middle-class. But it is likely to help persuade drug sellers that these calcium supplements must be essential for the under-nourished poor.

Sandoz point out that average calcium-intake is low in India, which it certainly is by comparison with most of Europe and North America. [10] They argue that their product provides a cheaper source of calcium in India than relatively high-priced dairy products: one litre of cow's milk costing Rupees 4-6 provides a similar amount of calcium to two tablets of Calcium-Sandoz, priced at Rupees 0.18. [11] But this comparison takes no account of other important nutrients in cow's milk. [12] Cow's milk is costly, but buffalo milk, with almost twice its calcium value, is readily available in Indian villages, and there are other local foods - particularly pulses and vegetables - which people could be encouraged to eat more of to boost their calcium- intake. [13]

These alternatives to medicines are masked by advertising campaigns. For example, promotion has opened a large market for vitamin and mineral supplements including extra calcium in Mexico, a country where people get plenty of calcium from *tortillas* which are soaked in lime. [14]

But to some extent the poor choose to buy expensive drugs, regardless of commercial and advertising pressures. Most people will readily believe that an expensive drug must be better than a cheaper one. If we feel ill - or a close relative does - we want to buy medicines. Whether the medicines are likely to serve any useful purpose is very much a secondary consideration. This dependence has obvious dangers, particularly where there are no controls on drug sales.

THE HAZARDS

All too often, there is a cruel contrast between the advertising claims and the reality of drug use in the Third World. Far from offering a "solution to illness", as an Ethiopian health planner points out, the random and dangerous use of powerful drugs has actually "brought about ill health". [15]

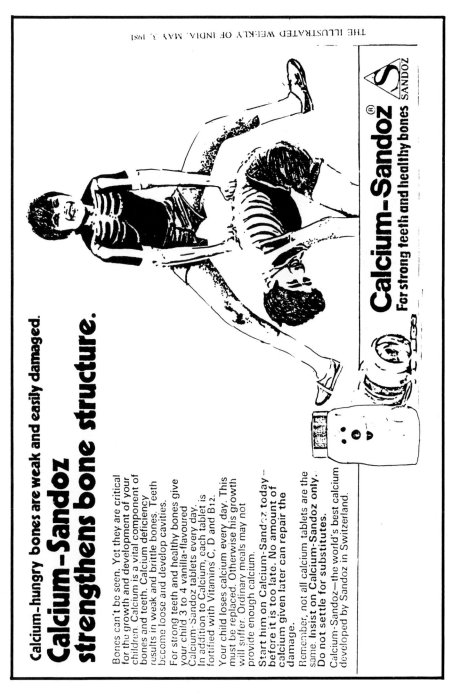

Calcium-hungry bones are weak and easily damaged.

Calcium–Sandoz strengthens bone structure.

Bones can't be seen. Yet they are critical for the growth and development of your children. Calcium is a vital component of bones and teeth. Calcium deficiency results in weak and brittle bones. Teeth become loose and develop cavities.

For strong teeth and healthy bones give your child 3 to 4 vanilla-flavoured Calcium-Sandoz tablets every day. In addition to Calcium, each tablet is fortified with Vitamins C, D and B12.

Your child loses calcium every day. This must be replaced. Otherwise his growth will suffer. Ordinary meals may not provide enough calcium.

Start him on Calcium-Sandoz today – before it is too late. No amount of calcium given later can repair the damage.

Remember, not all calcium tablets are the same. Insist on Calcium-Sandoz only. Do not settle for substitutes.

Calcium-Sandoz—the world's best calcium developed by Sandoz in Switzerland.

Calcium–Sandoz®
For strong teeth and healthy bones

SANDOZ

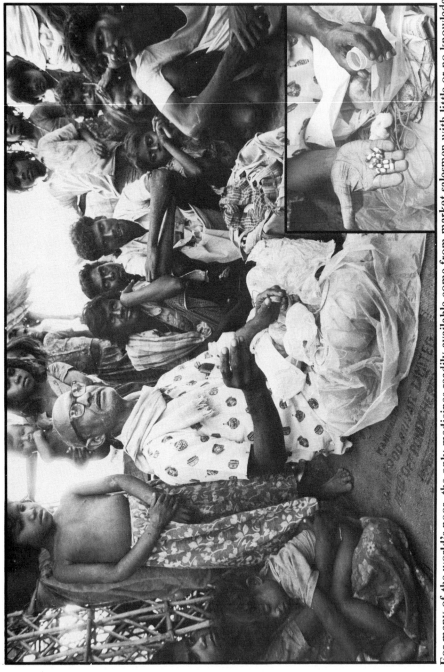

(Credit) Mike Wells.

For many of the world's poor, the only medicines readily available come from market salesmen with little or no knowledge of the ineffectiveness or potential dangers of some of their products.

The problem is that drugs are inherently 'unsafe'. According to the *British National Formulary,* "Almost any drug may produce unwanted or unexpected adverse reactions". [16] A professor of clinical pharmacy explains that "a drug's effects are like shot-gun pellets - some land on target, others do not", so "any drug produces some undesired effects along with the desired effects ..." [17] Consequently there are risks to be balanced against possible benefits in the use of any drug. In Britain, where the use of drugs is controlled by strict 'precription only' regulations, as many as one patient in ten is *reported* to suffer some adverse reaction to a prescription. Furthermore, a Cambridge Regius Professor of Medicine considers that the estimate of 6,000 deaths each year "associated with National Health Service prescriptions" is "unlikely to be an under-estimate". [18]

In developing countries where drug use is uncontrolled, the extent of drug-induced illness is impossible to measure. According to Dr. Silverman, "Among Latin American medical authorities - especially haematologists, pathologists and other experts - the damage caused by drugs is believed to be shockingly high". [19] But most people who take drugs in developing countries are not seen by doctors, let alone haematologists. In fact hardly any of the people prescribing and selling medicines in poor countries have any inkling of their possible dangerous side-effects and interactions with other drugs.

A French pharmacist round that 90% of pharmacies she visited in Mexico were staffed by unqualified sales assistants. All they knew about drugs they had learnt from visiting sales representatives. [20] They are fairly typical of drug sellers throughout the Third World, such as those observed by an anthropologist in El Salvador. "Pharmacy personnel in small towns have rarely received any formal training in the use of the products they sell. Some are skilful, but it is not uncommon for illiterate or semi-literate clerks or children to prescribe and dispense medications to customers seeking advice." [21]

The hazards are all too obvious. In Mitford market in Dacca, capital of Bangladesh, we bought one of the latest anti-cancer drugs over the counter. This drug which is used to treat lethal brain tumours, can have fatal side- effects. [22] The salesman assured us not only that it was "safe" but that it "cured all cancers". [23]

'PROBLEM' DRUGS

Manufacturers that we have approached about cases of misleading drug information and the marketing of harmful and non-essential products in poor countries invariably stress the differences in opinions and regulations that exist from one country to another. [24] For example, within Europe drugs considered too hazardous for sale in Britain and Scandinavian countries are still marketed in West Germany, Italy and other countries. Undoubtedly this complicates the issues as there can be as many opinions on the degree of risk of drugs as there are experts. [25]

But the 'differences' argument is advanced by companies to 'prove' that they are doing all that can reasonably be expected of them and that it is up to Third World governments both to decide which drugs they will allow onto the market, and to make sure they are used safely. But the argument needs to be turned on its head. Third World regulatory agencies rely on manufacturers for information on which to base their decisions. Inevitably manufacturers are in a position to convince governments that the advantages offered by their products outweigh possible hazards. As a result, drugs with known toxic side-effects are freely available in Third World countries. They are doled out to the unsuspecting often by illiterate sales assistants, quacks, even children, who can have no idea of the dangers, or that there may be 'safer' alternatives.

If anything the 'differences' - poverty and uncontrolled drug sales - put even more onus on manufacturers not to try to market drugs that can do more harm than good in developing countries, especially when they are not vital. Manufacturers are understandably sensitive about any singling out of individual 'problem' drugs - not least because all drugs carry some risk. But some carry more risk than others particularly in poor countries.

ANTIDIARRHOEALS

The dangers can readily be seen if we look at a number of antidiarrhoeal drugs widely sold in poor countries. According to WHO, diarrhoea is *the* major killer of children under three, particularly babies. [26] Two kinds of drugs are used to treat diarrhoea. One attacks the underlying infection causing the diarrhoea, the other stops only the *symptoms* of the infection, in other words, just the diarrhoea.

Any number of symptomatic antidiarrhoeals are marketed in the Third World. Amongst the most widely sold are Lomotil, manufactured by Searle, and the Ciba-Geigy products, Entero-Vioform and Mexaform. All are sold to treat young children of even very poor families. But experts, including Professor King and colleagues who compiled a WHO *Primary Child Care* manual for health workers, are adamant that "most children with diarrhoea don't need drugs". [27] They state that symtomatic drugs including diphenoxylate (the active ingredient of Lomotil) and Entero-Vioform "do not help children and are not necessary" ... "These drugs often *seem* to work with adults, because most adult patients with diarrhoea cure themselves. Many children have diarrhoea and you can waste much money giving them drugs which do not help." [28] (original emphasis)

Tragically, poor mothers are not aware of this. They *do* spend money on Lomotil, Entero-Vioform and Mexaform with the false assurance that these medicines will make the child better. No-one tells the mother that the immediate threat to her baby's life is not diarrhoea, but dehydration, which she can prevent with a home-made solution of water, salt and sugar.

Drug sellers through their ignorance, encourage mothers to believe that antidiarrhoeals will make the babies better. Manufacturers apear to have been doing very little to warn of the dangers. [29] A mother's false sense of security can lead to her baby's death.

98

LOMOTIL

But poor people are even less likely to be told that, apart from not being particularly helpful to their children, these comforting products also have hidden dangers. In the case of Lomotil (which contains diphenoxylate hydrochloride and atropine sulphate) the manufacturers warn British doctors that "Lomotil should be used with caution in young children", because "accidental overdosage may produce unconsciousness with respiratory depression, particularly in children, or atropine poisoning, or both". [30] These toxic reactions can be fatal. [31]

One doctor explains that the indiscriminate use of antidiarrhoeals in prolonged attacks of diarrhoea can run the risk of their acting as a "blindly harmful stopcock". [32] Lomotil stops diarrhoea from coming out, but to do that it also prevents the body from getting rid of the organism causing the infection. So Lomotil can make the infection last longer. [33] Although the child's body stops expelling fluid and vital electrolytes, these are not necessarily absorbed and may just be accumulating in the paralysed gut. This means that Lomotil can hide the seriousness of a child's condition, because it "can mask the signs of dehydration". [34] The dangers are potentially so great that experts urge doctors treating children to "avoid the potentially dangerous use of Lomotil for the treatment of diarrhoea". [35]

In recent years Third World prescribers have not been given the same warnings as British and American doctors. Since 1973 the US regulatory agency has stopped its use in children under two. [36] In Britain Lomotil is sold only on prescription, and Searle advises doctors that it "should not be given to children under one year old". [37] But in Third World countries, where there are no effective prescription controls, the manufacturers have recommended dosages for babies under a year old. The London-based action research unit, Social Audit, carried out an in-depth case-study and found that Lomotil has been recommended in India for babies "aged up to 3 months", and for Brazilian babies weighing "only 3kg (or some 6½ lbs) - a low-to-average birth weight". [38]

Lomotil has also been sold in poor countries without any warnings that it can be harmful to children. For example, in 1980 in North Yemen we bought packs of Lomotil *with neomycin* freely over the counter. Those packs, manufactured in High Wycombe, England, in May 1979, gave no precautions for use in children. This combination product with neomycin is even more expensive than Lomotil alone. Moreover, both WHO and the *British National Formulary* (1981) advise against the use of neomycin in treating diarrhoea. [39] Lomotil is also widely sold in Central America. The label of a small bottle purchased by OXFAM staff in the Dominican Republic in 1980 does give a warning in Spanish that the drug should be used "delicately". It also advises that in the event of an overdose the patient should be admitted to hospital. But there are no recommended *maximum* doses on the label.

In September 1981 Searle made the encouraging announcement that "in response to concerns expressed by Social Audit, Searle has decided to revise its product labelling to indicate clearly that Lomotil should be used for the adjunctive treatment of diarrhoea and is not recommended for use in children under two years of age provided these changes are acceptable to local regulatory bodies". [40]

Lomotil is a useful drug of convenience for the rich. But it can cost "up to 25 times more than other widely used symptomatic treatments for diarrhoea". [41] In response to the concern we have expressed that Lomotil is unlikely to represent 'value for money' for the poor, Searle have sent us the results of various clinical trials, but the reliability of some of these has been seriously called into question by Social Audit. [42] The hazards remain. How will illiterate drug sellers understand that Lomotil is only an "adjunctive treatment" without pictograms backed by an active health education campaign? [43]

CLIOQUINOL

Ciba-Geigy's antidiarrhoeals, Entero-Vioform and Mexaform, both containing clioquinol, are freely available over the counter in many developing countries. In most cases we found them on sale in foil strips, without instructions or warnings. Sales assistants in Bangladesh, India and North Yemen were obviously completely in the dark about the controversy that has surrounded the use of clioquinol since an 'epidemic' of drug-induced illness broke out in Japan in the 1960s. More than 10,000 people in Japan were victims of what came to be known as 'SMON' (sub-acute myelo-optic neuropathy). As a result of using clioquinol, they suffered numbness, weakness in the legs and eye damage. Some of the people who had taken prolonged high doses ended up in wheelchairs, others completely blind. [44] It has since been established that clioquinol can cause "toxic effects on the central nervous system". [45] The manufacturers of the most-widely sold clioquinol products, Ciba-Geigy and others, have paid compensation to victims in Japan and Europe. [46]

Entero-Vioform which was once sold over the counter in Britain "for the prevention and treatment of holiday diarrhoea" was effectively removed from the British market when all its licensed indications were withdrawn. [47] One antidiarrhoeal containing clioquinol was still listed in 1981 as available on a doctor's prescription, but doctors are warned: "Special precaution: avoid prolonged administration". [48] It has been withdrawn in other developed countries and the expert committee that decided on the WHO selection of essential drugs excluded clioquinol because they decided that the risks outweighed the benefits. [49] But some developing countries have included clioquinol specifically for use in amoebic dysentry as a three to four day course can be cheaper than treatment with antibiotics. [50]

Ciba-Geigy's UK-based Head of International Medical Liaison has assured us that the company is "making genuine attempts to ensure adequate literature and warnings are given about taking long courses or too many courses which could give rise to neurological symptoms. The problem is ensuring that this information reaches the patient." [51] From our research we know it clearly does not. Salesmen in North Yemen, India and Bangladesh whom we questioned about the safety of Entero-Vioform and Mexaform assured us that these drugs were "completely

100

safe'', as they urged us to buy handfuls of foil strips to treat ''all'' diarrhoea. They gave us vague and contradictory advice about the dosage we should take, and in many cases, no maximum dosage appeared on the packaging we received.

Ciba-Geigy is by no means the only manufacturer of antidiarrhoeals containing clioquinol which has not succeeded in ensuring that Third World patients and, in some cases, even doctors receive any warnings about prolonged use. In Bangladesh, for example, Fisons' local subsidiary is marketing Fistrep, a product containing 250mg of ''iodochlorhydroxyquinoline'' (ie clioquinol under its less well-known chemical name) and 100mg of streptomycin sulphate. The dose recommended for adults in the Bangladesh *Prescriber's Guide 79* (current in September 1980) was 1.5g daily. This means that even if they resisted the temptation to take more, *within a week* Bengali patients would have taken as much clioquinol as some of the Japanese SMON victims. [52] Fisons are not of course responsible for the entry in the Guide, but Fistrep has been selling in foil strips without warnings of the maximum dose.

At the moment there is no evidence to suggest that Bengalis are particularly susceptible to SMON. But nor is there any conclusive evidence to prove that they are any less susceptible than people in Japan, Sweden, or Britain. In the circumstances there is little room for complacency. [53] A remark recently attributed to the Managing Director of Fisons (Bangladesh) - if correctly reported - is particularly disturbing. He is reported to have expressed the view that ''We are businessmen first. First of all we want profits... we are oversensitive about reports from WHO. Restrictions on drugs and pesticides imposed in the US and Canada should not be applied in our country because our people are ethnically and biologically different from others.'' [54]

BAD INFORMATION MEANS DANGEROUS DRUG USE

It is inevitable that drug use will be even less safe in the Third World if manufacturers do not make sure that the people dispensing their products understand how they should be used. Getting the key information across to 'prescribers' with no medical training obviously presents major problems, particularly when so many are illiterate. A Swiss professor of pharmacology stresses that it is very difficult to balance the conflicting needs of Third World doctors, untrained drug sellers and illiterate patients, with the added complication of very limited space. Too much information can be as dangerous as too little. People may find it all too daunting and ignore all the warnings. [55]

In some cases, even with the best of intentions, manufacturers can end up detracting from the safe use of their products. In Third World countries it has become increasingly common to sell drugs in foil strips without cardboard packs or package inserts. This has the advantage of keeping down prices whilst still protecting drugs from humidity in tropical climates. But foil strips have the major disadvantage of allowing almost no space for vital information on dosage, and precautions for use.

The marketing manager of Fisons (Bangladesh) explained to us that manufacturers can come up against opposition when they attempt to make drug information more readily available. When Fisons consulted local doctors on whether they would like drug information to be in the local language, many were fiercely against the idea. The doctors' stated objection to the proposal was that it would encourage dangerous self-medication. [56] Clearly they take a dim view of any move that might make patients less dependent on them.

Similarly, in Central America some major foreign manufacturers are reported to have "eliminated the package inserts they used to include with their prescription products, purportedly in an effort to reduce the over-the-counter sale of these medications". [57] But this suppression of information had little impact on self-medication. If anything it made the situation worse. "The lack of package inserts describing indications for use, contra-indications, warnings and doses of medications led people to misuse products. For example one of the pharmacy owners was hospitalised as a result of an overdose of a product she took to treat a headache. The package contained no information regarding dose, very general indications for use and a label saying 'to be sold only with a physician's prescription'." [58]

In most developing countries a label that reads "to be dispensed on Doctor's prescription only" can be little more than decorative. Moreover, because drugs are so often prescribed by untrained people, the fact that package inserts are invariably written in technical jargon that is intelligible only to doctors and pharmacists drastically limits their usefulness. Warnings given in simple, direct language, or in picture form, could help encourage the safe use of drugs. At the moment, manufacturers in many cases are failing to put across information essential to the safe use of their products. In some cases the information given to Third World prescribers has been dangerously misleading.

The problems are illustrated by the way in which anabolic steroids have recently been promoted in poor countries. Their use is controversial and limited in developed countries, not least because they can cause serious toxic side-effects.

ANABOLIC STEROIDS

These drugs have not turned out to be as useful as was once hoped. [59] Their recommended uses have been shrinking so that in Britain and other developed countries they are now used for relatively few serious conditons including osteoporosis (bone disease), blood diseases such as aplastic anaemia, and chronic kidney failure "with varying degrees of success". [60] They are also given to women with breast cancer (though less so with modern surgery), people with chronic debilitating diseases, especially the elderly, and patients after major surgery to help build up body protein. [61] But a professor of clinical pharmacy stresses that it is "much more important to ensure that the patient takes a nourishing diet (high in protein)" than anabolic steroids. [62]

Anabolic steroids became popularly known as body-builders because of the publicity over their use by athletes. But the *British National Formulary* is adamant that "their use as body-builders or tonics is quite unjustified", not least because anabolic steroids have very nasty side-effects. [63] They can cause irreversible virilisation (hirsutism, enlargement of the clitoris and deepening of the voice). Most patients on anabolic steroids suffer some adverse effects to the liver, which can include jaundice and liver tumours. Another possible side effect is sodium retention causing oedema and heart failure. But experts stress that they can be particularly harmful to children: "The use of anabolic steroids to promote growth in underdeveloped children may lead to premature fusion of the ephiphyses and stunting of growth in adolescence." [64]

ORABOLIN DROPS

However, in Bangladesh the Dutch manufacturers Organon have been promoting a number of anabolic steroids specifically "for paediatric use in conditions like marasmus, malnutrition, poor weight gain, retarded growth, kwashiorkor etc.," listing one advantage after another without a word of warning about the hazards. Doctors are told, for example, that either one of Organon's two products Durabolin and Deca-Durabolin "stimulates appetite and ensures adequate food intake ... checks protein depletion ... increases resistance against infectious diseases [and] improves the general constitution and restores sense of well being". [65]

Dr. Schweiger, a British doctor working in a remote rural area of Bangladesh, drew our attention to the problem in 1980. A visiting Organon sales representative had specifically pointed out their anabolic steroid, Orabolin drops, because he knew the doctor was "working with malnourished children". [66] The insert on Orabolin from the Therapeutic Index of Organon (Bangladesh) is reproduced overleaf together with Organon's data sheet on Organon tablets for British doctors. (Orabolin Drops are not sold in Britain.)

Doctors in Bangladesh have been told that Orabolin is "a powerful anabolic agent" which is "exceptionally well tolerated, causes no fluid retention and is free from harmful effects on liver ... The raspberry flavoured liquid administered in drops is especially meant for younger children and infants." No warnings are given. [67]

Doctors in Britain are advised that Orabolin is "not recommended for children". Warnings include the fact that "anabolic steroids may cause fluid retention ...tumours of the liver have been reported occasionally", and that the development of tumours "cannot at present be excluded, and this should be considered when the use of this product is proposed, especially in young people who are not suffering from life-threatening disorders". [68]

In December 1981 Organon informed us that "It is our policy that promotion both verbal and written should be confined to indications as approved by the respective health authorities. It is therefore obligatory for local companies to have all material used for doctors' information approved by headquarters. Unfortunately sometimes the system does not work and something slips through. The printed material you saw, when in Bangladesh [i.e. September 1980] had not yet arrived (and consequently not approved) with Organon International. We

Organon

ORABOLIN
Tablets and Drops

Composition:
Tablets containing 2 mg. Ethylestrenol.
Drops containing 2 mg. Ethylestrenol per ml. aqueous solution.

Clinical Effects:
Ethylestrenol, the active principle of ORABOLIN, is a powerful anabolic agent which is fully effective when orally administered. Extensive tests have shown that ethylestrenol has an anabolic/androgenic ratio almost 20 times than that of methyltestosterone. In practice the small daily dose required. 0.05 mg. per Kg. body weight, ensures that the only clinical effect is anabolism.
ORABOLIN stimulates the appetite, promotes weight gain and in elderly debilitated patients produces a marked psychological improvement. Metabolic balance studies have shown that both nitrogen and calcium are retained during treatment, and that a negative nitrogen balance during corticosteroid therapy can be reversed. ORABOLIN is exceptionally well tolerated, causes no fluid retention and is free from harmful effects on liver and adrenals.
The raspberry flavoured liquid administered in drops is especially meant for younger children and infants.

Indication :
In adults :- Convalescence, weight loss, debility, osteoporosis, slow - healing fractures, during corticoid therapy, as an adjuvant after acute and chronic diseases.
In Children :- Retarded growth, lack of appetite and insufficient weight, nutritional disorders, failure to thrive and after infectious diseases.

Dosage :
Adults : 2 tablets daily
Children : According to body weight

Weight in Kg.	Drops per day
Less than 10 Kg.	5 drops
10-30 Kg.	1 drop/kg.
more than 30 kg.	30 drops.

Packing :
Bottles of 20 tablets.
Dropper-bottles of 5 ml.

ORABOLIN*

Presentation Ethylestrenol Tablets. Round, flat white tablets, diameter 9 mm, code-marked 'SB3' on one side, with 'Organon' and star on the reverse side.

Active ingredient: Ethylestrenol BP 2 mg per tablet.

Uses Ethylestrenol is an anabolic agent, the nitrogen and calcium retaining effects of which are fully effective when it is administered orally.

Dosage and administration Adults 1–2 tablets orally daily. Not recommended for children.

Contra-indications, warnings, etc Contra-indicated in pregnancy, prostatic carcinoma, breast carcinoma in the male and in severe disturbances of liver function.
Treatment should be discontinued if cholestatic jaundice appears or liver function tests become abnormal.
Tumours of the liver have been reported occasionally in patients subjected to prolonged treatment with C-17-alkylated androgenic-anabolic steroids. The possibility that these compounds may induce or enhance the development of hepatic tumours cannot at present be excluded and this should be considered when the use of this product is proposed, especially in young people.
Patients with myocardial or renal dysfunction, hypertension or epilepsy should be observed carefully, since anabolic steroids may cause fluid retention.
Skeletal maturation should be followed carefully when treating young people, since anabolic steroids in high dosages may accelerate this process.
Caution should be observed in young women whose cycles are not yet stabilised.
In diabetics, the need for insulin or other anti-diabetic drugs may be reduced.
When administered in the recommended dosages and for short periods of time (up to four weeks) side-effects may occur very rarely. Occasionally after high dosages, some liver function tests show abnormal values. These deviations, however, are transient and completely reversible after discontinuation of treatment. In some cases, particularly those treated with high dosages, nausea and some water retention may occur.
The possibility of menstrual disturbances exists, probably resulting from an inhibition of the secretion of gonadotrophins from the pituitary and/or from the occurrence of a progestational effect. In such cases the treatment should be discontinued or the dosage decreased.

Pharmaceutical precautions Protect from light.

Legal category POM.

Package quantities Bottles of 100 tablets.

Further information Nil.

Product licence number 0065/5043

Conflicting information on prescribing for children. Left, therapeutic information, Bangladesh; right, entry from data sheet for British doctors.

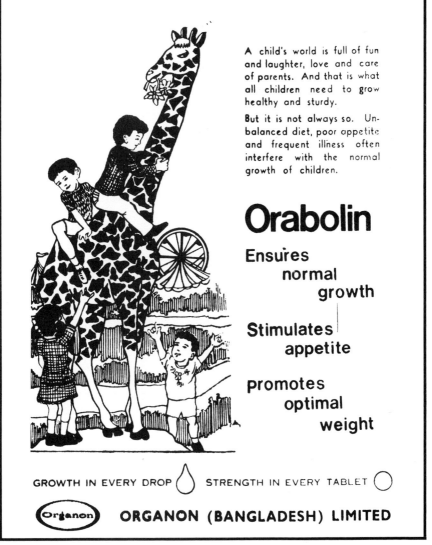

Advertisement which appeared in a magazine issued at a conference on The Role
of Rural Doctors in Child Care, at Dacca Children's Hospital in May 1981. The
conference was sponsored by WHO and the Bangladesh Ministry of Health.

have a rather strict product surveillance activity and also as a result of your information we have taken corrective measures with respect to Bangladesh, as well as other countries where this may have occurred.'' [69]

In January 1982 we wrote to Organon asking for a copy of the revised product entry. We did not receive this, but in April we were sent a copy of an Organon 'Product Safeguard' for Orabolin which the company advise us they distribute to doctors in Bangladesh. This contains 'warnings and precautions', but repeats that "Orabolin drops are especially suitable for use in children" without specifying any limitations on their use. [70]

ANAPOLON

Organon is not the only manufacturer to have been marketing anabolic steroids in Bangladesh as body-builders for children. The Bangladesh subsidiary of ICI produces an anabolic steroid, Anapolon (oxymetholone), under licence from Syntex. The advertisement on page 107 shows that ICI have promoted this to doctors as a "potent, *safe* anabolic agent" with "manifold uses" including to "promote growth in underdeveloped children". (our emphasis) A number of the claims made are directly contradicted by the Syntex UK data sheet. British doctors are warned that Anapolon in high doses "may lead to virilisation in ... pre-pubertal children" and that it can have "slight" virilising effects even in low doses. [71] The ICI Bangladesh advertisement claims "no effect on liver function". But the *British National Formulary* entry for Anapolon states that "jaundice and liver disturbances are common". [72]

The Chairman of ICI's Pharmaceutical Division has written with the reassurance that "I believe that your criticism of certain of the claims made does have substantial justification. I accept that the unqualified use of the word 'safe' is inappropriate - and more importantly, that the suggestion that the product be used in children who are under-developed as a result of malnourishment is open to criticism. Within the ICI international pharmaceutical operations, great care is taken to ensure that technical claims made for any ICI product are both medically and scientifically justified ... I find that Anapolon, being a product produced under licence and sold in only one country, has not been subject to the full rigours of that system. Steps have immediately been taken to withdraw all copies of that product leaflet..." [73]

In April 1982 Ciba-Geigy announced their decision to withdraw their anobolic steroid Dianabol worldwide. Dr. Burley advised us that Ciba had "come to the conclusion that the balance betweeen the use of the drug in certain medical conditions such as osteoporosis and anaemia is outweighed by the unfavourable side-effects when the drug is used either as a vitamin supplement or by athletes and others wishing to improve their performance". [74]

PAINKILLERS
When a decision is made to withdraw a drug in Europe or the US, the evidence suggests that it by no means follows that manufacturers will always voluntarily

ANAPOLON
OXYMETHOLONE

THE POTENT, SAFE ANABOLIC AGENT

● Restores weight loss

● Promotes utilisation of protein

● Stimulates appetite

● Speeds post-operative recovery and convalescence after illness

● Improves physical condition

● Induces sense of well-being

● Corrects de-calcification and relieves low back pain of osteoporosis especially in post-menopausal and senile women

● Promotes growth in underdeveloped children

● Non-virilising

● No fluid retention

● No effect on liver function

● Well tolerated at all ages

THE MANIFOLD USES OF 'ANAPOLON'
After debilitating diseases, muscle wasting states such as poliomyelitis and in bedridden patients. Malnutrition, carcinoma, arthritic conditions, asthenia, tuberculosis and sprue.
After severe infections.
After surgical operations.
After burns, fractures, injuries, etc.
During and after corticosteroid therapy to counteract excessive protein loss.
For children underdeveloped or debilitated as the result of illness or malnourishment.

DOSE :
Average course : Adults 1-2 tablets (5-10mg.) per day over 30-45 days.
Children ½ –1 tablet per day for 30 days.

PRESENTATION :
Scored Tablets of 5 mg. in packs of 25.

 ICI Bangladesh
Manufacturers Limited
9. Motijheel Commercial Area
Dacca - 2

Promotion of anabolic steroid for malnourished children, Bangladesh.

remove their product from the Third World market. The problems are illustrated by two chemically-related painkillers, whose use has recently either been controlled or completely stopped in a number of developed countries. By contrast, they continued to be widely marketed in Third World countries for over-the-counter sale, with no warnings of the dangers.

AMIDOPYRINE

For over 30 years amidopyrine has been known to cause agranulocytosis. This fatal blood disease kills by destroying the body's protective mechanism against infection - the white blood cells. As early as 1938 sales in the US were restricted to a doctor's prescription. In 1963 in response to the consensus of medical opinion, the drug was voluntarily withdrawn in Britain by one of its leading Swiss producers, today's Ciba-Geigy, (Ciba and Geigy merged in 1970). [75]

Amidopyrine is only one of a number of drugs, such as chloramphenicol, that can cause similar fatal toxic reactions. [76] But whereas chloramphenicol is an inexpensive life-saving drug, invaluable in typhoid epidemics, not only does amidopyrine not save lives, but it offers few advantages over other 'safer' painkillers. When the drug also came under suspicion of causing cancer, the Swiss drug regulatory authorities recommended its complete withdrawal. [77] In 1977 two Swiss manufacturers, Ciba-Geigy (which marketed four amidopyrine-based products) and Sandoz, with two, announced their intention to remove amidopyrine from all their formulations by the end of the year. [78] They were to be reformulated with prophyphenazone, a chemically-related drug.

Three years later, however, Ciba products containing amidopyrine were still being sold under the brand-names Cibalgin and Spasmo-Cibalgin in ten developing countries, and Portugal. In only one case was any warning given about the risk of fatal agranulocytosis. [79] The drug was still being used for minor pains including "painful conditions of all kinds e.g. headache, toothache, feverish colds, chills and influenza". [80] In December 1979 all six Ciba and Sandoz formulations were on sale over the counter in Mexico. [81] Ciba explain that they "did not think that the substitution of propyphenazone was urgent or demanded a product recall". [82] The reason for withdrawing amidopyrine was ostensibly the cancer risk, not agranulocytosis (which had been known about for so long). Consequently Ciba decided "to give priority to northern or non-tropical countries where nitrites are found in higher concentrations" because of the greater consumption of processed foods "such as sausages and hamburgers, but also beer". [83]

But it was not just a question of the old stocks that remained on pharmacy shelves in developing countries. As *The Lancet* reported in November 1981, "There is evidence that Ciba-Geigy has continued to manufacture preparations containing amidopyrine and that they have been selling off old stocks of preparations containing amidopyrine even after registering the new formulations". [84] Mexican trade statistics for 1978 show that Ciba imported 8,500 kilos of amidopyrine into the country, with 80% of the supply coming from Switzerland. [85]

Ciba-Geigy did successfully register the new formulation of Spasmo-Cibalgin without amidopyrine with the Philippines Food and Drugs Administration (FDA) in November 1978. But preparations with amidopyrine continued to be imported up to May 1978. [86] The old formulation of injectable Spasmo-Cibalgin was still in stock in a wholesale distributor's warehouse and was being sold to retail pharmacies in November 1980. A team from Dutch television which filmed these stocks interviewed the Managing Director of Ciba-Geigy Philippines who said that they had been told to deplete their existing stocks of the old formulation with the agreement of the Philippines FDA and Ciba headquarters in Basle. In November 1980 Dr. Arsenio Regala, the Philippines Food and Drugs Administrator, said he knew nothing of this arrangement. The Dutch film "Healthy Business" was shown in Europe at the beginning of 1981. Subsequently a 'to whom it may concern' letter dated 7 May 1981 arrived from the Philippines FDA saying that permission to use up old stocks of amidopyrine had in fact been granted, provided the manufacturers gave full information and warnings on the product labels. [87]

In September 1980 we purchased foil strips of Cibalgin over the counter in Bangalore in India. These contained amidopyrine and gave no dosage instructions or warnings. The manufacturing date appeared on each strip showing that they had been produced in Bombay in *February 1980.*

The delay in registering the new formulation of Cibalgin in India was apparently partly due to reluctance from the Indian Government. [88] Whereas amidopyrine was formulated locally, the new active ingredient, propyphenazone, would have to be imported. The Swiss companies were not alone in continuing to market amidopyrine. In 1981 there were reported to be 33 formulations on the Indian market alone. [89] The Central Drug Authority issued instructions to manufacturers in 1980 to withdraw amidopyrine "in a phased manner". But according to an Indian newspaper report in 1981 the Government "did not specify a deadline for the withdrawal and this seems to have been taken advantage of by the manufacturers and druggists". [90]

There is also evidence that at least one of the major manufacturers continued actively to promote sales of amidopyrine in a developing country two years after the drug's withdrawal had been announced in Switzerland. In 1979 a salesman for Ciba-Geigy was reported to be distributing free samples of Cibalgin in Maputo, the capital of Mozambique, dismissing fears over possible toxic side-effects as exaggerated. At that very time, a young British teacher was being rushed out of the country for emergency treatment, one of the few *recognised* victims of drug-induced illness in a Third World country. Carol Gates had been prescribed Cibalgin - for a headache. Without advanced medical treatment she would have died. [91]

Dr. Burley of Ciba-Geigy informs us: "I have never defended the lack of information in our literature about Cibalgin in Mozambique, and this matter was settled between Carol Gates and ourselves. Because of the very great publicity that surrounded the Carol Gates case, I think I was quite right to say that amidopyrine drew far more attention than perhaps it warranted. Anyway the situation is now unlikely to arise with aminophenazone (amidopyrine) again." [92] Dr.Burley explains that Ciba-Geigy stopped manufacture of all aminophenazone derivatives by December 1981.

DIPYRONE

Some of the most widely sold painkillers in the Third World today contain dipyrone, a drug that is chemically related to amidopyrine and can also cause fatal agranulocytosis in an estimated 0.57% of users. [93] Dipyrone has been described as "about as effective as aspirin". [94] The drug has been completely withdrawn from the market in Britain and the US on the grounds that "the incidence and risk of potentially fatal agranulocytosis ... far outweigh any benefit that can be derived from its use". [95]

The balance of risks, however, has been assessed very differently in West Germany, the home market of some of the leading manufacturers of these drugs. These include Hoechst, Boehringer Ingelheim, Asta-Werke and Merck, which all market dipyrone products in the Third World. In West Germany the widespread use of dipyrone and similar drugs for minor pains is highly controversial. At the beginning of 1982 an expert committee recommended that their use should be restricted to prescription only. Hoechst and other manufacturers oppose any new restrictions on the grounds that they are not justified by the risks. [96] At any rate West German doctors and pharmacists are well aware of the controversy and of the possible toxic side-effects, unlike many of their counterparts in developing countries.

According to UNCTAD at least ten different leading brands of painkillers containing dipyrone are marketed in the Third World. [97] In Mexico, for example, the eighth best-selling drug on the entire market, Hoechst's NeoMelubrina, contains it, as does the next most popular analgesic (by sales value and volume), Boehringer's Buscapina Compositum. [98] Consequently, thousands of patients in Mexico alone, who know nothing of the possible risks, may be unnecessarily exposed to danger when 'safer' alternatives exist. [99]

Health authorities may have difficulties in removing these and other products. In Bangladesh, for example, having assessed the dangers of the uncontrolled use of dipyrone, Drug Administration officials instructed manufacturers to remove products containing dipyrone from the market by 1980. This ban encountered local opposition. Subsequently another government department ruled that the ban need not take effect until the end of December 1982. [100]

INJECTIONS

There are some drugs that present a major health hazard in developing countries because they cannot be given safely by untrained drug sellers. One of the most striking examples is injectable drugs. Injections are very much in demand throughout the Third World. Many of the world's poor believe that tablets and pills are a second-rate substitute for an injection. Drug sellers are also keen on injections because they can charge customers both for the actual drug and for injecting it.

There are contrasting views on why injections are so popular. An OXFAM researcher writes from Upper Volta that injections are widely used. "This is a characteristic feature of Voltaique medical practice and the reasons seem complex. Originally injections were introduced by French doctors and probably became entirely associated with the new Western medicine. Pills, liquid, or ointments were similar to traditional medicine, while the needle was a complete novelty..." [101] In Africa as a whole from the 1950s the eradication of yaws by the use of injectable penicillin is reported to have made a deep and lasting impression. [102]

By contrast, Dr. Hassani in North Yemen attributes the popularity of injections to the traditional belief, common to most societies, that anything that makes you better must hurt. In Yemen treatments administered by traditional cuppers and burners can be very painful. Dr. Hassani explains that many of his patients insist on having injections of calcium gluconate. These can, and should, be given slowly and painlessly. But if he gives the injection correctly the patients complain that they have been cheated because they could not feel the 'difference'. So in Yemen doctors and drug sellers inject calcium fast. As another doctor points out - this practice can kill. [103]

The Yemenis' addiction to injections carries other unsuspected dangers, as a doctor working in a remote, mountainous area explains: "Many hormone injections and vitamin injections are given for 'gawi' (strength). These drugs are not known to be effective and in some cases are positively dangerous. Many a time we have seen a hormone preparation given to a woman because of a delayed period. The doctor had not examined her and in fact, often it was a brother, father or husband who had brought it to her. No one could read to see that one of the contra-indications was early pregnancy!" [104]

A recent report by the Institute of Development Studies in Britain on health services in rural Ghana showed that some health centres give injections to over 80% of patients. The over-use of chloroquine injections in particular was rampant. They were routinely given to adults who complained of fever but were not in a serious condition. These patients could have been treated with antimalarial tablets for a fraction the cost of the injections. Unnecessary injections can cost more than money. Young children routinely injected with chloroquine were needlessly exposed to the risk of sudden death from absorbing the drug too fast. [105]

Because the Ghanaian clinics gave so many injections, they were always short of syringes. So disposable syringes had to be rinsed out and reused. In some health units one needle was used for more than 20 patients. [106] Few untrained injection givers have any notion that if they hit the sciatic nerve, they can paralyse their patient's leg, or that an unsterile needle can cause painful abcesses or serum heptatitis. They are not aware that a dirty syringe can kill.

Manufacturers must be aware of the dangers, for back-room injections are routine and in some Third World countries it is a common sight for ordinary people to be buying syringes and vials for home injections. In Bangladesh Fisons' subsidiary has produced an instruction leaflet in Bengali on how to give an injection safely

111

and Pfizer showed a documentary there on the subject. [107] But few injection givers come into contact with helpful advice. In the home of one poor family in North Yemen we witnessed a home injection of procaine-penicillin and streptomycin which one woman gave another for a cut thumb which had already been well daubed and protected from infection with gentian violet. Before giving the injection the woman unwrapped the disposable syringe and left it on the floor. She made no attempt to cleanse her cousin's arm. This injection of two antibiotics to forestall a possible infection carried dangers undreamt of by these Yemenis.

ANTIBIOTICS AND DRUG RESISTANCE

The combined injection was of two key drugs, penicillin and streptomycin. These are relatively inexpensive and therefore used as *first line* drugs for attacking a range of bacterial infections. Streptomycin is particularly useful for TB. But if these antibiotics are over-used the bacteria they attack quickly build up resistance. Bacteria can make themselves resistant to streptomycin very fast, so the drug becomes useless for TB sufferers. They then end up paying for more costly *second-line* antibiotics. Drug resistance presents problems everywhere. But it can make the difference between life and death in poor countries.

An Indian doctor explains that the use of streptomycin "in combination with penicillin [and] chloramphenicol for ordinary infections is creating increasing problems for developing countries like ours. Primary resistance of tuberculosis to streptomycin which is one of the first-line drugs is a calamity. We can't afford expensive second-line drugs. Further infection of individuals with resistant tuberculous mycobacteria helps in making the situation worse." [108] A doctor in Bangladesh confirms that "patients are very likely to die as a result of this".[109]

Despite the obvious dangers, in many Third World countries manufacturers are marketing products containing streptomycin and other first-line antituberculous drugs for trivial, unnecessary uses. For example, UNCTAD reports that many cough and cold remedies containing streptomycin are sold in Nepal, a country where almost a quarter of child deaths are caused by TB. [110]

These antibiotic mixtures are more irrational than they may at first appear. Antibiotics attack *bacteria*. Colds are caused by *viruses*. So it is futile to take an antibiotic for a cold. It is also pointless, and even self-defeating to take antibiotics as a routine treatment for diarrhoea. The *British National Formulary* stresses that "most cases of diarrhoea are not bacterial in origin", but "even when a bacterial cause is suspected, antibiotics ... should be *avoided* ... because they may prolong rather than shorten the time taken to control diarrhoea and carrier states". [111] (original emphasis)

Yet antibiotics are commonly taken for diarrhoea and non-bacterial infections all over the Third World. One drug store owner in a large village in Bangladesh told us that he *always* recommends the antibiotic Sumycin (tetracycline syrup) for young children suffering from diarrhoea. Not surprisingly, it is his best selling product and he orders it frequently. He said that the sales representative for the manufacturers, Squibb, has never mentioned on his monthly visits that tetracycline should not be used indiscriminately for any attack of diarrhoea. Nor had the drug store owner ever heard that he should not sell tetracycline for young children or pregnant women. The Sumycin packs he sold gave none of the warnings that must be given in developed countries. [112] Squibb Bangladesh assure us they have never promoted Sumycin for the treatment of diarrhoea and have promised to investigate the retailer in question. [113]

In the Bangladesh *Prescriber's Guide* (current in September 1980) doctors are informed that Upjohn's antibiotic Lincocin (licomycin) is particulary useful for treating a number of conditions including "acne vulgaris". [114] The *British National Formulary,* referring to licomycin, stresses that "These antibiotics have a very limited use because of their serious side-effects". [115]Upjohn inform us that they do not recommend Lincocin for "acne vulgaris" in any country. They point out that they have no editorial control over guides like the *Bangladesh Prescriber's Guide,* and that they will attempt to have the indication removed from the Guide. [116] But the scale of the problem of over-use of potentially dangerous antibiotics is enormous. In 1978, Lincocin was the second best selling drug on the *entire* Mexican market. [117]

Some rich world manufacturers appear to have actively encouraged the misuse of powerful and potentially dangerous antibiotics for mild infections. For example in North Yemen the Swiss company, Rivopharm, has marketed Rivomycin Strepto (a combination of chloramphenicol and dihydrostreptomycin) indicating that the drug can be given to infants for "common diarrhoea". [118]No mention is made of "the liability of chloramphenicol to produce life-threatening toxic effects, particularly bone-marrow aplasia..." which in the authoritative words of *Martindale* (the pharmacists' 'bible') means that the drug "should never be given for minor infections". [119] It was recommended by a Yemeni pharmacist to the author (along with Entero-Vioform) for a mild attack of diarrhoea.

Rivopharm wrote to us on 11 February 1982 stating: "We strongly object and we are at a loss to understand the basis of your statement that 'Rivopharm appears to be actively encouraging the misuse of two powerful and potentially dangerous antibiotics'. We believe that you overlooked the clear and distinct statement (in English and French) [not Arabic - author's comment] on the Rivomycin Strepto outer carton ... that the product is 'to be dispensed on medical prescription'." [120] This statement was confirmed in a further letter of 8 April 1982. But by 17 May there was an apparent change of heart and a more encouraging response from Rivopharm. "We would like to communicate to you that the leaflet insert of Rivomycin Strepto is under examination and revision, as part of our regular revision procedure. This revision will be done with the view to change the leaflet and in particular to delete the words 'common diarrhoea', which may be misleading as you have rightly indicated." [121]

However greater impetus to drug misuse of this sort comes from local manufacturers. For instance, in Bangladesh one of the leading local companies has recommended the use of ampicillin for influenza, coughs, infantile diarrhoea, boils, even hepatitis (for which there is at present no known drug cure). [122].

As a result all the key *first-line* antibiotics are used irrationally throughout the Third World. The pattern seems to be, when in doubt, prescribe an antibiotic. A pharmacist in Bangladesh will recommend a penicillin injection for a baby with nappy rash. Hospital doctors in North Yemen will give penicillin injections to a breast-feeding mother with sore nipples. In Bangladesh a young boy knocked down by a motorised rickshaw is prescribed tetracycline (and half a dozen other drugs) for mild concussion. Even in remote areas of the Amazon, poorly trained health workers have been distributing tetracycline capsules with apparent total disregard for the problems of drug resistance. [123]

The extent of the over-use of antibiotics is illustrated by the records of drug consumption from just one health station in Ethiopia over a *three month* period. During that time a total of about 100 patients consumed the entire stock of 500 vials of procaine-penicillin, 500 vials of streptomycin, 4,000 capsules of tetracycline and 2,000 capsules of chloramphenicol. The patients' records show that some were given streptomycin for coughs, and others simultaneous course of three antibiotics (chloramphenicol, penicillin and streptomycin) for bronchitis. [124]

Since both manufacturers and prescribers give too much encouragement to the indiscriminate use of antibiotics, it is hardly surprising that ordinary people have come to see antibiotics as panaceas. When her child falls ill, a poor woman in Bangladesh may well try to save money by going straight to the pharmacy, by-passing the doctor. She remembers that last time the child was ill, the doctor prescribed ampicillin or penicillin syrup, and the baby recovered quickly. This time, no matter what is wrong with the child, she buys the same antibiotic. As soon as the baby seems better, she stops giving it the medicine to save some for next time. [125]

Most of the Third World poor (and many in the rich world) have no idea that it is dangerous to take just a few capsules of an antibiotic, or break off a course of treatment as soon as you begin to feel better. An incomplete course enables the bacteria to build up resistance and makes outbreaks of drug-resistant disease a virtual certainty.

In developing countries antibiotics are sold loose on market stalls without packs or instructions - often illegally. In the open markets in Upper Volta antibiotic capsules are displayed on huge trays alongside assortments of equally colourful sweets. They cost about 5p for three and people will buy a single capsule to cure a headache or stomach pain. [126] Antibiotics are even sold in incomplete courses by the pharmacies. In Nepal, for instance, a health worker reports that it is an everyday occurrence to see people buying two or three capsules of chloramphenicol or tetracycline when a child has diarrhoea or is feverish. [127] In a number of African countries, people take the odd penicillin or ampicillin capsule as a blanket protection against illness, particularly venereal disease. [128]

The inevitable result of this random medication is that reports of drug resistance are coming in thick and fast from all over the Third World. Since 1972 there have been reports of chloramphenicol-resistant strains of typhoid from a growing

114

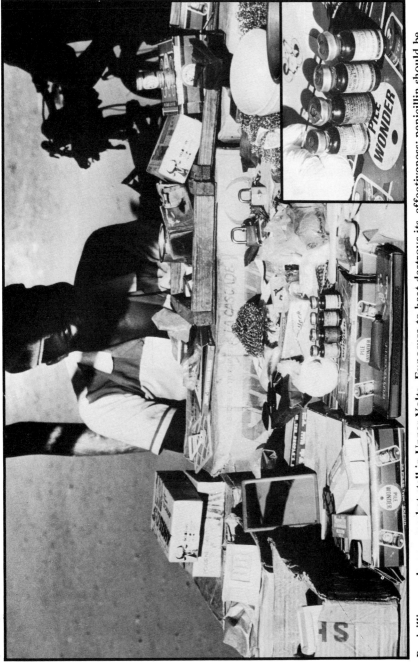

(Credit) Leigh Hart.

Penicillin on sale on a market stall in Upper Volta. Exposure to heat destroys its effectiveness; penicillin should be refrigerated.

number of Indian states. One research institute in India found that 690 out of 822 salmonella strains they were able to identify were resistant to at least one antibiotic and some were resistant to three or more. An outbreak of drug resistant disease led to the closure of the entire paediatric unit of a hospital in Bangalore, and another strain of salmonella, resistant to five antibiotics, lasted 20 months and killed over 80 babies in Delhi hospitals. [129]

The most serious epidemics of drug-resistant disease to date have been reported from Central America. In 1969 an epidemic of Shiga dysentery killed 12,500 people in Guatemala and 2,000 more in El Salvador. The disease was resistant to chloramphenicol, tetracycline, streptomycin and sulphonamide drugs. Three years later there was an outbreak of typhoid affecting over 6,000 people in Mexico. As with the strain of typhoid reported in India that year, the drug of choice, chloramphenicol, proved useless. At the start of the epidemic there was a high fatality rate with one in seven dying before doctors realised that trying to treat the sick with chloramphenicol was futile. [130]

The growing scale of antibiotics resistance has alarmed the experts. At a conference in 1979 the Dean of the London School of Hygiene and Tropical Medicine called for action: "The widespread use of antibiotics, even by quite poor people in poor countries must be discouraged by controlling their availability, as individual benefits are likely only by chance and disadvantages to the community are a certainty." [131]

Much of the onus falls on Third World governments to introduce controls, but little can be achieved without the active cooperation of the rich world. This fact was highlighted by US experts in the aftermath of the Mexican typhoid epidemic. They attributed part of the onus for the deaths caused by drug resistance to manufacturers who had been promoting chloramphenicol for trivial uses. In a statement to the US Senate, Professor Lee of the University of California stated his belief that "the problem is related to the promotional practices of the drug companies. It is serious and it can affect not only the residents of the countries involved and all those who visit there as well, but people who have never travelled to Latin America." [132]

Drug resistance can provide manufacturers with an incentive to carry out further research to develop new products. [133] But to the consumer - above all the poor Third World consumer - drug resistance is disastrous, because it pushes up the cost of life-saving treatments. The threat of drug-resistant disease emphasises the impossibility of shifting responsibility for responsible drug marketing entirely on to the shoulders of Third World governments.

116

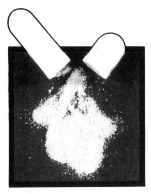

CHAPTER 7

TRADITIONAL MEDICINE

IF HUMAN history were telescoped into a day, modern medicines would put in an appearance only in the last few seconds. Over thousands of years different societies have evolved ways of coping with illness and people have relied on plants and other substances believed to have medicinal powers. These traditional health care systems have survived even the rapid incursions of modernisation.

In the Third World today, about three-quarters of the population still rely on traditional medicine - precisely the proportion of people denied access to modern medical care. [1]Indigenous medicine is the major source of health care for many of the rural poor. It is estimated that the village population of India spends ten times more consulting local healers than the Government spends on health services. [2] In one area of the State of Uttar Pradesh served by a primary health care centre, there were known to be 110 folk healers. They made up 86% of all health practitioners in the area. [3]

Even in the towns, where health centres are more accessible, the poor often consult a traditional healer first. A survey of mothers taking their children to a clinic in the capital of Bangladesh revealed that over half went to a traditional healer before attempting to get help from a doctor or health centre. [4] This seems to be partly out of habit, and partly because of the prohibitive cost of modern medicine. An OXFAM researcher in Upper Volta points out that the minimum daily wage in the capital in 1980 was about 90p, but many workers were in fact earning much less. "This group treads between traditional and western medicines. For some ailments: headaches, skin conditions, certain fevers, or hepatitis, where the indigenous medicines are recognised as effective, the traditional healer will be visited first. A consultation and the medicine usually made from leaves or roots, can cost between 9 pence and 36 pence; whereas seeing a nurse, even at a free clinic, will often entail buying medicines at a much higher cost. Seeing a nurse privately costs between 90p and £1.80, and visiting a doctor by appointment costs between £1.80 and £3.60." [5]

There has been a recent surge of interest in traditional medicine. In Europe and North America homeopathy, acupuncture and other alternative health systems have increasingly won acceptance, to the point where acupuncture is now part of the curriculum in some US medical schools. [6] Since committing themselves to the target behind the WHO slogan "Health for all by the year 2000" (which really means health services for all) Third World governments have also begun to reappraise the potential of traditional medicine. Dr. Hye, whilst Director of Drug Administration in Bangladesh, explained their thinking: "In recent years, there has been a world-wide search for new approaches to health and health care to close the gap between the 'haves' and 'have-nots' ... and attain a minimum level of health for all citizens within the limitation of a country's own resources. In this context, the utilisation of traditional systems of medicine, which have a long history of practice, utility and know-how ... is obviously a useful approach in attaining the goal of primary health care for all." [7]

WHO has lent its stamp of respectability to indigenous medicine, urging Third World governments not to "rely exclusively on western-type medicine or western-trained physicians in attempting to provide health care for all their people", but aim for a "synthesis ... between the best of modern with the best of traditional medicine". [8]

GOOD AND BAD PRACTICES

Attitudes to traditional medicine are often polarised between contemptuous dismissal and idealised overstatement of its advantages. As with *allopathic* (or conventional modern) medicine, there are of course both negative and positive sides to traditional systems. Some local remedies are simple and effective and enable people to be self-reliant. For example, in Bangladesh people make the most of wood apples *(aegle mermalos)* that grow wild throughout the country. When diarrhoeal disease is at its height in the monsoon season, the raw green fruit can be boiled with sugar and used to treat diarrhoea. In the dry season, the ripe fruit has the opposite effect, acting as a laxative. [9]

Dr. Klouda, OXFAM Medical Adviser, reports from Tanzania that the usefulness of traditional healers is as varied as their healing methods. "The healers' role in society has been greatly romanticised. There is a broad spectrum of such people - from idiots, to charlatans, to people just starting, to the very- experienced, to members of a family who happen to have dealt with some illness before. Some are generalists and some specialise in herbs, or bone-setting, or psychiatry, or social medicine, or magic or witchcraft, or poisoning. Some are a very great benefit - especially because of their personal knowlege of families, the background causes of poor health and their individual attention to their patients." [10]

Amongst the most helpful local practitioners are the traditional midwives. WHO estimates that these women help with as many as two-thirds of all births in some countries. [11] They are experienced and they give invaluable psychological reassurance. But some of their practices are very harmful, particularly the widespread tradition of applying cow-dung after cutting the umbilical cord. This is responsible for many cases of neo-natal tetanus.

Other local healers' practices are at best dubious and sometimes positively dangerous. Dr. Klouda cites the example of a colleague in Tanzania who "was nearly killed by a drug that partly destroyed his kidneys's tubules". He had been prescribed this remedy by a traditional healer for "weakness" after a bout of malaria. [12] From Bangladesh, a *kobiraj* (one type of local healer) is reported to have slit open the swollen legs of a malnourished child, to reduce the swelling. The child ended up with septicaemia, in addition to malnutrition. This was also the fate of another child with kwashiorkor, after a *kobiraj* had made slits in the skin across her stomach. [13]

REASSURING RITUALS

Traditional healers often wield a great deal of power in their community. Like the white-coated doctor, they are treated with reverence, even fear. In fact there are as many parallels as differences between the role performed by the traditional healer and the doctor. Doctors and healers everywhere tend to build up a mystique around their healing abilities and limit their role to treating patients. Few attempt to stimulate patients' awareness or encourage them to take more responsibility for their own health. Referring to health practitioners in India, one doctor writes that the "obscurantism of indigenous systems and the elitist mysticism of western medicine serve one common interest, that is to prevent people's participation in them in order to further their commercial interests". [14]

Most illness is self-limiting, so the majority of sick people will eventually recover, whether they are treated or not. But medical intervention can speed up the process, through the physical and psychological effects of healers and the drugs they prescribe. A doctor in the Philippines points out that "basically there is no difference betweeen the doctor and the [local] *herbolario* in terms of the psychological effects of the rituals they perform". He juxtaposes their different but essentially similar rituals:

Patient A "regularly goes to the *herbolario* for his treatment. Every time he goes to the *herbolario,* the *herbolario* will blow on his head, place saliva on his shoulders, recite prayers in front of him and surround the place with incense while the patient sips a herbal decoction ..."

Patient B "regularly sees his doctor and during his visits, the doctor will take his pulse first, put a thermometer in his mouth, get his blood pressure and make him lie down while listening to his heart beat through a stethoscope. Then he is given a prescription to buy the necessary medicines ..." [15]

There are also strong similarities in the psychological effects of the drugs they prescribe. The oldest herbal remedy can have a placebo effect equal to the latest patented drug. The most obvious difference between traditional and modern drugs is that whereas the latter are tested for safety and efficacy, very few traditional remedies have ever been scientifically screened. Of course this does not mean that all modern drugs are particularly safe or effective, or intrinsically "better" than herbal medicines, especially in the treatment of minor ailments. But there is no doubt that herbal medicines cannot compete with modern drugs in the treatment of most communicable diseases, TB for example, or of serious conditions like diabetes. [16]

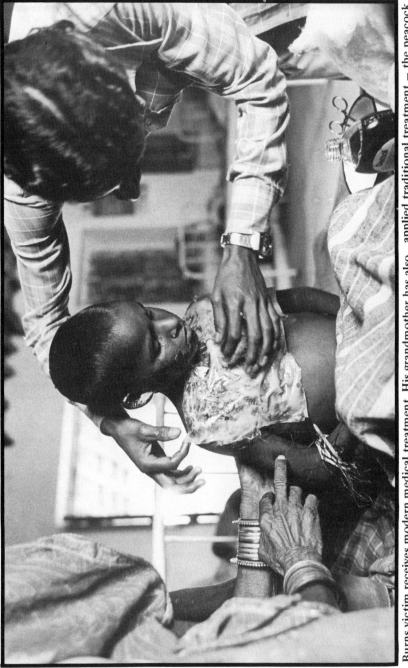

Burns victim receives modern medical treatment. His grandmother has also applied traditional treatment – the peacock feather around the boy's arm.

HERBAL MEDICINES

There is a rich variety of herbal medicines worldwide. The written records of Ayurveda, just one of the ancient systems, contain more than 8,000 herbal recipes. Some date back some 5,000 years, but according to WHO the same recipes are used in India today by about half a million healers. [17] A single local shrub can be put to very versatile uses. Neem, for instance, is a tree that grows all over the Indian sub-continent. The juice of fresh neem leaves with a little salt is used to treat thread worms and ascaris, and the ripe fruit can be decocted and used for urinary troubles. Neem is thought to have antiseptic properties and broken bones are bandaged with camphorated lint soaked in a neem decoction. Neem oil can be applied to skin to treat scabies. The sap is used for stomach troubles, the bark for sores, and tender Neem leaves for dysentery. [18]

In a world increasingly dominated by Western cultural values, it is easy to forget just how much modern medicine owes to traditional medicine. The wealth of knowledge of medicinal plants built up over centuries in Asia, Africa and Latin America has been tapped by the modern drug industry as the basis for a number of key drugs. Digitalis (from foxglove) has been used for centuries to treat heart failure and still provides the raw materials for a number of modern heart drugs. The snake-root, *rauwolfia serpentina,* was sold in bazaars in India 3,000 years ago for snakebites and as a calmative. From the 1940s, reserpine was extracted from *rauwolfia serpentina* and is still used to treat high blood pressure. Curare, from wourali root, was first used by South American indians as a paralysing arrow poison. One of its active alkaloids is now an important muscle relaxant in modern surgery. The Incas used cinchona bark to reduce fever. This is rich in quinine, one of the first modern antimalarials. Quinine remains important, particularly with the emergence of malaria strains resistant to more recent drugs, such as chloroquine. Quinine is also used for muscle cramp. In China the medicinal value of the ephedra plant has been known for over 5,000 years. Today the alkaloid ephedrine is used to treat asthma. [19]

As modern drug production got underway in Europe and America, some poorer nations were used as an important source of raw materials. An UNCTAD study describes the pattern of pharmaceutical trade established. "In conformity with colonial economic relationships of the time, British pharmaceutical manufacturers opened trading branches and agencies in India and kept India as a preserve for their finished products until the 1940s. British manufacturers and traders shipped out from India chemical raw materials (such as cinchona bark, *nux vomica* seeds, poppy pods etc) and shipped back to India extracts and other medical preparations for general prescriptions." [20]

PLANT-BASED DRUG INDUSTRY

Even today with advanced technology, it can still be cheaper to manufacture drugs from a plant extract, rather than synthesising them entirely from chemicals. The Third World continues to provide drug manufacturers with valuable raw materials. A number of hormonal contraceptives are made from diosgenin, an active ingredient extracted from dioscorea, a plant that grows wild in many parts of Asia. Two major American manufacturers, Searle and Wyeth, now have factories in Southern India and Kashmir to produce the chemical intermediates from dioscorea. These are then exported to the US and Europe to be processed into the actual contraceptive pills, some of which will end up back on the Indian market. [21]

Other examples of plants growing in developing countries that are processed into modern drugs include *vinca rosea* (rose periwinkle) the source of the modern drug vincristine, used to treat acute leukaemia.   Portulaca oleracea   another traditional medicinal plant that grows wild in the Philippines, where it is known as gualisman, contains the active ingredients of the modern drugs noradrenaline (for low blood pressure) and dopamine (for treating heart failure). [22] The continuing importance of plant sources to the modern drug industry is stressed by an Indian analyst who comments: "Today more than half the prescriptions written by American physicians are estimated to contain a plant-derived drug - a drug that has either been extracted from a plant, or one that has been synthesised to duplicate (or improve on) a plant substance." [23]

FACTORY-PRODUCED HERBAL MEDICINES

A growing number of developing countries are now keen to exploit the potential of natural plant resources. Amongst them, Tanzania, Nigeria and Burma all have national programmes to build up plant-based drug production, already successfully established in China and Vietnam.

In some countries private manufacturers have launched into the commercial production of herbal medicines, free from the controls imposed on manufacturers of allopathic drugs. In Bangladesh, for example, traditional Ayurvedic, Unani and homeopathic drugs are all exempt from any controls under existing drug legislation. [24] The lack of controls can seriously endanger health, as the President of the British Pharmaceutical Society has recently warned. He cited the fact that "tests on medicines imported into Singapore ... showed that 38 out of 140 samples were contaminated with dangerous amounts of toxic metals - one sample contained 20,000 times the permissible level of mercury and several had 1,000 times that of arsenic". [25] Some officials responsible for drug control have recognised that, in the words of the then Bangladesh Director of Drug Administration, "the precautions observed in the manufacture and distribution of traditional medicinal products should be, as far as possible, similar to those followed for modern allopathic drugs". [26]

Because the potential hazards are great, it has been argued that traditional medicines should be put through the same elaborate clinical pharmacological trials and processing as modern drugs. [27] Partly in response, new research institutes are planned for a number of Third World capitals, including Dacca, where the Bangladesh Government has allocated over £4 million for a such an institute. Research scientists are keen to establish the efficacy of local medicinal plants by extracting their 'active principle' or 'pure compound'. Technical back-up has been provided to a number of countries by agencies such as UNIDO, as for example in the form of a mobile demonstration and training unit equipped to extract the active ingredients from plants. [28]

The process of vetting and refining herbal medicines by modern scientific methods can be every bit as expensive, however, as developing new drugs. The cost of extracting the active ingredient and formulation into modern dosage forms can destroy the advantages of herbal medicines by pricing them out of the reach of the poor. As Dr. Hye, then Director of Drug Administration in Bangladesh, explained: "Mechanisation of production and commercialisation of distribution have been observed to increase prices of traditional medicines at times far beyond that of comparable modern drugs." [29] This has been the experience in China where communes have found themselves paying as much for factory-produced herbal medicines as they do for modern drugs. Consequently, many communes choose to keep the costs down by mixing their own traditional remedies from medicinal plants grown on the communes. [30]

Many Third World governments are fully aware of the pitfalls. Representatives of the Asian governments attending a WHO meeting in Delhi in 1980, agreed on the importance of seeing that "the supposedly low cost of traditional drugs and remedies, which is one of the major advantages of their use, is not lost in commercialisation and in the enthusiasm to put them in modern pharmaceutical dosage forms". [31] Furthermore at the first UN meeting on the production of herbal drugs, held in Lucknow, India, in 1978, participants from a range of Third World countries agreed that it is not always necessary to go through the expensive process of extracting the active principle from a medicinal plant, because there is no real *medical* need to do so. In most cases, the patient can make do with a standardised extract, which can be produced cheaply by simple extraction and purification. [32]

LOCAL SELF-RELIANCE

In fact, the best way to ensure that traditional medicines are used to the best advantage of the Third World poor is very similar to the approach that WHO urges poor countries to adopt in using modern drugs. At the 1980 Delhi meeting it was agreed that the Third World's policy on traditional remedies should be "to make a proper selection of traditional drugs of established efficacy and safety for use in primary health care". [33]

The process of cataloguing and evaluating traditional medicines has to be carried out, not in research laboratories, but in the rural areas where their use has been observed over centuries. This empirical knowledge has been passed by word of mouth from one generation to another but is now increasingly threatened by the pressures of the modern world. In India, for example, concerted efforts are now being made to catalogue the medicinal plants known to the tribal people, who make up nearly a tenth of the population. But it is feared that already much of their knowledge has been lost. [34]

The same dangers are apparent throughout the Third World as tribal people are forced to change their lifestyles. Under the pressures of social and economic change, more people are being forced from their lands or changing their style of cultivation. A former health minister of North Vietnam has warned of a threat common to many Third World countries. "We are exploiting our forests and reafforesting on a very big scale. Within a few dozen years many so-called wild species will have disappeared and our pharmacopeia will be greatly impoverished." [35]

The need to make a proper evaluation of traditional medicine is seen by many in the Third World as one element in a much wider cultural and social process of achieving self-reliance. Dr. Galvez-Tan in the Philippines explains: "Medicinal plants can be one of the alternatives for our people to use. But many people will still ask the question - 'Do medicinal plants really have a basis enough to warrant their widespread use again?' The answer is yes. It is from the ancient herbs that our modern pharmacopeias have developed... The scepticism regarding herbal medicines can be traced to our cultural 'miseducation'. We have always been taught that the practices of our *herbolarios* and *hilots* are quackery and unscientific. We were led to believe that anything that comes from the 'West is best'. We have failed to recognise the beauty of our own indigenous science and culture." [36]

GRASS ROOTS INTEGRATION

To serve the needs of the poor, there has to be a concerted attempt to capitalise on the best of both traditional and modern medicine by integrating the two systems at the primary health care level.

This integration is already taking place. For example in India allopathic doctors and health workers have incorporated Ayurvedic principles on diet, meditation and exercise into their practice. Moreover, research in one Indian community reveals the extent to which indigenous healers look to modern drugs, with these prescribed to 80% of their patients. [37] Integration between these two systems has of course been consciously and successfully achieved in China.

But in contrast to China, the problem remains that a model integration of the best of traditional and modern primary health care systems may still do little to improve health if merely grafted onto political and economic structures that perpetuate poverty. There is even some evidence that indigenous healers working in joint clinics with modern health workers in India may effectively be catering mainly for a more educated minority, and treating conditions that are not primary health care priorities. [38]

Nonetheless, three clear advantages can be seen in attempting to create grass roots integration. The first is stressed by WHO: "A sudden change from traditional to modern medicine causes negative attitudes in the population towards the organised health services. This leads to under-utilization of these services and to competition between them and traditional medicine." Traditional medicine has the advantage of "high consumer approval", so if traditional practitioners are seen working alongside modern health workers, patients will be encouraged to make use of the new primary health care facilities. [39]

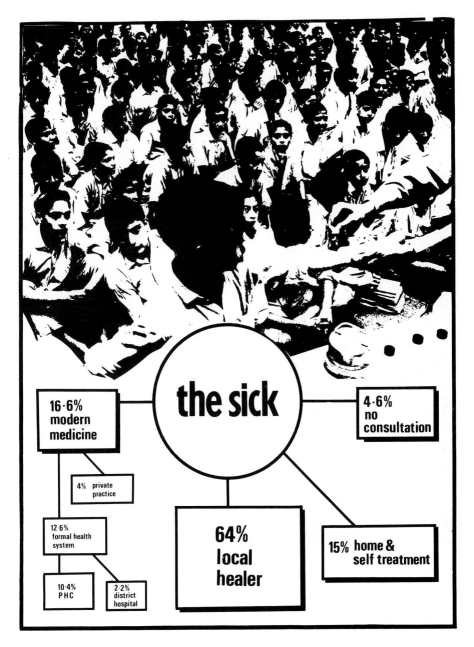

Where the sick turn for treatment in India.

125

A survey in Sri Lanka reveals that a quarter of traditional healers and 40% of college-trained Ayurvedic healers already refer patients to modern health practitioners. [40] It is hoped that with joint Ayurvedic/allopathic clinics patients will benefit from choice in whom they consult, and can be referred to the more suitable source of treatment - for example modern drug therapy for TB, but the Ayurvedic healer for stress and other psychological problems. A pilot joint-clinic was set up in Kandy, Sri Lanka in 1980 and similar clinics already operate in parts of India.

The second advantage is that modern practitioners can benefit from the knowledge and experience of indigenous healers, particularly in the use of herbal medicines that can provide simple and readily available treatments.

The Director of the Centre for Scientific Research into Plant Medicine in Ghana has attributed the past failure of many plant-screening programmes to the fact that no attempt was made to learn from local healers. [41] A growing number of people trained in modern medicine have recognised the wisdom of this approach. One doctor in India recently set up a 'self-reliant alternatives to western medicines' project to tap existing knowledge about herbal medicines and put it to good use. Working from a base at a people's health project, in the State of Maharashtra, Dr. Dhruv Mankad is making contact with individuals and groups that have a special knowlege of local medicine and homeopathy. His aim is to compile a list of herbal remedies and establish which are the most successful by testing them out in clinical practice. The results, claiming or disproving the usefulness of local remedies, will then be spread as far afield as possible to benefit the poor. [42]

Another project in India, run by the Apeksha Homeopathic Society, aims to make homeopathic medicines widely available to poor villagers. Homeopathy has limitations in tackling the diseases of poverty, because the system does not focus attention on the social causes of ill health. But homeopathic medicines do offer some clear advantages over modern drugs in the treatment of the mass of self-limiting illnesses. They provide similar psychological reassurance at much less cost and are potentially far less dangerous than modern medicines. [43]

Thirdly, integration of modern and traditional practices has the advantge of maximising available skills and improving traditional practices to safeguard health. For example, a study of the comparative performance of trained and untrained traditional midwives in India revealed that: "Deliveries performed by trained traditional birth assistants resulted in a considerably lower percentage of complications due to neonatal tetanus (2.8% versus 8.9%) and other infections (20% versus 73.2%)." [44]

A project in Raymah, an isolated and mountainous region of North Yemen, is specifically designed to try to make the best of the health care already provided to local people. Volunteers from the British Organisation for Community Development are attempting to change the emphasis of the health care provided by both the *saheen* (local "health" men) and the *jidaat* (traditional midwives). Training sessions aim to increase the local practitioners' awareness of the social

126

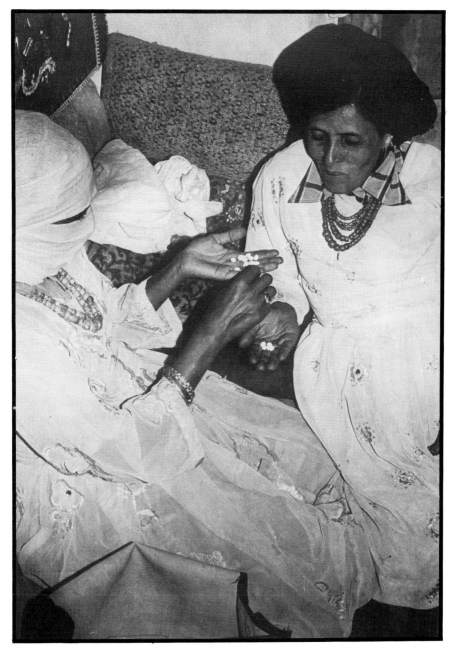

A traditional Jiddah in the Yemen provides antenatal care, following training in the basics of modern midwifery.

causes of ill health, and the dangers of over-medication with potentially harmful and expensive drugs. Both the *saheen* and the *jidaat* are encouraged to see their role as being one of service to the community and to act as health promoters by giving advice on hygiene and better nutrition. They are also taught how to use a limited range of basic drugs and prepare other appropriate treatments such as simple oral rehydration fluid. [45]

In some ways, it would be a simpler task to import new health workers whose attitudes have been entirely formed by the principles of modern primary health care. After visiting the project, Dr. Lusty, OXFAM's Medical Adviser, commented: "A case can be made for ignoring the *saheen* and concentrating on training a new cadre but to do this is to ignore the situation as it stands. The *saheen* are carrying the main burden of health care in the rural areas: anything that can be done to raise the standard of their work will have immediate results." [46] This is as true of the traditional healers in one mountain area of North Yemen, as it is of local healers responding to the needs of communities throughout the Third World.

In the next chapter we look at other positive and imaginative schemes to improve the health of local communities, and provide them with basic modern drugs.

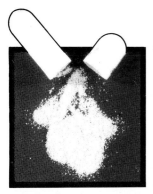

CHAPTER 8

TRAIL-BLAZERS
Small-scale Solutions

POOR PEOPLE suffer most ill health, but benefit least from modern health care and life-saving drugs. The Third World market is flooded with unnecessary and overpriced medicines which poor people make great sacrifices to buy, unaware that their uncontrolled use is wasteful and dangerous. That is our diagnosis of the problems.

Before identifying some of the policy options open to Third World governments in tackling these problems, we shall focus now on what is being achieved nearer the grass-roots. Some of the small-scale projects we shall describe are acting as trail-blazers for programmes now being adopted on a national scale. OXFAM's involvement with these and many other health projects, has taught us about the problems the poor confront. Watching the progress of these projects over some years, and learning from friends and colleagues in the villages, we have seen that improvements can be achieved with persistence. But we also have been forced to the realisation that some of the more intractable problems for the Third World poor cannot be tackled locally. In the case of medicines, action must also be taken in the rich drug-producing nations, where many of the market pressures originate.

GONOSHASTHAYA KENDRA
One of the most exciting projects in which OXFAM participates is Gonoshasthaya Kendra (the People's Health Centre) in Savar, a rural district about twenty miles from the capital of Bangladesh. [1] The project was set up in 1972 by Dr. Zafrullah Chowdhury and a group of medical colleagues who had worked together treating casualties and refugees during the country's struggle for independence in 1971. Their first objective was to set up community-based health services for the 200,000 people living in the villages of Savar.

From the outset the emphasis was on prevention. The team at Gonoshasthaya Kendra were committed to stopping their centre from becoming nothing more than "community disease centre". [2] They became increasingly aware that health care alone could do little to improve health without an attack on poverty. So the scope of the project was extended to include schemes for agricultural credit, literacy and vocational training. Both the wide range of community development work at Gonoshasthaya Kendra and the project's bold new initiative in establishing a modern drug factory are important because, by themselves, attempts to improve the supply of essential drugs could have little impact on health.

Health promotion is carried out by teams of paramedics who are given a year's training, partly at the base health centre and partly out in the villages. There are now over 60 paramedics who divide their work between the villages, four sub-centres and the main centre. The paramedics are able to handle the majority of common illness including diarrhoea and dysentery, scabies, upper respiratory tract infections, night blindness, worms, anaemia and 'body pain', which is mostly backache.

Difficult cases are referred to the four doctors at the main centre, who supervise the paramedics' work and carry out surgery. But most of the out-patients who come to the centre are seen by the paramedics who also carry out some straightforward operations. For instance, 85% of tubectomies are performed by the paramedics, with a lower complication rate than the doctors. In the villages, the paramedics make house-to-house visits to encourage disease prevention and keep an eye on the health of mothers and young children who are most at risk. Children are vaccinated free of charge and women of child-bearing age are immunised against tetanus. The paramedics carry vaccines in thermos flasks, in addition to a small number of basic drugs.

Drugs are only used when they are essential. Prevention comes first. For example, to help prevent diarrhoeal disease, women are encouraged to use tubewell water for cooking and drinking. They are also shown that instead of buying expensive antidiarrhoeals, they can make a homemade rehydration solution, *lobon-gur,* from *lobon* (salt) and *gur* (molasses) - ingredients which are easy to get hold of locally. Rather than routinely handing out vitamin A capsules, the paramedics try to convince mothers to include plenty of green vegetables in the family diet. If medicines are necessary, the paramedic will wait while parents give children their medicine, to make sure they understand the correct dose.

As this basic health care is now helping to ensure a better survival rate for children, the paramedics are in a better position to offer advice to mothers on birth control, and monitor the use of contraceptives, particularly the pill. The injectable contraceptive, Depo-Provera (medroxyprogesterone acetate) was used on the project, but although it was popular, its use has been abandoned because of fears over the unknown degree of risk. Close monitoring of the women who received Depo-Provera revealed that over an eight-month period, eleven women suffered such severe bleeding that they had to be admitted as in-patients. The health team at Gonoshasthaya Kendra have contacts in the health field all over the world, so they are at an unusual advantage in keeping themselves informed about the controversy in Europe and the US, over the use of Depo-Provera. However, after stopping use of the drug, the health team openly expressed their uncertainty, as to whether "we have helped our women or not".[3]

The traditional village midwives, the *dais*, have also been incorporated into the health team as far as possible. They are trained to use more hygienic methods for deliveries, and are also involved in family planning.

The project can claim to have made an impact on health. For example, there has

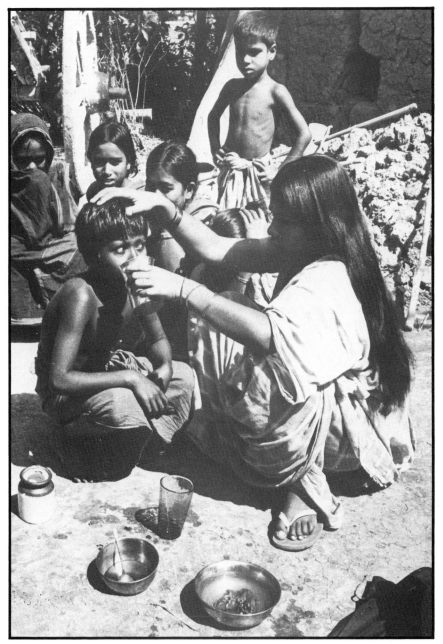

A health worker in Bangladesh teaches villagers the importance of oral
rehydration in the treatment of diarrhoea.

been a definite fall in the incidence of severe dehydration, and of skin diseases such as scabies. The birth rate in the project area is now about a third less than that for the rest of the country, and whereas the infant mortality rate in Savar is now about 120 deaths for every 1,000 babies born, the national rate is 140 deaths, and higher still in some rural areas.

But the Gonoshsthaya Kendra team are the first to acknowledge that their health activities can only be seen as a qualified success. They have had difficulty encouraging active community participation in village health, so outsiders still play a key role as health promoters in the villages. Originally, health volunteers were recruited from the Savar villages, but they showed little commitment and were replaced by the full-time paramedics. Many of the paramedics are young, unmarried women from outside Savar. As unmarried women in a traditional Muslim society, they cannot live alone so they have to be based at the centre, not in the villages. The fact that they are outsiders also means that many move on to live and work in other areas, leading to a fairly high drop-out rate.

Many of the villagers have little time for the paramedics who go round the villages. They prefer to walk all the way to the main centre, or a sub-centre, where they assume the services must be better. Village health committees were set up to encourage people to take an active interest in health and participate in running the sub-centres, but these initiatives were blocked by apathy and political constraints. As a result the better-off, more powerful people in the community have been able to manipulate the health committees to their advantage.

This highlights the major obstacles the poor face in attempting to improve their health. Real progress is held back by the social and economic forces underpinning poverty. The poor are ultimately at the mercy of whoever owns the land they work, and controls water supplies and credit. In the words of the woman in charge of Bhatsala People's Health Centre (which is modelled on the Savar project): "The poor feel that lack of food is the root of their health problems. A change in their ability to produce enough food is necessary for any change in the health status." [4]

To free the poor from the oppression of the landowners and the money lenders, the team at Gonoshasthaya Kendra set up Gono Krishi Khamar (or the People's Farm). This scheme aims to increase food production by trying out new farming methods, and to make credit available to poor landless farmers through a credit cooperative. Initially, some local landowners used intimidation to try to destroy the credit cooperative. Now it is firmly established, but the intimidation continues. The landowners have been taking advantage of the fact that the landless poor can obtain credit from the cooperative. So they have increased their charges for supplying water from the tubewells, which were installed under a joint Government and UNICEF programme. These tubewells were of course intended to benefit the whole community, but the powerful managed to wangle things so that the wells were dug on *their* land.

132

If people are to be able to get access to water, land and credit to grow enough food to be healthy, it is vital that they should be in a position to defend their rights in the face of harrassment from the powerful, usually educated people in the community. To this end the People's School has been set up at Savar to educate the children, who in turn help with adult literacy classes for their parents.

A further serious obstacle to better health is the fact that the women are held back from playing an active role in improving hygiene and nutrition both by their lack of education and their low status in the community. Their oppression is being actively challenged at Gonoshasthaya Kendra. Most of the paramedics are women, who are visibly seen to be challenging convention as they set off for work in the villages on their bicycles. But village women are also participating in literacy classes, and acquiring radically new vocational skills to enable them to gain some independence and more equality. They are learning shoe-making, bakery, sewing, carpentry, welding and other skilled manual jobs that have been strictly male preserves.

GONOSHASTHAYA PHARMACEUTICALS LIMITED

One of the tasks recently accomplished by the women in the project workshop is the construction of all the metal window-frames for the project's brand new pharmaceutical factory. [5] The factory started production in May 1981 with the formulation of the first batches of ampicillin and paracetamol.

It is an ambitious step for Gonoshasthaya Kendra, a charitable trust, to have set up a sizeable commercial operation to manufacture drugs in rural Bangladesh. But the team at Gonoshasthaya Kendra had strong motivation, having experienced the difficulties of obtaining inexpensive, good quality generics, with the local market dominated by the subsidiaries of big research-based manufacturers. As the team at Gonoshasthaya Kendra explain: "The project experience, and especially the problem of getting good and cheap medicines to the people ... led to thinking about a pharmaceutical factory based on four principles: low prices, quality, manufacture of essential drugs only and responsible marketing." [6]

Gonoshasthaya Pharmaceuticals Limited (GPL) is unique in Bangladesh and probably in the Third World in being a private company with its production entirely geared to meeting the needs of the people. All the shares in the company are owned by the charitable trust and under its charter profits are limited to 10-15% (after payment of duties and bank charges). Half of the profits will be ploughed back into the company to expand production, reduce prices further and fund research. The remainder will be used to fund health and development projects.

Over the first three years of production, the factory will build up to formulating a range of about 30 drugs all included in the WHO Selection of Essential Drugs. Every effort will be made to keep prices down by purchasing raw materials by competitive tender on the world market. Despite its initial high overheads, the retail prices of GPL's drugs are considerably lower than those of equivalent products on the local market. Comparative prices are illustrated in the table below, which also shows GPL's deliberate policy of setting different profit margins - lowest on the drugs considered most useful.

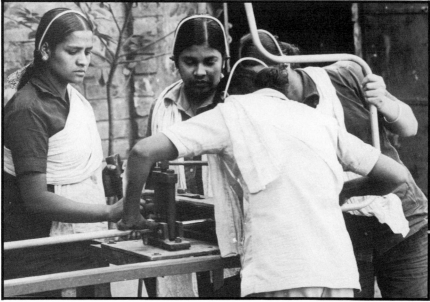

Women workers at Gonoshasthaya Pharmaceuticals Ltd. have been trained in technical skills. Here components are prepared for the factory.

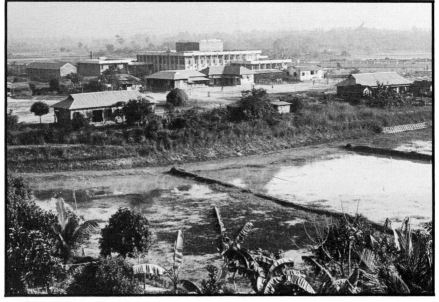

GPL's factory has been built in a rural setting. Some of the profits are to be ploughed back into rural development work.

COMPARATIVE RETAIL PRICES BETWEEN GONOSHASTHAYA PHARMACEUTICALS LIMITED (GPL) AND OTHER MANUFACTURERS IN BANGLADESH, APRIL 1982

Drugs	Unit cost to GPL	GPL Profit	Maximum retail prices per capsule/tablet in paisa (100 paise = 1 taka)	
			GPL	OTHERS
ampicillin (250mg)	76.2	6.57%	100	Hoechst 186 Square 175 Beecham 169
tetracycline (250mg)	38.4	5.26%	50	Squibb 110 Pfizer 106 Albert David 77
metronidazole (250mg)	25.6	22.7%	40	BPI 79 (200 mg tab) Square 65
paracetamol (500mg)	11.7	3.41%	15	Fisons 24 Square 25
diazepam (5mg)	7.1	36.6%	12.5	Roche 55 Square 30
frusemide	26	85.6%	60	Hoechst 125

Source: Chowdhury & Chowdhury, "Essential Drugs for the Poor" (see ref. 5)

Prices will not be kept low at the expense of quality. GPL is a modern factory, with quality control facilities comparable to the local big name producers. GPL aims to be competitive by going for large-scale production, taking advantage of modern machinery, production and management techniques. The factory has 42,000 sq ft of floor space, making it one of the largest in Bangladesh. It was built with capital provided mainly by the Dutch charity NOVIB, a loan from the Bangladesh Shilpa (Industrial) Bank and further contributions from OXFAM and Christian Aid. [7] Although GPL has had to rely on foreign donor agencies to provide the initial capital and the International Dispensary Association in Holland for technical assistance, the underlying objective of the project is self-reliance. Designs for the factory building, air-conditioning and machinery lay-out were all planned and executed by Bangladeshis. Similarly, the production, quality control and marketing managers are all Bangladeshis who have gained valuable experience in the past working for big foreign manufacturers.

There are plans to carry out research into using locally available raw materials as excipients (the non-medicinal ingredients like starch that are mixed with the

135

active ingredient to make up a medicine). Attempts are also planned to develop better dosage forms to suit local conditions - for instance, to take account of the nutritional status of the poor, and humidity during the long months of the monsoon. This sort of research tailored to meet local needs is largely neglected by the bigger foreign-owned companies. Patents on both processes and products are protected by law in Bangladesh. But Dr. Chowdhury stresses that GPL would not want to patent any new process discovered because they do not believe in "the monopoly of knowledge". [8]

To achieve greater self-reliance and leave their operations less vulnerable to external pressures, the team at GPL are keen to expand into the more complex production of raw materials. These would have to be produced on a large scale to make the operation cost-effective. But the main difficulty to be confronted would be in obtaining the necessary technology. This is seen as an important wider objective behind setting up the factory.

In January 1982, GPL marked its official opening by hosting a conference on Technology Transfer to the Third World, with participants from many different countries. Previously, the team had explained: "Gonoshasthaya Kendra is not only interested in proving its ability to set up this particular pharmaceutical factory, but sees this effort as a learning situation for a genuine transfer of technology to the Third World. This is not achieved by multinationals bringing in complete blueprints which give no opportunity for training and experience of local manpower ... We hope that our work will demonstrate possibilities for such self-reliance ... Most important of all, transfer of technology does not itself mean improvement for the poor. To find ways which guarantee that industrialisation can be controlled by the poor masses of Bangladesh rather than becoming an instrument of oppression, is one of the main goals of GPL". [9]

The unskilled labour force is drawn from the villages of Savar and skilled labour from the capital. Most of the unskilled and semi-skilled production work is being carried out by local women who received a year's special training before the factory started production.

In its first year of operation GPL has faced technical difficulties particularly with production interrupted by power cuts and damage to equipment caused by fluctuations in the electrical current. They have also experienced management problems. The original production manager broke his two year contract after five months to go and work with WHO in Jordan, after GPL had funded a three months' training period for him in Europe. The factory was late in starting production because of bureaucratic delays in obtaining its initial raw materials import licence. But now that it is producing good quality, low cost drugs the major problem GPL faces is in ensuring that these drugs actually reach the poor for whom they were intended.

GPL expects to sell about 60-70% of its production to the government health services and the voluntary health sector. This distribution through organised health services is seen as "the safest and quickest way to channel the benefits of cheap drugs to the people most in need". [10] The remainder will be sold on the open market. This raises a major problem for GPL in trying to prevent middlemen from stealing the advantages intended for the poor by jacking up the prices. According to Dr. Chowdhury cases of retailers charging more than the maximum retail price for GPL products have already been reported. He comments: "A lack of confidence in anything that comes from Bangladesh itself is part of our sad colonial heritage, and pharmacists, having heard something of Dutch financing, charge excessive prices claiming that this is a new 'Bilati' (European) medicine." [11]

The team at GPL are well aware that past attempts to promote the use of cheap generics have failed because doubts about their quality are easily whipped up in the minds of doctors and patients. GPL has its own sales representatives to promote its products to doctors and pharmacists, but priority is also given to the need to popularise wider health issues. This is done through the health project's monthly magazine, "Mashik Gonoshasthaya", printed on its own presses. The magazine is written in simple Bengali and aims to be lively and informative. It covers many health issues including appropriate non-drug treatments and warns against the socially damaging effects of existing drug sales and over-medication. 15,000 copies of the magazine are distributed each month.

A drug company's success depends to a great extent on its reputation with doctors. So there are plans to invite doctors and pharmacists to visit Savar to see for themselves that GPL drugs are produced in a modern, efficient factory. This will be an extension of visits arranged in the past for groups of medical students with the aim of exposing them to village reality and the radical approach to health care adopted at the People's Health Centre. This is all tantamount to a vist to Mars for most middle class medical students after the secluded anatomy sessions at medical school, but it is crucial in influencing the attitudes of the country's future doctors to accept a new direction in health services to benefit the mass of the people.

The drug factory is an exciting new venture. Local drug company managers that we interviewed in 1980 told us that they did not see GPL as a threat to their market because the potential demand for drugs is so great, with the planned expansion of primary health care facilities. Certainly, if it is to succeed and offer a model for voluntary agencies in other countries to follow, GPL will need to count on the active goodwill of the rich world manufacturers who are in a position to threaten its future viability.

GPL has already experienced the problems of trying to challenge existing market power. In 1981 the Government invited manufacturers to quote their prices to supply ampicillin. In the previous year, a local state-owned manufacturer supplied the drug at 99 paisa a capsule. In 1981 GPL tendered to supply ampicillin at 93 paisa, based on raw material prices quoted to them by a local trading company. The day after GPL had submitted its bid, the trading company revised its quotation for the raw material which would have allowed GPL to supply the finished drug at 5 to 17 paisa less.

137

Dr. Chowdhury takes up the sequence of events: "We did not win the tender. It went to a national company which had bid at 80 paisa per capsule. The retail price of the same company's ampicillin is 159 paisa. For the Government this was the cheapest ampicillin they had ever purchased and giving credit where credit is due, some officials thanked us, requesting us to keep up the good work." [12]

VOLUNTARY HEALTH ORGANISATIONS

The voluntary health organisations in both India and Bangladesh have set up associations to look after their members' interests and act as forums for discussion and information sharing on a broad range of health issues. Both use their own monthly newsletters, seminars and training workshops to exchange ideas and information. For instance, women health workers attending a workshop in Bangladesh were able to pool ideas on how to handle the problem of uneducated villagers who take a whole course of tablets at once because they do not understand the instructions. [13]

The voluntary health sector in India is very big, providing a third of organised health services in the country. Although the public health service infrastructure covers most of the population, in the rural areas there is a desperate shortage both of personnel and resources. Funds allocated to medicines for primary health care were increased by tenfold in 1975, but still account for only 6p a head. [14] The Voluntary Health Association of India (VHAI) collects and disseminates information and advice to both health personnel and patients. As VHAI explains: "Education and awareness as to how to avoid disease and then how to handle it appropriately at the lowest possible cost is the crux of our approach in low-cost appropriate health care." [15]

To help reduce costs, VHAI is encouraging its members to standardise prescribing for specific health problems and prescribe only single-ingredient drugs by generic name. For example tetracycline formulated with vitamin C is widely sold in India, but costs twice as much as straight tetracycline. One member, the Deenabandu Medical Mission in Tamil Nadu in the south, has found that by rationalising prescribing along these lines, and using herbal medicines as the first line of treatment, overall health care costs can be reduced by almost a third. [16]

VHAI is also keen to influence the attitudes of the general public to discourage the over-use of medicines. So they stress to patients the dangers of misusing injections, tonics and steroids and try to encourage people to adopt a positive attitude of "self-responsibility" towards their health. [17]

The difficulties of obtaining regular supplies of reliable drugs at competitive prices is shared by members of both associations. In Bangladesh The Voluntary Health Services Society (VHSS) has been collecting information on comparative prices of drugs on the local market. The intention is to issue price guides to help members and avoid duplicated effort on market intelligence work. VHSS has also succeeded in reducing drug costs by organising pooled procurement for its members. For example, it was able to bulk-buy mebendazole (deworming tablets) from a local manufacturer and pay only half the standard wholesale price. [18] In future, its members' needs will increasingly be met by Gonoshasthaya Pharmaceuticals Limited.

138

VHAI is also taking practical steps to help its members obtain the drugs they need, by negotiating a ten year contract with a small manufacturer in the State of Maharashtra. The manufacturer is being asked to formulate 50 essential drugs, gearing production and distribution to the specific needs of VHAI's members. Costs will be kept down by ensuring that raw materials are purchased at competitive prices, and because the scheme will cut out additional promotional costs. [19]

NEPAL HILL DRUG SCHEME

The problems of drug distribution are acute in Nepal, one of the world's poorest countries, where the rugged, mountainous terrain makes transport extremely difficult. Only half of the country's health posts are accessible by road, so drugs and other supplies have to be carried on foot. These distribution problems and the very small drug budget allocated to the health posts means that drug supplies, which are delivered only once a year, will usually last no more than about 3 to 4 months. [20]

This means that for most of the year patients are forced to buy the drugs prescribed for them in the health posts out in the private drug stores, which often charge exorbitant prices and stock a mass of unnecessary drugs. With only 25 trained pharmacists in the whole country in 1979, most pharmacies are staffed by totally untrained sales assistants, who may have little understanding or interest in drugs, beyond their sales potential. [21]

The Hill Drug Scheme was set up in eastern Nepal in 1969 with two objectives. Primarily it aimed to improve the supply of low-priced essential drugs to the areas covered, and to encourage safer drug use by giving retailers some basic training. The success of the scheme hinged on its attempts to persuade selected retailers to sell drugs more as a service to the community than as a means of making as much profit as possible.

The project is coordinated by the Britain Nepal Medical Trust which bulk-buys drugs both from the Nepalese manufacturers, Royal Drugs Limited, and from companies in India. The drugs are then supplied to villages where there are government health workers trained to prescribe them and distributed through retailers specially selected with the help of local officials on the *panchayats* (village or town councils). The retailers receive some basic training and undertake to dispense only the essential drugs supplied to them. They also agreee to sell the medicines at fixed prices, with a set 10% mark-up. The scheme was intended to provide a back-up to health workers, allowing them to refer patients to these retailers in the knowledge that they would not be overcharged or sold unnecessary medicines. [22] In fact health workers have not shown a great deal of interest.

Over a dozen retailers have participated in the scheme at any one time and sold medicines at much lower prices than the bazaars. But the scheme has had only limited success. Its major problem is that retailers stand to make far less money selling the limited range of basic drugs at fixed prices, than they would from stocking the mass of over-the-counter remedies on sale in the bazaars. So it has been very hard to find retailers with both the necessary capital and the motivation to participate in the scheme. A recent project report explains: "Ideally the retailer is someone with an interest in medicine, an interest in community service and the ability to manage finances (ie pay in advance for drugs on the shelf). However, this community-minded capital *wallah* is an endangered species." [23] Almost invariably the retailers have to be given their stock on credit. Recovering money from them has proved a time-consuming and expensive process.

On balance the Hill Drug Scheme strategy of trying to improve drug availability through the private sector has not been as successful as hoped. In the words of Dr. Cassels, Medical Director of the Britain Nepal Medical Trust, "... all too often the retailers' need to make a profit has been incompatible with the patients' need to obtain medicines cheaply." [24]

BHOJPUR DRUG SCHEME

In 1980 a new model was tried, this time to increase drug supply within the health services. Dr. Cassels stresses that the Nepalese Government is in no position to provide more free medicines. "With costs rising and more and more new health posts being opened every year the effective medicine budget per health post is in fact going down." [25] The new scheme pioneered in the Bhojpur district of eastern Nepal is modelled on the fixed prescription charge that patients in Britain are asked to pay for National Health Service prescriptions. Hospital and health post patients in Bhojpur who had previously received medicines free must now pay a prescription fee of Rupees 2 (8p).

Exemptions were made for TB, leprosy and antimalarial drugs, and for patients suffering from "chronic diseases" who would not be expected to pay more than once every three months. The Health Post Committees were made responsible for collecting the prescription fees which go into a central fund to buy more medicines from an agreed list. The advantage for patients is that, whereas before they were forced to pay high prices in the bazaars when stocks of free government drugs ran out, now there should be regular drug supplies at the health posts.

The scheme is intended to be self-financing. In its first year, income from prescription fees only covered about one third of the cost of drugs bought by the Britain Nepal Medical Trust which had to make up the deficit. But subsequent analysis of why the scheme ran at a loss has been valuable in highlighting specific problems in drug use in the health service. Amongst these, over-prescribing was a major problem, with health post patients receiving an average of 3.7 items on the one prescription fee. Some expensive items, particularly antibiotics, were over-used, as were costly proprietary preparations like cough mixtures. About 20% of patients complaining of the same symptom as on their last visit were given prescriptions without a charge, because the "chronic illness" exemption had not been clearly defined. The standard fee was also unrealistically low to cover the cost of drugs for in- patients, averaging Rupees 27.68. [26]

140

Solutions have been proposed to make the scheme pay for itself and these now await approval by the Nepalese health authorities. The major change proposed is that the prescription fee should be replaced by a charge for each item prescribed. A drug manual has been prepared to help prevent over-prescribing and misuse of antibiotics. Items on the list considered disproportionately expensive will in future be available only at cost price. Measures are proposed to stop repeat prescriptions being given free to patients who are not chronically sick and a daily charge for in-patients is proposed.

If the Bhojpur Drug Scheme can be made economically viable and remain acceptable to patients and health workers, it could be more widely adopted throughout Nepal. But the major concern of all involved is to ensure that the scheme continues to make treatment accessible the whole population - especially the poorest. [27]

VILLAGE THEATRE IN MEXICO

Nothing can be done to stop poor people wasting money on medicines that are arguably useless or potentially harmful, unless *they* can be convinced that 'wonder drugs' are not all they may seem. It is all the more necessary to make the poor aware of the problems in countries where medicines are widely promoted over the radio, as happens in Mexico.

In the mountainous state of Sinaloa, Project Piaxtla aims to involve the *campesinos* (farmworkers) and their families in helping set up their own health care network. As part of the project's educational work, the village health team in Ajoya found an imaginative and entertaining way of using health festivals to get their message across. They helped to organise improvised theatre skits to draw local people into identifying with 'real life' situations at the same time as stimulating their awareness of the issues. David Werner, author of *Where There is no Doctor* and director of Project Piaxtla, explains: "We have come to believe strongly that education and awareness- raising is essential to the process of demystification and sensible use of medications." [28]

The health workers in Ajoya performed one sketch aimed at opening people's eyes to the overuse and misuse of medicines. The following is David Werner's translation of the health workers' play, which conveys something of the universal experience of the Third World poor: [29]

> It is nearly dawn. The rooster crows: "Cock-a-doodle-doo."
> (The rooster is actually a health worker in costume). The old man and his wife stir in bed, as they usually wake up early in the morning. Beside the bed is an enormous 'radio' with a sign that reads 'Radio Deception'. Hidden inside the radio is an actor.

> Old Dona Luisa turns on the radio. There are the sounds of country music. Then the voice from the radio says: "Good morning to you all. The last song was dedicated to Juanita Torres in Ajoya, Sinaloa. And now before we play more country

141

favourites, a word from the Drug Company: 'Are you feeling weak and tired? Do you find it hard to wake up in the morning? You may be suffering from *tired blood*. What you need are the new *Vita-Meyerhov* vitamin pills. You'll wake up every morning feeling like dancing. Remember, Vita-Meyerhov'.''

As Dona Luisa gets up and begins to make maize tortillas for breakfast, the music and advertisements continue. But look. Her husband, Don Lino, is still in bed. He feels too weak to get up.

Finally Dona Luisa coaxes him out of bed and gives him a cup of coffee. He asks what there is for breakfast. She answers: ''Just tortillas. You know that's all we have.''

Just then, they hear a knock on the door. (Bang, bang, bang.) It is their neighbour who makes his living by selling medicines that he buys in the city.

Today he is selling Vita-Meyerhov. Old Luisa is excited because she just heard about Vita-Meyerhov on the radio. She is sure that it will make her husband wake up strong and eager to work, like before. The salesman tells them the bottle is worth 300 pesos [over £6]. But since they are such good friends, he will let them have it for only 150 pesos.

But the old couple only have 50 pesos. So they have to sell their 2 chickens at 50 pesos each in order to pay for the vitamins.

As their neighbour, the salesman, walks away with the chickens, the couple eagerly talk about how wonderful things will be when old Lino's health is restored.

The next scene takes place a few weeks later. Again it is dawn, the rooster crows: ''Cock-a-doodle-doo'', and Dona Luisa turns on the radio. The beat of ranchero music drifts out into the silent dawn. The radio announcer wishes a good morning to all, and goes on with more praise for the products from the Drug Company. While the radio announcer is praising the miraculous Vita-Meyerhov, we see that old Lino is too weak to get out of bed by himself. His wife tries to pull him out.

Lino, tries to get up, but falls to the ground. Dona Luisa cannot lift him up herself.

Frightened, she runs out to get help from the village health worker. The health worker comes running.

Between them, Dona Luisa and the health worker lift old Lino back onto the bed. The health worker figures out that his weakness comes from not eating well. The family has barely enough maize to make tortillas, and none to trade for beans.

142

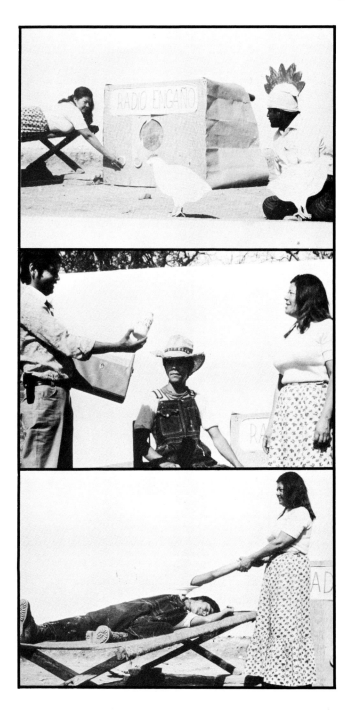

143

They sold their last two chickens to buy the Vita-Meyerhov vitamins.

The health worker explains that the eggs from those chickens would have helped Lino much more than the vitamin pills. But Dona Luisa is not easily convinced. She thinks that her husband should be given 'artificial life' (Intra-Venous (IV) solution). The health worker tells her that this is just sugar water; it would be safer and cheaper for Lino simply to mix sugar and water, and drink it. But what the old man really needs is more and better food. Maybe their neighbours can get together and help them out with the food problem. He will speak with them.

After the village health worker leaves, the old man and his wife talk things over. They are not sure they trust the young health worker. "What does he know? He is just a villager like us. We saw him when he was born. An ugly baby at that." They decide to get Miss Ivy, the nurse, to give Lino some IV solution.

So that afternoon, Miss Ivy comes to the house. (To make the play more entertaining, the role of Miss Ivy is played by the same young man who plays the health worker. He has to change costumes quickly.) Nurse Ivy gives Lino an intravenous solution. He says he feels a little stronger already.

Because they do not have much money, the old couple give the nurse their prize rooster in partial pay for her services. But they will still owe her money.

The next morning when old Luisa wakes up, she notices that old Lino has a fever and seems very ill. She cannot wake him.

She runs to get the village health worker. He comes right away. He asks what could have happened to cause this sudden turn for the worse. Dona Luisa admits that they did not follow his advice and instead gave Lino IV solution.

The health worker examines Lino and finds that he is in critical condition, probably because of a blood infection introduced with the IV solution. He runs back to the health post to get antibiotics to fight the infection.

But before the health worker can return with the medicine, Lino dies. The lesson is painfully clear:

Food, not medicine, is the key to good health - especially for people who are weak and hungry. Do not waste your money on vitamins advertised on the radio.

Buy food - not vitamins.

And do not use IV solutions to gain strength.

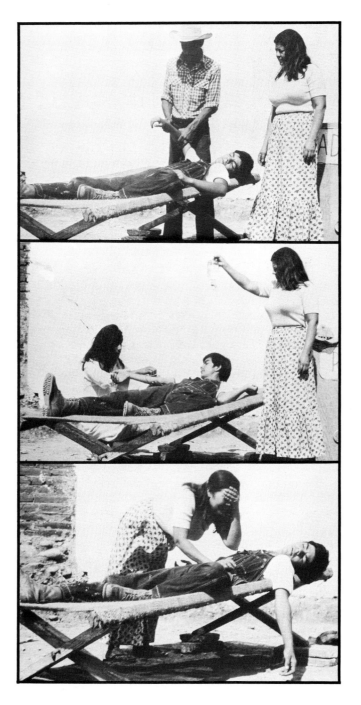

145

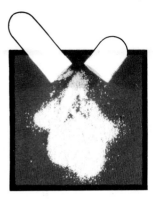

CHAPTER 9

HEALTHY SOLUTIONS
Third World National
and Regional Policies

IN EARLIER chapters we focused on policies and practices that harm the poor and inevitably facilitate the misuse of drugs. Of course, the picture is not uniformly bleak. Third World policy-makers are acutely aware of the problems. Some, notably in Sri Lanka, Mozambique and a variety of other countries, have pioneered constructive solutions. In this chapter, we look at some of them.

This means that there are workable blue-prints to revolutionise drug policies to benefit the poor. Health planners in other developing countries can adapt them to suit local needs. They can also call on technical assistance from UN agencies like WHO, UNCTAD and UNIDO, that have helped devise many of the new strategies. Already these policies have led to major improvements. For example, the use of generic names, restricted drug lists and buying by competitive tender have succeeded in cutting costs massively and increasing supplies of vital drugs. On the face of it, it may seem incomprehensible that such obviously advantageous policies have not been universally adopted.

Yet there are powerful obstacles to change. The crucial one is lack of political will. In the words of a senior WHO official: "Some authorities consider drugs simply as consumer products which are subject to the laws of supply and demand." [1] Consequently, their drug policies relate more closely to the needs of industrial and trade development than health development. [2] In many developing countries health ministries are notoriously weak, compared with the more influential ministries of commerce. But, if health-centred drug policies are to stand any chance of being adopted, WHO and industry commentators stress that health ministries must have bargaining power. [3]

Most governments are under pressure not to rationalise their drug policies. As the senior WHO official observed, "Pressure groups have arisen - particularly among certain pharmaceutical industries and in sections of the medical professions - which would prefer to see the status quo maintained". [4] Local and foreign business interests lobby hard for any rationalisation to be confined to the public sector, leaving the vast private market largely uncontrolled. [5]

In some cases policy-makers may themselves oppose changes. An anthropologist's observations on one African country could apply more widely: "It seems probable that the delay in the adoption of the WHO directives concerning cheap essential

146

medicines is also due to the fact that influential people will lose attractive privileges when foreign pharmaceutical firms are forced to deliver medicines in a way which is commercially unattractive.'' [6]

Despite the obstacles, many developing countries have introduced some controls on both the public and private sectors. These range from 'paper tigers' - that look good but change nothing - to measures that are actively enforced. We shall focus here on some of the key policy options open to developing countries. But WHO stresses that individual measures have only a limited chance of success. The countries that have most successfully tackled problems of drug supply, use and distribution are those that have adopted comprehensive national drug policies, giving clear priority to essential drugs for primary health care. [7]

MAJORITY HEALTH SERVICES

Among the countries that have made the most impressive achievements in reaching virtually the entire population with health services are China, Cuba and Vietnam, and the less well-publicised success stories of Sri Lanka and Papua New Guinea. Their approach has varied a great deal. For instance, whereas Cuba opted for what one observer has described as a ''super-professionalised and centralised approach to health care'', [8] China, Vietnam and Sri Lanka, with proportionately far fewer doctors, have set up decentralised services run by community-based paramedics.

On the communes in China, for example, where about 850 million of the population live, health care is provided by 'barefoot doctors' (or village health workers) chosen by the commune, which pays for their training. Workers have been paying about one-twentieth of their average monthly income for free medical treatment, and a small prescription charge for medicines. [9] This puts the richer production brigades in a position to afford better services. But it does not rule out the possibility of a poor brigade getting help from a richer one, if for exmple one worker has rheumatoid arthritis and needs constant and costly injections. [10]

Papua New Guinea has also succeeded in setting up decentralised health services with a referral system. In contrast to China, it has a population of under 3 million. But it has major communication problems with its people divided into different ethnic and language groups, living in scattered and isolated settlements separated by rugged mountains and jungle. These difficulties mean that about 10% of the people still have no easy access to health care facilities, as they live some 2-3 hours' walk from the nearest aid post. [11] The health services are organised into various tiers starting with the aid post, which serves a community of about 2,000 people. The orderlies who run the aid posts receive 1-3 years' training and can handle 95% of the problems brought to them. More complicated cases are referred to the nearest health centre, which acts as a referral point for a population of 10,000 to 50,000. They are staffed by orderlies and nurses who work under the supervision of a health extension officer. Any patient needing an operation or complicated in- patient treatment can be admitted to the provincial hospital. Treatment is given free at the aid posts and most of the health centres. There are hospital charges, but these are waived for children, the old and the poor. [12]

Up until independence in 1975, health spending in Mozambique had been allocated almost exclusively to expensive curative services for the urban elite. Since then there has been a radical reallocation of priorities and health resources. For example, whereas 47% of the national drug budget was once consumed by the central teaching hospital, it now receives only 10%. Priority is given to preventing disease. But because of the need for essential drugs, spending on drugs rose five times, in real terms, in the five years after independence. [13]

Mozambique stands out as having developed and implemented a comprehensive drugs policy to support its overall health strategy. Within months of independence all drug policy-making was centralised under the Technical Committee for Therapeutics and Pharmacy which immediately started work rooting out wasteful and unnecessary drugs. [14]

ESSENTIAL DRUG LISTS

Countless WHO reports have concluded that the single most important measure needed to cut costs and ensure that drugs are used effectively is to limit the number available to those "most necessary for the health care of the majority of the population". [15]

As early as 1959 Sri Lanka acted to rationalise prescribing in the public sector. Under the impetus of serious economic problems and resulting drug shortages, the Government restricted all health service prescriptions to the 500 drugs on the Ceylon Hospital Formulary. [16] Mozambique introduced similar legislation and its more restrictive National Formulary in 1977 - the same year that WHO produced its first model list of essential drugs. Since then a growing number of countries have made their own selections of essential drugs based on local needs. At the last count, in April 1982, 70 countries had restricted drug lists. [17]

Many of these lists, however, represent little more than policy goals because they have yet to be strictly enforced. Virtually all are intended to apply only to the public sector. Moreover, even in the public sector only a minority of countries have rationalised drug use to the same extent as Mozambique where doctors need special permission to prescribe a non-formulary drug. [18] In many cases controls on government purchases can be circumvented. Just one example is the situation in Mexico, where company sales representatives can still promote their products and distribute free samples in the hospitals. As a result doctors put pressure on hospital administrators to buy drugs not included in the country's 'Cuadro basico' - its list of 426 essential drugs. [19]

Limited lists can only reduce drug costs if they are backed by an efficient purchasing system. In Brazil the central procurement agency, CEME, bases its purchases on a restricted list and has succeeded in buying drugs at under 50% of local commercial prices. [20] A report of the United Nations Centre for Transnational Corporations (UNCTC) describes this system as a trade-off in which the government agency "applies its list to a restricted market, and the private sector collaborates by providing it with drugs at preferential prices ... as long as the richer markets are left unaffected". [21] The obvious advantage of the system is that essential drugs

148

are secured cheaply for some of the poorest. But only a minority benefit from these free drugs - an estimated 9% of Brazil's population in 1973. Meanwhile the majority of the poor are still vulnerable to high prices and non-esssential products in the private market. [22]

These shortcomings, common to many countries, are no argument against the importance of limited drug lists. They underline the need for curbs on promotional pressures and for controls to apply also to the private market.

Sri Lanka, Mozambique and Afghanistan are exceptional in having taken measures to restrict both the health services and the private market to a selection of essential drugs. [23] In Sri Lanka the National Formulary Committee reviewed 4,000 drugs imported for use in the private sector in 1962 and recommended that they should be reduced to 2,100. After a major policy review in 1971 import licences were withdrawn from all but 600 approved drugs. This rationalisation of the private market was achieved by removing all irrational combination drugs, products of doubtful efficacy and unacceptable safety hazards and brands of almost identical drugs. [24]

Private medical practice was banned in Mozambique immediately after independence, and the number of drugs granted import licences was cut from 13,000 to 2,600. This selection was further reduced with the removal of drugs considered either non-essential or unnecessarily expensive. Now only the 355 drugs included in the 1980 National Formulary are routinely supplied and prescribed. [25]

SAFER, MORE EFFECTIVE DRUG USE

Limited drug selections have major advantages in encouraging the safe and effective use of medicines. Many health authorities draw up much shorter lists of drugs that can be safely and effectively used by paramedics. For example, Bangladesh has selected 31 drugs for primary health care use and in Sri Lanka no more than 60 drugs are dispensed at rural clinics. In Mozambique the *agentes polyvalentes,* paramedics with only primary school education and 6 months' training, are restricted to using about 50 drugs. [26]

With fewer medicines in use it becomes a more manageable task for governments to ensure that health workers and doctors receive vital drug information. For example, the 1981 *Proposed Essential Drug List for Zimbabwe* includes details of cost-effective treatments for common diseases and specific guidance on the use of some categories of drugs like antibiotics. [27] Peru has compiled information sheets on each basic drug and a number of countries have developed standard treatment schedules. Mozambique's *Therapeutic Guide* sets out the first-line treatment for TB as a combination of streptomycin, isoniazid and thiacetazone. Only if this fails should the second-line treatment of rifampicin and ethambutol be given, as it costs 8 times more. Health workers are also urged to avoid expensive syrups and drops unless they are strictly necessary as these preparations can cost 20 times more than tablets. [28]

GENERIC NAMES

Many governments have seen the advantages of buying drugs by generic name. Very few have attempted to make generic prescribing or labelling compulsory. The Hathi Committee, which reported to the Indian Government in 1975, recommended phased abolition of brand names as one element of comprehensive new drug policies. The Committee suggested that initially generic names should be made compulsory for 13 drugs. [29] In the event, it was not until 1980 that the Indian Government moved to ban brand names for 5 drugs. [30]

After the setting up of the State Pharmaceuticals Corporation in Sri Lanka in 1971, the use of generic names, already enforced in the public sector, was extended to the private sector. Manufacturers were obliged to label their products with generic names in bold type. Brand names could appear in lettering only half the size. Exceptions were made for some patented products imported in small quantities. However, after a change of Government in 1977, the enforcement of generic names was relaxed and some major manufacturers reverted to their old style of labelling, as illustrated opposite. [31]

In Afghanistan legislation introduced in 1979 compelled private wholesalers to import only generic drugs listed in the national formulary. Brand name products could only be imported if no generic equivalents were available and in these cases the state buying agency carried out the transactions. [32]

In 1972 the Government of Pakistan made generic names compulsory. But the policy was reversed four years later after a mass of substandard drugs flooded onto the market. A subsequent investigation by the Pakistan Monopoly Control Authority disproved claims that there had been anything wrong with the generics policy itself, only with its implementation. The policy failed because quality control checks were totally inadequate and little was done to convince doctors of the advantages of generic prescribing. [33]

These advantages are clear to prescribers in countries where quality control works efficiently. In Papua New Guinea, for example, generics are bought on competitive tender and undergo strict quality control testing in laboratories in Australia, before being imported into the country. One doctor in Papua New Guinea comments: "Perhaps the major advantage is that we are not canvassed or otherwise bothered by reps and drug advertising. It leads to clear thinking and better prescribing to use only generic names." [34] There are similar reports from Mozambique. [35]

CENTRALISED PROCUREMENT

A 1979 report summarising the results of a survey of drug policies in Asia, Africa and Latin America, instigated by the Non-Aligned Movement and other developing countries, concluded that, "In spite of the availability of good quality drugs at much cheaper prices, many developing countries are tied to traditional sources of supply - namely, the transnational corporations. This is mainly due to the fear that these companies may retaliate. There is inadequate appreciation that it is within their power to formulate new policies, which when implemented would enable them to reduce their imports bill by as much as 50% or more." [36]

Sri Lanka insisted on packaging emphasising generic names until a change of government in 1977. Left, post-1977 packaging; right, pre-1977 packaging.

Sri Lanka was the first country to prove that the drug import bill could be cut dramatically when it pioneered its system of bulk purchasing through a centralised government agency. Initially the Sri Lankan system was limited to drugs imported for the health services. But a major drug policy review in 1971/72 identified the need to stop the massive wastage of valuable foreign exchange caused by private importers paying high prices to monopoly suppliers. Wide disparities were discovered between the private importers' prices and those that the Government was paying for the same drugs by buying by generic name on worldwide, competitive tender - in other words, by 'shopping around' for the best price, after inviting a range of manufacturers to compete for an order. [37]

During 1972/73 the State Pharmaceutical Corporation (SPC) began a phased takeover of drug imports that had previously been carried out by 134 private importers. The prices paid by the private importers in the first half of 1972 were later compared with those paid by the SPC for the same drugs in the second half of the year. This showed that centralised purchasing achieved a 40% overall saving on the cost of importing just 52 drugs. For example, chloroquine had previously been imported from six different suppliers. After choosing from a variety of quotes, the SPC bought chloroquine from Sterling UK at *less than half* the price paid earlier to another manufacturer by the private importers. [38]

The SPC only accepted the cheapest offer for 11 of the 52 drugs. It lacked the quality control facilities to test drugs offered at exceptionally low prices by unknown suppliers. So Sri Lanka continued to buy from the research-based manufacturers, but at far lower prices. The experience proved that it was possible to challenge the market power of leading manufacturers. In the words of SPC Chairman, Dr. Bibile, ''The results demonstrate the kind of foreign- exchange savings that accrue to a developing country when it establishes a state buying agency and adopts an open-tender procedure for purchasing. It places the agency in a strong bargaining position and compels competition even among the transnational corporations which had previously monopolised the market.'' [39]

Encouraged by Sri Lanka's success, a number of countries have since set up national procurement agencies to bulk buy drugs on the world market. In most cases these public tenders are used to buy drugs only for the health services, not for the private market as happened in Sri Lanka. [40] Centralised procurement has been particularly successful in Costa Rica, where the Social Security Agency is estimated to have saved the country £17.6 million in 1978 alone. The policy has contributed to the Social Security Agency's success in increasing its ability to meet the people's drug needs from 46.8% in 1970 to 81.5% in 1976. [41]

Previously the Costa Rican Government's ability to buy the cheapest reliable generics was seriously hampered by laws protecting patents. But its bargaining power has increased with reforms in patent laws enacted after a dispute over the result of a 1978 tender. At the time a foreign manufacturer filed a case against the Costa Rican agency for deciding to buy from a generics producer instead of paying the much higher price for its own patented product. [42]

The 1979 report on the results of a survey of 14 Third World countries found that many are still paying very high prices, even though they buy drugs by competitive tender. The survey revealed that "At present a large part of drug purchases of developing countries follow relatively primitive tendering procedures, if at all, with litle available information concerning alternative suppliers, quality and costs of the product". [43]

A senior scientist working on the WHO Drug Action Programme confirms that, whereas it appears very logical and straightforward to suggest that poor countries should buy drugs on international tender, at least for the public sector, it is hard to "imagine how they can buy through international tender without a proper means of communication outside their own country". [44] Very few developing countries share Cuba's advantages in having both sophisticated quality control facilities and a market intelligence network operating in major drug producing countries. [45]

Mozambique's centralised procurement agency, Medimoc, for example, has worked under the limitation of poor quality control facilities. These are being improved, but it has also experienced difficulties in keeping up with demand, partly as a result of transport delays and partly because manufacturers often require an advance payment in dollars. Tenders are made annually and it can be a year before the drugs actually arrive. In the meantime international currency fluctuations can contribute to dramatic price rises which may make it necessary to reorder. [46] But despite the problems, Medimoc has achieved excellent results. Prices paid in 1979 were similar to, or up to 20% less than 1975 prices, without any adjustment for inflation. In some cases prices have dropped substantiallly. For example the 1979 prices for methyldopa, cotrimoxazole and frusemide were respectively 72%, 44% and 7% of 1975 prices. [47]

LOCAL PRODUCTION

Developing countries at very different stages of industrial development have taken active steps to reduce their dependence on imported drugs. Their strategies range from attempts to obtain the drugs they need by influencing what subsidiaries of foreign companies produce locally, to building up local production under public ownership.

In India the Hathi Committee advocated in 1975 that foreign subsidiaries should be stopped from merely carrying out formulation and packing, particularly of over-the-counter remedies like vitamin tonics and cough mixtures. The Committee urged that they should be actively encouraged to set up bulk drug production and bring valuable technology into the country. [48] Since then a succession of carrot and stick measures have aimed to implement this policy. The 1978/79 New Drugs Policy stipulates that manufacturers which only produce finished drugs will have to reduce their foreign ownership, but those prepared to produce bulk drugs can keep up to 74% foreign equity, depending on how many they produce and the sophistication of the technology they import. [49]

To date this policy has not led to the expected rise in bulk drug production, and the new policies have been heavily criticised by the industry which blames over-regulation for holding back growth in this area. [50] Nevertheless, in contrast to most developing countries, India has a sizeable state owned drug industry which produces predominantly bulk drugs. Both public and private Indian companies now export drugs and production technology. [51]

Very few developing countries have as much bargaining power as India in dealing with subsidiaries of the transnationals. Bangladesh, for example, has up till now had little success in persuading foreign manufacturers to produce more bulk drugs locally. Foreign companies that set up local production whilst the country was part of Pakistan were allowed to do so on condition that they produced some raw materials as well as finished drugs. However, because the terms of their undertaking were left extremely vague, some manufacturers have been able to dodge the issue, justifying their reluctance to set up bulk drugs production on the grounds that it would be uneconomical. [52]

This apparent impasse has encouraged a number of countries, including Bangladesh, to look to government-controlled production as the best solution to guaranteeing supplies of essential drugs for public health needs. In Bangladesh the Government's existing formulation plant at Tejgaon is being expanded and there are plans to set up new production units to produce raw materials. [53]

In the small African state of Lesotho the Government has established local production with technical support from the International Dispensary Association, a non-profit making organization. The Lesotho Dispensary Association, set up in 1977, satisfies Lesotho's needs for basic drugs and is now expanding its production to supply neighbouring countries. [54]

Some countries have already succeeded in setting up large-scale state-controlled production. China, which is now reported to be virtually self-sufficient in drugs and a sizeable exporter, is an obvious example. [55] In Cuba the situation before the 1959 revolution closely resembled that of many developing countries today. Cuba was dependent on imports from foreign manufacturers for 80% of its drug requirements. A recent UNCTAD study shows that now the Cuban state-owned industry supplies over 80% of the country's needs. Like India, Cuba has also developed its own technology to produce some bulk drugs. [56]

Less well-known is what the UNCTC has recently described as the Egyptian Government's "remarkable achievement in moving the country from being dependent on imports for 80% of its drug needs (in 1963) to producing 83% of total demand locally" (in 1980). [57] The public sector alone can now meet nearly 70% of total requirement.

Egypt's achievement can be directly attributed to the comprehensive drugs policy pursued by successive Governments since all but two drug companies were nationalised in 1962/63. The first step taken was to centralise policy-making on imports, production and distribution under one state agency. A drug research and control centre was set up to carry out quality control and production research.

Priority was given to training scientists and engineers, estimated to number about 22,000 in 1978. Production in the public sector is now closely integrated with seven factories engaged in formulation, one producing basic chemicals and other packaging materials. Any raw materials that cannot be produced locally are imported by the state trading corporation. [58]

The Egyptian drug industry is still dependent on foreign manufacturers for production equipment and chemical intermediates. Foreign expertise is needed to produce some speciality drugs which are produced under licensing agreements or joint ventures with some major research-based companies. But because of the size and market power of the nationalised industry, Egypt is in a better bargaining position than most developing countries to obtain technology on favourable terms. [59]

DISTRIBUTION

Many developing countries are attempting to improve *public* drug distribution through extending the primary health care infrastructure. But the logistics of transport, storage and administrative back-up remain problematic in most.

Some countries have set up efficient distribution systems ensuring that public dispensaries receive the drugs they require. In Papua New Guinea, for example, detailed procedures have been established to avoid wastage. The aid posts and health centres supply information to one of six regional stores on their requirements and current stocks. The pharmacist in charge of the regional store then sends in a printed order form for the region's requirements to the central medical store, giving a stock-in-hand figure for every item on the list. This allows the central store to make an accurate assessment of the country's overall needs and prepare tenders. [60]

The extent to which governments control *private* drug distribution is heavily influenced both by political considerations and the availability of drugs through the public sector. For example, after the expulsion of the French in 1954, North Vietnam imposed strict controls on private retailers. Despite the controls, overcharging by drug sellers was widespread because of the serious shortage of drugs. Decentralised health services had already been established during the nine year struggle for independence, so the state system could provide people with an alternative to buying drugs over the counter. Consequently the Government decided to ban all private drug sales and incorporate existing pharmacies into the state system. A Vietnamese doctor explains: "The pharmacists' interests were taken into consideration, but the people's interests were to be the first consideration." [61]

The difficulties of controlling private drug distribution in non-socialist countries can be considerable. Many countries have laws banning over-the-counter sales of drugs that should be sold on prescription. In practice, these are virtually impossible to enforce. Attempts have been made to control private sales by issuing licences only to qualified pharmacists. This is the case in El Salvador where licences to sell drugs are restricted to pharmacists or *idoneos* (salesmen with a formal

155

qualification in drug use). In practice these controls are easily by-passed, as an anthropologist observed: "Licensed pharmacists or *idoneos* often appear at the store only to sign the appropriate documents for the renewal of the pharmacy licence, in early January, and thereafter simply to pick up their pay checks on a monthly basis. Their time is spent pursuing other business interests." [62]

Another policy option considered by some governments is to limit the range of drugs that untrained retailers can sell, in much the same way as restricting paramedics to an agreed list. This system has been adopted in Mozambique. [63] But regulatory authorities in most developing countries have little more than a handful of drug inspectors. It would be an impossible task for them to monitor the vast number of scattered retailers, not to mention illegal traders. So most have concentrated any efforts made on trying to control the drugs that come onto the local market.

DRUG REGISTRATION
In the rich world stringent controls are applied to new drugs before they can be marketed. In Britain, for example, the main objective of licensing procedures is to ensure that the usefulness of drugs outweighs their possible hazards and that they are effective for each use recommended by the manufacturer. Criteria of cost-effectiveness, vital to poor countries, are not taken into consideration in allowing a new drug onto the market.

Most developing countries operate some, often minimal, registration procedures. Few regulatory authorities in the Third World are in a position to evaluate the evidence produced by manufacturers to support their claims. Few have access to unbiased scientific evaluations, much less facilities to make their own clinical trials. They have to rely on regulatory decisions taken in Europe and the US. These are often contradictory, but should keep dangerous or ineffective drugs off the market. However, they offer poor countries no guarantee that a new drug represents value for money in meeting their specific needs.

The registration system operated in Cuba before the 1959 revolution illustrates the problems faced by other developing countries today. This is described in a recent UNCTAD report as "merely a bureaucratic formality with a firm presenting a large volume of information, which no one read, and then making the required payment of excise taxes as well as other irregular payments." [64]

Today the Cuban National Formulary Commission makes a detailed evaluation before any new drug is approved for use in the country. Controlled clinical trials are carried out to assess whether the new drug has clear medical advantages over cheaper drugs already on the market. According to the UNCTAD report, the experience of the Cuban regulatory authorities has shown that disregarding "the subjective factors introduced by commercial propaganda, ... when economic studies are made, it is found that in the majority of cases, the cost per treatment with the new drug is four to ten times higher than with the one in current usage, with more or less the same effectiveness". [65]

156

New drugs are not the only problem. Most regulatory authorities are confronted with the existence of a mass of similar and non-essential products that have already been licensed for sale. In April 1982, the Mexican Government announced new regulations designed to make it easier to cancel existing licences. Whereas product registrations used to be valid indefinitely, they will now be subject to review every three years. If the manufacturer does not apply for a product to be re-registered, its existing licence will automatically lapse. In future the Mexican regulatory authorities will also have new criteria on which they may decide to cancel registration. These include evidence that the manufacturer's original registration documents were misleading, and any cases where combination products have no clear advantages over single-ingredient drugs. [66]

The major constraint on effective registration systems is often that the regulatory authorities lack the powers to enforce their decisions. For example, according to the 1979 Annual Report of the Supreme Board of Drug Control in North Yemen, on occasions their procedures have been completely by- passed. Manufacturers have approached other apparently more sympathetic departments to get permission to market their drugs. [67]

IMPORT AND PRICE CONTROLS

A considerable number of Third World governments apply some form of controls on the prices of finished drugs. Some try to prevent retailers from overcharging by compelling manufacturers to print the maximum retail prices on the packs. This measure is enforced in North Yemen and Pakistan. [68] Some governments have been particularly successful in keeping down prices. Egypt, for example, applies strict controls to all drug prices. [69]

Over the last ten years successive Indian Governments have introduced a variety of measures in attempts to peg the prices of finished drugs. With about 15,000 formulations on the market, the Government has been forced to implement selective controls. One scheme was based on regulating the prices of some of the market leaders' products. But the drug price index continued to rise. According to a recent case study by the UNCTC these controls proved ineffective because they covered only about one-third of the manufacturers' products. "Apparently, pharmaceutical firms took advantage of the loopholes in the (Drug Price Control) Order and increased the prices of unregulated drugs to compensate for the controls. Also, the price of imported raw materials and intermediates remained largely outside the purview of the new controls." [70]

The main difficulty faced by governments attempting to control prices of finished drugs manufactured locally is that they are seldom in a position to evaluate manufacturers' figures on their production costs. Drug control agencies throughout the world have problems in assessing transfer prices for chemical intermediates and bulk drugs.

Amongst developing countries, the Colombian Government made what the UNCTC described as "pioneering efforts to monitor transfer pricing and detect abuses." [71] The process began some years ago when a Colombian economist

157

compared the import prices that parent companies charged their Colombian subsidiaries with prices at which the same intermediates could be bought on the world market. He found that, on average, transnationals were overcharging by 155%. In some cases their transfer prices were up to 50 times higher than the cost of the same intermediate from other sources. [72]

Fines were imposed on the companies found to be overcharging and a Government agency was set the task of systematically collecting price information from world market sources to check against the transnational companies' invoices. According to UNCTC this monitoring by the Colombian Government led to "a significant reduction of over-invoicing practices and a corresponding decline in the price of finished drugs". [73]

Sri Lanka tried a different strategy to tackle high transfer prices. Policymakers decided that the most effective way to keep down prices of imported raw materials would be to centralise procurement under Government control. In the face of strong industry opposition, the State Pharmaceutical Corporation (SPC) took over raw materials imports in 1973. It achieved major savings over the cost of raw materials imported in the previous year. For example, the SPC bought chlorpheniramine from Halewood UK for only 13% of the price Glaxo had charged its Sri Lankan subsidiary for the same drug the previous year. Some manufacturers dropped their *own* prices massively from one year to the next. For instance Beecham reduced the price to its subsidiary for cloxacillin and ampicillin to respectively only 22% and 17% of their previous transfer prices. [74]

The Sri Lankan State Pharmaceutical Corporation monopoly over raw materials imports was reversed with the change of Government in 1977. But according to Professor Lionel, Head of the Colombo University Pharmacology Department, private imports continue to be closely monitored by the Government and the SPC's low prices provide an incentive to local manufacturers to keep their prices down. Moreover, Professor Lionel explained that there are now fewer shortages than when the SPC was the sole importer and private sector prices are much lower than in countries where controls are weak or non-existent. [75]

In attempting to control transfer pricing, the Indian Government has fixed the prices of eight critical chemical intermediates which it keeps under review. The state-owned Chemical Pharmaceutical Corporation (CPC) also has a monopoly on importing some of the most important bulk drugs. These are then distributed for formulation to both private and state-owned companies. In its 1981 report the UNCTC states that the Indian CPC has made significant savings by buying bulk drugs on competitive tender. Moreover, "By supplying foreign subsidiaries, it has prevented them from importing bulk drugs from their parent companies at prices fixed by these companies. It has also ensured the regular supply of important drugs to indigenous companies." [76]

CONTROLS ON MARKETING PRACTICES

A government that introduces comprehensive drug policies, bans private medicine and restricts doctors to prescribing from the national formulary may find there is little need to introduce controls on marketing practices. In these circumstances manufacturers may abandon promotional activities as they stand little chance of influencing doctors' prescribing habits. This has been the experience of Mozambique, where only a few manufacturers still have local sales representatives. Most Mozambican doctors are committed to the new direction of health policy and have little time for visiting sales reps. [77]

But where the private market still flourishes and doctors are free to prescribe any drug they choose, controls on marketing practices are essential. However, despite the need, only a minority of Third World governments have adopted measures comparable to those enforced in Europe and the US. The UNCTC singles out Egypt as a country that has adopted "effective regulations on marketing practices". Some controls are stricter than in developed countries. "Although brand name products ... are allowed on the Egyptian market, advertisements are confined to professional journals and samples to professional bodies. No advertisements are allowed for over-the-counter products. Information on each drug is checked for accuracy by a government agency." [78]

The Costa Rican Government has also introduced strict controls on the promotion of both prescription-only and over-the-counter medicines. Sanctions against companies that break the rules have been written into the legislation, so that a company violating advertising standards can either be fined or have the registration of its products revoked. [79]

A number of countries have tried to ensure a balanced flow of information to prescribers. In Sri Lanka, government doctors are sent a quarterly publication, *The Prescriber,* started in 1966 by the National Formulary Committee. *The Prescriber* aims to combat the effects of manufacturers' promotion, for instance by providing comparative assessments of new products as against much cheaper, well-established drugs. [80]

HEALTH EDUCATION
Currently one of the most neglected areas of policy appears to be government attempts to impress on people that there are *alternatives* to medicines. Most governments carry out some limited health education work. In Costa Rica, for example, the Ministry of Health has prepared special leaflets for the public warning against self-medication. [81] But few governments take advantage of the potential of mass-media advertising campaigns on popular mobilisation to promote preventive health. One of the exceptions is the Sandinista Government in Nicaragua which has organised *'Jornadas Populares de Salud'* - 'days of mass mobilisation' - as part of its strategy for getting people to take more responsibility for their own health. [82]

* * * * *

Mozambique and Sri Lanka are amongst the countries that have adopted the most comprehensive policy changes. The political climate in Mozambique, a socialist country, has been crucial to the Government's success in challenging doctors'

159

prescribing freedom. In most other countries this is vigorously defended. Members of the country's Portuguese medical establishment who might have opposed the new drug policy left Mozambique after independence. Professor Mazargao of the Technical Committee for Therapeutics and Pharmacy stresses that the limited drug list can only be implemented "through political understanding. It cannot be compulsory, it must be understood." [83]

By contrast, in Sri Lanka the programme of rationalisation was carried out "in the face of much opposition from the pharmaceutical industry and their agents in Sri Lanka. Some of this opposition was channeled through doctors even up to the Formulary Committee", according to Dr. Bibile, who was Chairman of the State Pharmaceuticals Corporation. [84] But the positive results of the policies adopted in Sri Lanka are clear. Whereas other Asian countries such as Bangladesh and Nepal were spending 44% of their health budgets on drugs in 1976, but only covering a minority of their population, Sri Lanka was able to meet about 80% of its people's needs. Moreover, according to a 1979 WHO report, "In Sri Lanka the expenditure on drugs constitutes about 7.5% of the total health expenditure, probably reflecting the strict control exercised by the state on drugs allowed to be used in state medical institutions and in the private sector". [85]

But the majority of developing countries have yet to implement significant controls in the drugs field. The difficulties, not least their unequal relationship with the big foreign manufacturers, have led a growing number of developing countries to look for strength in numbers. Neighbouring countries have joined forces to analyse common problems and mobilise their pooled resources in achieving solutions. In the words of Dr. Mahler, Director General of WHO, "Nothing will work more in this area than the joint effort of countries to exchange technologies, information and experiences and jointly boost their bargaining positions". [86]

REGIONAL COOPERATION

Developing countries are actively cooperating over joint drug policies within a number of political, economic and regional groupings. Many of these regional initiatives are backed with financial and technical support from the UN agencies. Under the broad umbrella of the Non-Aligned Movement a succession of resolutions has been passed calling for comprehensive policy changes to be implemented. At their meeting in Colombo in 1976, the Non-Aligned countries agreed to start work on setting up new regional cooperative pharmaceutical production and technology centres, known by their acronym, COPPTECs. Each region would have its own COPPTEC to coordinate regional policy, exchange of information, pooled procurement and the setting up of local production. [87]

To date many of the proposed regional initiatives, including the COPPTECs, are still in their planning stages. It is obviously unrealistic to expect countries in the same region which may have major political differences to implement joint policies without considerable difficulties. But countries of every political complexion are increasingly stressing the need for positive action within regions and sub-regions, a mood underlined by delegates to the May 1982 World Health Assembly. [88]

160

Some common market groupings have already achieved consensus on regional priorities, notably the Caribbean countries in CARICOM, the Andean Pact countries and the member states of the West African Economic Community. There is considerable overlap between these initiatives and work coordinated within the WHO regions. Just one example of the positive results is that the Caribbean countries have now set up pooled procurement procedures and have a new regional drug testing laboratory in Jamaica. Similarly, both the Andean Pact countries and 33 African member states of WHO have drawn up a regional list of essential drugs as a concrete basis for joint purchasing and production. [89]

Besides providing a forum for exchanging information and agreeing joint strategies, regional meetings give individual countries a more forceful and unified voice in making demands on the UN system. For example, at a workshop in Abidjan in October 1981, 17 francophone African states called for the setting up of a revolving fund to help countries acquire drugs. They also urged WHO and UNCTAD to work together in drawing up an international code of pharmaceutical marketing practices, covering promotion, prices, distribution, research and development and transfer of technology. [90]

Developing countries see regional cooperation as an important means to strengthen their hand in obtaining the drugs they need. But they are acutely aware that even mutual support cannot entirely remove their dependence on the major manufacturers. It is the rich world that controls the key area of drug technology. At a meeting in Harare in April 1982 the Zimbabwean Minister of Health expressed the fears of some Third World policy makers in forceful terms: "Self-sufficiency in Africa can only be achieved by concerted group action in rationalising and coordinating the extension of our own manufacturing capacity, avoiding unnecessary competition and complementing each other in the variety of our products. Of course, this is not going to be allowed to succeed by the giants of the pharmaceutical industry in the developed world. Technology will be denied, royalties will rise and some of us will be made dumping grounds for cheap preparations which will throttle our nascent pharmaceutical manufacturing industry. Our awareness of these problems will make it that much easier for us to avoid the pitfalls of the 'divide and rule' philosophy of the multinationals." [91]

Are these fears justified by the attitudes and policies of rich world governments and manufactures? In the next chapter we examine the developed countries' response to the Third World's desire for change.

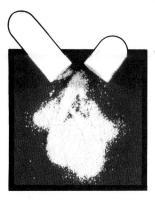

CHAPTER 10

HELP OR HINDRANCE?
The Rich World's Response

"The 'haves' are rarely willing to relinquish their control and their resources and share them with the 'have-nots'." (The Brandt Report)

THE BRANDT REPORT has documented the inflexibility of rich world institutions in the face of the problems confronting the Third World poor. [1] Poverty is condemned but it is also tolerated. Rich world interests oppose changes in the world economy that might offer some hope for the poor, but challenge the dominance of the rich. Poor people are central to any analysis of the problems of the Third World. But when it comes to the solutions, the poor are almost invariably shifted backstage. Their interests tend to be lumped together with those of Third World governments and the powerful people in their societies, who may be as unenthusiastic about change that threatens their position as their counterparts in the rich world.

The solutions to the problems affecting the poor that concern us here - the lack of essential drugs and harmful marketing practices - cannot be separated from these wider political and economic issues. But in this chapter we focus on rich world attitudes in relation to Third World drug policies and the role of rich world governments, manufacturers and international and non-governmental organisations.

INTERNATIONAL ORGANISATIONS
The UN agencies most actively involved in helping to plan and implement drug policies appropriate to the needs of developing countries are WHO, UNCTAD, UNIDO and UNICEF. [2] Apart from the fact that these organisations have their headquarters in Geneva, Vienna and Paris, it may seem strange to include them in a chapter on the rich world's response to the Third World's needs. After all, developing countries far outnumber developed nations amongst the 157 member states of WHO. But their inclusion here *is* appropriate.

The UN agencies are in the unenviable position of having to perform a balancing act in response to the conflicting demands and pressures imposed on them by very different governments. Their policies are, however, unlikely to succeed unless they are backed by the economic muscle-power of the rich industrialised countries. WHO officials are acutely aware that where health issues overlap with industrial and trade policies the whole area rapidly becomes a political minefield. They have to bear in mind that major drug producers may be few in number, but they can control the purse strings. Over half the total annual WHO budget is made up of contributions from just half a dozen leading drug manufacturing countries (the US, West Germany, Japan, France, Britain and Italy). The United States alone contributes almost a quarter of WHO's entire budget. [3]

The other obvious weakness inherent in the UN system is that WHO and other agencies can do little more than make recommendations. If governments choose not to act on them, UN agencies can do nothng besides issue polite reminders. For example, Dr. Halfdan Mahler, Director General of WHO, pointed out to member states attending the 1980 World Health Assembly that they were not making good use of the technical assistance available to them to serve their people's most pressing needs. [4]

Thousands of pages of enlightened analysis of Third World drug problems have been written and filed away in cubic metres of reports. Similarly countless resolutions urging governments to act on WHO recommendations have been adopted by the World Health Assembly, but never translated into action. Not surprisingly all the paperwork and the resolutions have made almost no impact on the lives of the Third World poor. In some developing countries shortages of essential drugs are becoming more acute despite the false impression created by government reports to WHO that everything is under control.

WHO has traditionally concerned itself with the technical and professional aspects of drug use. It has played an important role in disseminating drug information. [5] But its focus of attention on drug policies shifted in the mid-seventies, soon after Dr. Mahler became Director General. WHO then grasped the nettle and began to emphasise the underlying social and economic issues. For example, in addressing the World Health Assembly in 1975, Dr. Mahler denounced inconsistent standards in drug marketing practices between developed and developing countries as "unethical and detrimental to health". [6]

Dr. Mahler went on to point out that WHO had already made "a significant contribution towards assisting countries in improving drug quality, safety and efficacy". But he stressed that "It is now important to assist countries also in formulating and implementing national drug policies. The question is not merely technical, but also political and ethical, involving governmental responsibilities as well as the global social responsibility of the parmaceutical industry with regard to both the availability of existing essential drugs and the development of better ones." [7]

These wider social and economic issues have always concerned the relatively newer UN agencies, UNCTAD and UNIDO, which were set up during the 1960s expressly in response to problems generated by the growth of trade and industry. [8]

UNCTAD has worked closely both with individual governments and at regional level in documenting the problems and drawing up new drug policies to counteract them. UNCTAD officials emphasise the need for poor countries to sever their dependence on monopoly suppliers. They advocate bulk-purchasing on competitive tender; revision (or suspension) of patent restrictions, and less restrictive terms for the transfer of essential drug technology from rich to poor. In contrast to WHO, UNCTAD stresses that it is unrealistic not to include the private drug market in any rationalisation. The volume of private sales makes this essential to protect the interests of the majority. [9]

UNIDO has carried out feasibility studies and provided technical assistance to a number of countries in setting up local production of finished drugs. UNIDO is also involved in projects to establish the production of bulk drugs using multi-purpose plants. [10] UNICEF shares WHO's close involvement in extending primary health care services and has its own drug procurement operation based in Copenhagen. Essential drugs are bought in bulk and re-sold to developing countries well below market prices. [11]

UNICEF, UNCTAD, UNIDO and other UN agencies are also all collaborating with WHO on different aspects of the WHO Action Programme on Essential Drugs, which is now the most comprehensive international programme on Third World drug policies. [12] The Action Programme emerged under the aegis of Dr. Mahler and the first significant step towards its adoption was taken in 1978 when the World Health Assembly passed a resolution (WHA31.32) urging member states to adopt essential drug lists, generic names and other measures including tougher drug legislation. The resolution also mandated WHO to cooperate with other UN agencies in assisting member states to adopt new drug policies and continue discussions with drug manufacturers on the supply of essential drugs. WHO also received a mandate to evolve strategies for reducing drug prices and to develop a code of drug marketing practice. [13]

The first major evaluation of progress on the Action Programme took place four years later - at the May 1982 World Health Assembly. [14] The delegate from Ghana echoed the views of other member states in referring to the Action Programme as "one of the most exciting developments in the international health field". [15] But many delegates felt there had been rather more talk than action on the programme and some were particularly critical that dialogue with industry had been both so protracted and so unproductive. This view was expressed more forcefully by the Algerian delegate. He was highly sceptical about industry's motivation in switching from opposition to the concept of 'essential' drugs to a desire to participate and referred to the industry as "a new Trojan horse" inside the Action Programme. [16]

The feeling that the industry's involvement needed to be approached with caution grew during the course of the Assembly. Delegates had earlier been promised concrete details of the terms under which manufacturers would be prepared to supply essential drugs to developing countries. [17] In the event delegates received no written clarification of the industry's well-publicised offer to supply essential drugs for public use in poor countries under "favourable conditions", although the offer had been made through the industry's international representative body three years previously. [18]

A number of West German manufacturers made the first approach to WHO as early as 1977. At the time the pharmaceutical newsletter *SCRIP* quoted a leading German industrialist as saying: "But they ⌈ poor countries ⌉ must understand that they can't get everything free, and must not attempt to undermine our patent and trade-mark positions which are essential for the industry's profitability and existence." [19] The clear implication was that as *quid pro quo* for special prices for their health services, Third World governments would have to respect patents and brand names (against the recommendations of UN agencies). To date this assumption has not been publicly ruled out by the industry. When Dr. Vischer, President of the International Federation of Pharmaceutical Manufacturers Associations (IFPMA), addressed the 1982 World Health Assembly to clarify industry's position, he left delegates still uncertain about whether the industry's offer really held out any tangible benefits for the majority of developing countries. Dr. Vischer explained that "the words 'favourable conditions' " meant "quite simply ... a *preparedness* to supply drugs to the countries taking part in the Drug Action Programme at *non-commercial* prices". [20] (our emphasis) Readers who have seen the striking differences in drug prices (documented in Chapter 4 of this book) will share the bemusement of delegates to the World Health Assembly as to what is so "favourable" about a "preparedness" to negotiate on "non-commercial" prices.

Dr. Vischer went on to say that until countries were clearer about their drug requirements (quantities, pack sizes, labelling, time-scale for orders) he suggested "that it would not be helpful to speculate on how the term 'favourable conditions' should be interpreted in terms of actual prices". [21] So three years on from when the offer was originally made discussions with industry had yet to yield concrete results in the form of drugs for the world's poor.

The deadlock was a classic chicken-and-egg situation. Industry (understandably) could not quote prices until it had a concrete order to go on. WHO, for its part, rightly had no intention of endorsing a deal for the world's poorest countries without being sure that it would be to their advantage. However, we understand that in 1981, when industry was asked to quote its prices for the specific needs of one African country, Rwanda, the prices they came up with averaged out at more or less the same as those Rwanda was already paying *without* having to agree to any special terms. [22]

Consequently, if lower prices were to be made conditional on their agreeing to recognise patents and brand names, most developing countries would probably do better bargaining for themselves by buying on competitive tender. That was certainly the conclusion of a number of delegates at the 1982 World Health Assembly. Brazil, for example, pointed out that by buying drugs on competitive tender for health service requirements, the Government never paid more than 50% of local commercial prices. [23]

A number of the poorest countries expressed their uneasiness at the prospect of any long term agreements they might have to strike with powerful drug producers. These would reinforce their dependence and leave them highly vulnerable to future

165

market whims. Some thought that a policy whereby individual countries made agreements with manufacturers on a one-to-one basis also ran counter to some of the key aims of the Action Programme, above all the need to build up collective self-reliance through local production and regional cooperation. [24] The consensus reached in discussion on the Action Programme indicated that WHO should give less priority to Geneva-based discussions with industry and concentrate on its role as a "catalyst" for positive new policies in the Third World itself. [25] This was summed up in the strongly-worded resolution passed by the 1982 World Health Assembly which urged that the Action Programme should be enforced "in its entirety" and that WHO's Regional Offices should see that the programme is "vigorously pursued" in developing countries. [26]

The fact that delegates wanted the Action Programme to be implemented "in its entirety" is crucial in ensuring future progress on a WHO code of marketing practice (WHO was mandated to start work on a code in May 1978). A number of delegates wanted to know why no progress had been reported on the code. Countries of very different political complexions pressed for what the Chilean delegate described as "dynamic legislation ... as a defence against certain unethical practices of some producers". [27] Cuba, Burundi, Romania, and Samoa all raised the question of a WHO code. But the most forceful intervention on the need for a WHO-sponsored international code was made by the Dutch delegation. The Netherlands urged that a code was necessary "to prevent serious problems in which the good name of our organisation (WHO) might be at stake", having previously cited problems including "misinformation, incorrect advertisements, ineffective products, the introduction of inappropriate technologies and ... a possible move from essential drugs to non-essential drugs in the programme". [28]

Although a number of delegations gave priority to the need for a code, immediate prospects of a code being introduced at the May 1983 World Health Assembly are not good. Senior WHO officials make no secret of the fact that influential member states are firmly opposed to any international regulations on drug marketing. The organisation is still feeling the shock waves after the adoption of the International Code of Marketing of Breast-milk Substitutes in 1981 in the face of strong opposition from the United States. [29] WHO officials feel that a code on drugs would be too much of a political hot potato for the organisation in present circumstances. Some see the 'threat' of a WHO code as a useful Sword of Damocles to encourage industry's cooperation. Their fear is that attempts to push through a code would encourage such fierce opposition that the future of the entire Action Programme might be in jeopardy. It is a gamble they will not take without concerted pressure from more member states than have so far pushed for a code publicly.

For its part, the US Government has left no room for doubt about its views on the matter. During the discussion at the 1982 World Health Assembly the US delegate strongly objected to a draft resolution on the marketing of breast milk substitutes. (This was put forward to improve enforcement of the 1981 code.) The Americans were particularly unhappy with a reference stating that the code "was designed to *regulate* these marketing practices". (our emphasis) The US delegation was unsuccessful in quashing the 1982 follow-up resolution but they did get the wording changed to read that the Code had been "intended to, *inter alia,* deal with these marketing practices." [30]

On the issue of a pharmaceuticals code, the US delegate to the January 1982 meeting of the WHO Executive Board stated that he himself "did not think it would be constructive to give that matter (the question of a WHO Code) any further consideration particularly in view of the fact that the Director-General was shortly to be engaging in consultations with the representatives of the International Federation of Pharmaceuticals Manufacturers Associations. It was important not to take any steps which might jeopardise the outcome of those consultations." [31] His words were echoed by the US delegate at the May 1982 Assembly who expressed the hope that the Assembly would "take no action that might damage that cooperative relationship and prove counterproductive regarding the supply of essential drugs to countries where they were most needed." [32] Other US officials have recently been more explicit in referring to the code as "irrevocably opposed by the US". [33]

RICH WORLD GOVERNMENTS

Most governments of drug-producing nations have a decidedly ambiguous relationship with the local drug industry. This is particularly true of major drug-exporting countries such as Britain. [34] An industry-funded publication refers to the "dual and seemingly conflicting functions" of the British Department of Health and Social Security (DHSS) and explains: "On the one hand, its role could be seen as that of a regulatory authority with direct controls over the development, marketing and promotion of drugs..." but "on the other hand, the DHSS is the sponsoring department for the industry and is, therefore, keen to assist the latter's performance, especially in the field of exports." [35]

EXPORT CONTROLS

Before a new drug can be marketed in Britain, manufacturers have to obtain a product licence from the Government. These licences are made conditional on the drug being approved by the Committee on Safety of Medicines, which makes a thorough check on the safety, quality and efficacy of each new drug. But when it comes to drugs produced for export the regulatory functions of Government appear to be overshadowed by a desire to achieve a healthy export balance. Drug exports are specifically exempted from these controls. [36] The same is true in other major drug producing nations, such as Switzerland and France, which have also excluded drugs for export from regulatory controls. [37]

This gives exporters *carte blanche* to export drugs that have been withdrawn at home because they proved unsafe or ineffective. Effectively there is nothing to stop overseas sales of drugs that would never have been licensed for sale on the home market. In the words of a US Congressman, "under current law, companies can pretty much export whatever they can convince ... people abroad to buy". [38]

In most developing countries controls are notoriously weak - if not non- existent. As a result patients and consumers in poor countries are left highly vulnerable to questionable practices. The full extent of the problem is impossible to gauge because governments of exporting nations are reluctant to release details of exactly which products get exported where. [39] Trade secrecy is well defended by governments and manufacturers alike.

When questioned about the different standards applied to drug exports, rich world governments advance essentially the same arguments. For example, successive British Governments have all stressed that factors such as disease patterns, climate, diet and the availability of health services vary so much from one country to another that regulatory decisons taken in Britain would have little relevance to the requirements of developing countries. Consequently, as a civil servant explains, ''The United Kingdom has long argued that the only effective and appropriate method of controlling the safety and efficacy of medicines is for the less developed countries to develop their own procedures for control''. [40]

Does this mean that if a British manufacturer goes on marketing an unsafe drug after it has been removed from the home market, the British Government feels under no compulsion to do anything? And would this apply even to the marketing of drugs with known toxic side-effects in poor countries where they will inevitably be sold without a doctor's prescription? When these questions were raised in the British Parliament in 1979 Government spokesmen were adamant. ''It is for the governments of the Third World to decide whether they will permit that to happen … there is a limit to what Her Majesty's Government can do.'' [41]

The response was negative, albeit realistic in view of the difficulties for a national government in attempting to control the activities of transnational companies. But the absence of export controls is also presented in a positive light - in terms of the need for exporters to respect each country's right to choose. In the words of a spokesman for a former British Government, ''Is it not reasonable to question whether we have the right to deny a foreign government the right to make their own decision on the basis of their own expertise on the circumstances prevailing in the country?'' [42] A corollary to this freedom of choice argument is that policy statements usually imply that developing countries are also opposed to tighter export controls.

The arguments sound persuasive. After all, interference smacks of neo-colonialism. But looking at the argument in the light of the needs of poor countries it is not true that people in the Third World are happy with the existing situation where the onus falls on them to sift out hazardous and ineffective drugs. In fact there is a growing body of Third World opinion urging exporting nations to take an active role in safeguarding the health of people in developing countries. One illustration of this is the joint ''Declaration on the Export of Hazardous Substances and Facilities'' issued by participants from nine developing countries who attended an international seminar in Malaysia in 1980. The Penang Declaration urges that ''there should be no distinction between domestic and foreign consumers; so that if a hazardous substance or production facility is banned, disapproved or restricted in any country, the presumption will be that it will be treated equivalently for export purposes.'' [43] The Declaration also stipulates that governments should only allow the export of a banned product to go ahead in exceptional circumstances, after the exporters or the government of the importing country have made a special case that the benefits expected from the hazardous product would outweigh its health risks. [44]

An attempt to introduce export legislation along these lines was made in the United States in 1980 when Congressman Barnes presented a bill to Congress on the Export of Hazardous Products. It sought to shift the burden of proof so that a case would have to be made in favour of rather than against the export of a product banned or restricted in the US. [45] Not only has Congressman Barnes' bill been abandoned, but in May 1982 the Reagan administration was considering lifting a 44 year old prohibition on the export of unapproved drugs. [46] However there is a fundamental weakness in controls that apply only to exports from major drug producing nations. They can do nothing to stop manufacturers from producing banned or obsolete drugs in factories overseas.

INFORMATION POLICIES

The major fallacy in rich world complacency about the Third World's 'freedom of choice' is that this freedom can only be illusory unless regulatory agencies and drug prescribers receive a good flow of accurate and balanced drug information.

When the question of the need for manufacturers to give full information to Third World prescribers was raised in the British Parliament in 1979, the Government expressed a decidedly optimistic view of information provision in developing countries. In the words of one Government spokesman, "It is *likely* that many governments supply information to their doctors reflecting the licensed status of products in the United Kingdom and in turn, the promotional literature used in the United Kingdom, which must conform to that approved status ..." [47] (our emphasis) Rich world health officials imply that the poor world's needs are already adequately covered by existing sources of drug information that can be tapped by their regulatory authorities. For example, British health officials point to the British Pharmacopoeia, and other national quality specifications, which can provide a reference framework on formulation and quality. [48]

A number of major drug producing nations, including the US, UK, Japan and Italy, are participating in a WHO Certification Scheme set up to give importing nations some guarantee of the quality and reliability of drugs on the world market. [49] Governments that join the scheme undertake to monitor the quality of drugs produced locally and importers can ask for a certificate indicating whether a particular drug is licensed for sale on the home market. But the scheme is not as comprehensive as it might be. WHO itself points out it provides no guarantee of the quality of drugs once they reach their destination. [50] Moreover, it is being under-used. Some key drug exporters such as Switzerland and West Germany

169

were not among the original signatories, and by May 1982 less than half the WHO member countries had agreed to participate. [51] Some exporters would not agree to comply with all the terms of the scheme. Britain, for example, undertook to certify only the quality (not safety and efficacy) of drug exports, in accordance with the Medicines Act. [52]

Governments of drug-producing nations also stress that WHO is already collecting and disseminating drug information useful to developing countries. They also point out that Third World regulatory agencies can always consult reference books and their better-equipped counterparts in developed countries for assistance in evaluating drugs. [53] But the existing mechanisms are totally inadequate to meet the needs of the regulatory agencies throughout the Third World. Data-collection and dissemination on new products, adverse reactions and drugs withdrawn from the world market is handled by only a couple of scientists at WHO headquarters. WHO also runs a computerised system to collect details of drug adverse reactions in Uppsala in Sweden. But hardly any developing countries are amongst the two dozen nations to whom information is currently being circulated, despite the fact that more developing countries would like to participate if they were allowed to. [54]

Some recent initiatives to give more support to developing countries in improving their regulatory systems have been coordinated within the European Region of WHO. These proposals have had most active backing from the Nordic countries (Norway, Denmark, Sweden and Iceland). Some have met with opposition from other European Governments, notably those of Switzerland, West Germany, France and Britain. [55]

One recent initiative was a series of discussions between regulatory authorities from developed and developing countries held in Rome. Referring to one of the aims behind the meetings ("to propose a scheme for cooperation in registration and drug control between developed and developing countries") a senior WHO official felt the need to describe the intention as "innocent" when he addressed an audience including representatives of the US drug industry. [56] A proposal that has been fiercely resisted by governments of a number of influential drug producing nations is to establish a Drug Evaluation Unit in Copenhagen. Amongst other functions, this would assist developing countries by providing reliable and impartial assessments on new drugs. Industry may be keen to see more uniformity in drug registration procedures which would cut their costs, but there is concerted opposition to any suggestion of supra-national evaluations of new drugs. [57]

In assessing new drugs the question whether they are really *needed* is central to poor countries. But amongst developed countries, the Norwegian Government is exceptional in including a "test of need" for new drugs. [58] Most governments in the rich world are unanimous in opposing the concept of "need" becoming a criteria for assessing new drugs. [59] Inevitably this limits the relevance and usefulness of their regulatory decisions as a guide to Third World health authorities.

170

The prospects of rich world governments putting the interests of developing countries before their trade balances are not optimistic. However, one encouraging sign is a statement made somewhat surprisingly by the West German delegate to the 1982 World Health Assembly. Dr. Gaudich is reported to have said that "the industrialized countries of the European Region should really direct their efforts to ensuring that no drugs were exported which were not admitted in the country of origin and that patient information was of the same quality in the exporting and in the importing country, particularly in regard to drug safety and such matters as contra-indications, warnings and precautions to be taken ". [60]

TECHNICAL ASSISTANCE

Rich world governments are of course contributing valuable technical assistance to developing countries in the field of drug production, management and training. For example, the Italian Government has recently allocated $15 million (£8.3m) specifically to the WHO Action Programme on Essential Drugs. [61] According to a recent WHO report, the Norwegian, Dutch, Swedish, Danish, French, West German, Swiss and US Governments are all helping to finance projects to improve the supply of essential drugs in developing countries. [62]

Under the British aid programme funds were allocated to finance medical sciences training for over 1,000 students from developing countries in 1980. [63] Special training of official inspectors for medicines control has also been arranged jointly between the British Government medicines inspectorate and the law department of the Pharmaceutical Society of Great Britain. [64]

In addition to their proportionately large contributions to WHO and other international agencies, governments of rich drug producing nations all allocate considerable official development aid funds to health-related projects. For example, an estimated 8% to 10% of the total British aid programme was allocated to health aid in 1980. This means that developing countries benefited from between £69 and £86 million in health aid. [65] In the same year Britain benefited from sales revenue on over £404 million worth of pharmaceutical exports to developing countries (including the relatively rich oil-producing states). [66]

Some aid funds are allocated to projects directly related to the needs of the poor - such as the training of village health workers. But the vast majority (over two-thirds of total British official development assistance in 1980) was either fully or partially tied to the purchase of British goods and services. [67] In some cases poor countries have been encouraged to buy expensive capital equipment and high-technology machinery at the expense of the basic services relevant to the needs of the poor majority. The non-governmental organisations are increasingly putting pressure on rich world governments fundamentally to reappraise the *quality* of official aid and ensure that aid benefits the Third World poor instead of adding to their deprivation. [68]

Rich world governments have generally been slow to respond to initiatives that would put the interests of poor consumers before those of rich world manufacturers. But in 1981 governments of all the industrialised countries (with the sole exception of the United States) showed their willingness to take a stand to safeguard the health of the world's poor by voting for the International Code of Marketing of Breast-milk Substitutes. In the build-up to the World Health Assembly vote, the British and other Governments showed their readiness to listen and to be swayed both by the body of professional opinion and pressure from the general public and supporters of aid agencies and other non-governmental organisations.

NON-GOVERNMENTAL ORGANISATIONS

An assortment of very different organisations share an active interest in the supply and marketing of pharmaceuticals in developing countries. The views of the manufacturers are represented both by national and international industry associations whose main function is to bring pressure to bear to defend their members' interests. Similarly, the lobby on behalf of patients and consumers (particularly the Third World poor) is actively pursuing changes in current drug marketing practices. The activities of lobbyists based in the rich world need to be looked at alongside those of Third World pressure groups because they work closely together. We look first at a number of charitable organisations based in developed countries, that are involved in supplying drugs to charities in developing countries.

ECHO

ECHO (the acronym for Equipment to Charity Hospitals Overseas) in Britain, and Action Medeor, in West Germany, are both non-profit-making organisations that supply essential drugs to charity and mission hospitals throughout the Third World. We shall concentrate on ECHO, the larger of these two similar, but unconnected organisations.

ECHO was set up in 1966 on the inspiration of the Burtons, a husband and wife team, after they returned from carrying out medical misionary work in Africa. Whilst in Africa they had experienced the chronic shortages of basic medical equipment. Back in Britain, they launched an imaginative scheme to collect obsolete, but perfectly serviceable, hospital equipment and send it to poor countries where it would be put to good use.

Today the renovation of used hospital equipment is a relatively small part of ECHO's operations. But the supply of new equipment, worth just under £1 million in 1980, has grown to the extent that ECHO now has a Technical Department to provide a back-up service to customers and adapt equipment so that it can use solar energy systems. Standard equipment is either bought at competitive prices, or ECHO commissions small manufacturers to produce specific items, like operating tables, to very simple, highly cost-conscious designs.

In the early 1970s ECHO carried out research into its customers' needs and found that most were facing problems with the escalating cost of basic drugs. Peggy Burton explains the background to ECHO's decision to supply drugs: "In 1974 the worldwide supply of drugs to mission hospitals was still critical. Inflation fanned the flames created by world poverty and need. The questionnaire we circulated threw up enormous demands, especially in the basic generic, life-saving drugs such an antibiotics, anti-leprosy, anti-tubercular and anti-malarial drugs. For example, a mission on the Ivory Coast spent £15,000 on drugs in 1973; for the same amount of drugs in 1974 it spent £26,000. In 1975, the same drugs would cost nearly £40,000. ECHO set itself the task of reducing the expenditure to the 1973 level."[69]

ECHO soon found itself handling large drug orders, particularly when aid agencies like OXFAM needed emergency supplies for disaster relief work. Demand rose, so that in 1977 a budget of £224,000 was specifically allocated for drug purchases that year. By 1980 ECHO's annual drugs turnover had leapt to £2 million. The scale of ECHO's operations is illustrated by the fact that it has held stocks of up to a third of total world production of the vital anti-leprosy drug, dapsone, ready to turn round orders within 7 to 14 days.

ECHO supplies a range of 120 basic generic drugs which it buys both from British generics manufacturers and increasingly from Pharmamed, a non-profit-making factory in Malta. Pharmamed was set up by the International Dispensary Association (IDA), with funds from the Dutch Development Bank. In 1981 its production was 600-700 million tablets a year, which were sold to ECHO, IDA, Action Medeor and other non-profit-making drug suppliers in Europe. [70]

ECHO sells only good quality generics (to British Pharmacopeia standards) and offers its customers considerable savings on the cost of equivalent brand name products. According to Dr. Burton, ECHO's Medical Director, "The price saving is in the range of the generic drug being anything from one-quarter to one-tenth of the price of the exact equivalent advertised product". He adds that "the argument the multinationals used to give that their ethical products were superior to the generic, has no real basis in scientific fact ..." [71]

A number of research-based manufacturers have shown their readiness to collaborate with ECHO. Some are charging ECHO specially reduced prices for a few of their patented products that are particularly relevant to Third World needs, but normally prohibitively expensive. For example, ECHO has bought rifampicin from Ciba-Geigy (under its brand name Rimactane) at a quarter the commercial price in Britain. This obviously helps the mission hospitals. For manufacturers, ECHO offers the advantages of regular, sizeable orders.

ECHO has recently produced its own Pharmaceutical Data Sheet Compendium. This booklet gives a simple description of how to use each of the basic generic drugs supplied. It is aimed at nurses and health workers who may not be aware of the existence of simple generic equivalents to brand-name products. Dr. Burton explains, "we have found that this information is rarely available to the users of simple basic generic drugs, whereas the multinational companies flood the world with literature concerning their advertised ethical drugs". [73] At the receiving end, some hospitals are translating the data sheets into local languages so that they will be of use to people working in village dispensaries.

173

AID AGENCIES

Amongst ECHO's biggest customers are aid agencies such as OXFAM, particularly when emergency drug supplies are provided in disaster situations, but also when drugs are supplied as part of the main core of small-scale development work. Recently, as we have seen, some of the biggest European aid agencies, notably NOVIB, have put up funds to help create self-reliance in drug supplies with the building of Gonoshasthaya Pharmaceuticals factory in Bangladesh. Aid agencies are also compaigning for drug policies to benefit the poor.

But there is also a negative side to aid agencies' involvement in drug supply. Like manufacturers, some have created problems by exporting a mass of drugs that poor countries do not want, or need. The problems have been particularly acute in disaster situations where human and physical resources are stretched to the limit. For example, during the disastrous floods in Bangladesh in 1974, a motley collection of medicines and samples, scrambled together by generous and well-intentioned donors, poured into the country. The physical effort of picking through the drugs to sort out the useful from the useless was a sheer waste of the overworked doctors' time. A former Director of Drug Administration in Bangladesh stresses that this sort of philanthropy which remains blind to real need can be positively harmful. [74]

OXFAM staff and health teams experienced a similar situation during the height of the Kampuchean emergency in 1979, when random drug donations from all over the world created chaos. [75]

But it is not only in emergencies that unsolicited gifts of medicines can cause serious problems. According to a Government official in Upper Volta, "The most uncontrolled section of imported medicines are the gifts from governments and aid agencies. These gifts are accepted without quibble or question and of course many of them will be, at the very least, inappropriate. There are also problems for the nurses or dispensers in actually administering these free medicines, since they come from various countries of origin, and of course have differing strengths. There may also be the temptation for the nurses to hand out these free medicines to patients, not because they are suitable treatments, but because they are all that is available." [76]

HEALTH PROFESSIONALS

Individuals and groups of health workers, nurses, doctors and pharmacists in developed countries are increasingly expressing concern over the scale of the problems faced by their counterparts in poor countries. Many come up against similar dilemmas in their everyday work - particularly the heavy dependence on drugs which is perpetuated by promotion and patient demand.

One example of a group of health professionals which is taking an active interest in the specific problems of drug use in developing countries is the International Pharmaceutical Federation (known as FIP). FIP has set up a special Third World project, which is co-ordinated by Professor D'Arcy, Head of the Pharmacy Department at Queen's University, in Northern Ireland. The first objective was to discover the key problems that lend themselves to technical solutions. FIP members would then offer their services to Third World health authorities as consultants on pharmacy training, drug storage and transportation and technical aspects of setting up local production. FIP planned to make specific recommendations to WHO based on the information gathered from the national pharmaceutical associations in various Third World countries. But Professor D'Arcy believes that in addition to the technical problems, "FIP must also tackle the problems *from home* by setting up a more active dialogue with the industry on the special needs of the Third World". [77] (our emphasis)

A number of European and American non-governmental medical groups have acted to fill the vacuum created by the lack of objective information on the safety and efficacy of new and existing drugs. In Britain, the *Drug and Therapeutics Bulletin,* edited by Dr. Andrew Herxheimer and written by general practitioners and specialists, discusses appropriate treatments and reviews manufacturers' claims for their products. The bulletin was started in 1963 and initially sent to doctors on a subscription basis. Since 1980, the Government has paid for it to be distributed to all doctors in Britain. The UK Consumers Association, which publishes the bulletin, also offers free subscriptions to Third World health officials and prescribers. [78]

A number of professional groups and individual doctors both in developed and developing countries have produced reports highlighting abuses in drug marketing and use in the Third World. The intention behind these studies has been to inform professional and public opinion and encourage positive corrective from governments and drug manufacturers. [79]

A recent example of the growing alarm shared by scientists and health professionals at the worldwide misuse of drugs is the "Statement Regarding Worldwide Antibiotic Misuse" issued by participants attending a conference on bacteriology in the Dominican Republic in 1981. The signatories, mainly from the developed but also from developing countries, set up the Alliance for the Prudent Use of Antibiotics (APUA). As a first step they intend to press for national and international committees to issue guidelines on the prudent use of antibiotics and to lobby for "proper standards of advertising and dispensing" of antibiotics to be adhered to worldwide. [80]

TRADE UNIONS

The Geneva-based International Federation of Chemical and General Workers Unions has a longstanding interest in drug marketing practices. In Britain, officials of the General and Municipal Workers Union (GMWU) have been particularly active in exploring new policies to benefit people in the Third World.

175

HEALTH ACTION INTERNATIONAL (HAI)

Health Action International was launched in Geneva in May 1981, at the end of an international seminar on Pharmaceuticals, attended by participants from 27 developing and developed countries. [81] HAI is a network of over 50 development action, consumer and other public interest groups and organisations. Its founder members include development agencies such as OXFAM, the International Organisation of Consumer Unions and organisations of health professionals such as the Voluntary Health Association of India. Each member has different priorities and specific areas of interest, but all share both a common interest in health and medicine in developing countries, and a commitment to achieving positive changes.

Amongst the North American and European groups, one of the most active HAI members is the London-based action-research unit Social Audit, which has produced a number of publications documenting discrepancies in drug marketing practices. [82] In 1981 Social Audit released the first of a planned series of 'anti-advertisements' aimed at encouraging Third World prescribers in particular to be sceptical in approaching manufacturers' claims for their products. The first of these anti-advertisements, *WHO says Lomotil has no value?* is reproduced opposite. By focussing on a specific product, Social Audit were instrumental in getting the manufacturers to agree to change their labelling worldwide. [83] But Social Audit stress that this specific case-study into one drug raises far-reaching issues of corporate responsibility and the impact of uncontrolled practices in developing countries. [84]

Consumer organisations in a variety of developing countries form a key part of HAI's international membership. The Regional Office for Asia and the Pacific of the International Organisation of Consumer Unions (IOCU) acts as HAI's clearing house and the editorial office of *HAI News*. IOCU and its associated organisations in a large number of developing countries do not confine themselves to the 'narrow' issues popularly associated with 'consumerism' in developed countries. As Anwar Fazal, President of IOCU emphasises, "The consumer movement is an integral part of the development process and is therefore even more important for developing countries. The consumer movement concerns economic justice … it concerns human rights … it concerns action and change." [85]

These HAI members are thus concerned with medicines in the broad context of poverty and health. For example, the Consumers' Association of Penang (CAP) has been actively campaigning on the pharmaceuticals issue for some years. CAP has focussed on inconsistent standards in drug marketing - as one aspect of how the rich world takes advantage of the poor. CAP has lobbied against double standards in marketing by creating public awareness and pushing for the withdrawal of hazardous drugs. But the problems are also tackled in the villages through health education to make poor people aware of alternatives to unnecessary and potentially dangerous drugs. [86]

The World Health Organization says:
"A number of medicines, which are of no value and are even dangerous, are often given to treat diarrhoea. Money and time are wasted in their use." So . . .

WHO says LOMOTIL has NO VALUE?

LOMOTIL (diphenoxylate/atropine) is made by the US multinational drug company, G.D. Searle; and promoted to physicians all over the world in terms such as "established success", "good tolerance", "excellent value" and "ideal for every situation". This leaflet — prepared and published by Social Audit Ltd., and friends* — calls into question these claims.

LOMOTIL may be of value in giving *symptomatic* relief for non-specific "travellers' diarrhoea" in adults. But experts say Lomotil — and other products like it [2] — have little or no place in the treatment of young children — especially in developing countries, where infective diarrhoeas are the major cause of death in children aged under three.[1] Lomotil's limitations include:

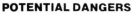

POTENTIAL DANGERS
"Lomotil, which is widely used in the treatment of diarrhoea in the paediatric age group, is dangerous and unwarranted . . . we urge that all physicians treating infants and children avoid the potentially dangerous use of Lomotil for the treatment of diarrhoea."
(Clinical Notes [1974])[3]

"Lomotil can relieve the symptoms of acute gastroenteritis in children, but it can also mask the signs of dehydration and cause fatal toxic reactions . . . use of this combination for treatment of diarrhoea in children is hazardous."
(The Medical Letter [1980])[4]

"Lomotil is a dangerous combination of drugs contra-indicated for children under 2 years of age and probably never indicated in childhood diarrhoea."
(Pediatrics [1980])[5]

QUESTIONABLE USEFULNESS
"The use of Lomotil as an antidiarrhoeal agent in children is difficult to justify . . . we doubt if it has any place in the treatment of diarrhoea in children."
(Arch. of Dis. in Child. [1979])[6]

"A diarrhoea that needs 4 such tablets to be cured would probably have been cured without it too. A more prolonged diarrhoea needs proper investigation and specific therapy rather than a blindly harmful stopcock."
(Leb. Med. J. [1974])[7]

ECONOMIC WASTE
Lomotil costs up to 25 times more than other widely-used symptomatic treatments for diarrhoea.
(AMREF [1980])[8]

"Lomotil (no value)." (WHO [1976])[1]

177

IOCU's Regional Office, which is also based in Penang, has drawn up a Consumer Action/Research Kit identifying 44 "problem" drugs to act as a guide for groups in other developing countries that want to carry out their own action-research to stop sales of unnecessary and harmful drugs. [87] IOCU is also setting up a *Consumer Interpol,* grouping together about 120 organisations in 50 countries covering every continent. Members and various documentation centres in developed countries will feed information into a central data bank on regulatory decisions taken to withdraw or restrict the use of potentially harmful products. News of these decisions will then be disseminated to local groups in developing countries. Armed with this information, they will lobby their own governments to adopt similar restrictions. When plans for a *Consumer Interpol* were first drawn up, its purpose was described as fighting "deceptive and unfair trade practices" that have a "particularly severe impact on the most disadvantaged consumers". [88] The project has received financial backing from the Dutch Government.

For the majority of HAI members the immediate objective is to campaign against double standards in marketing practices. HAI's longer term aims are to press for health-centred drug policies to benefit the world's poor. Central to this strategy are attempts to publicise and encourage public support for bold Third World initiatives for better drug use. HAI is also lobbying for meaningful international controls on drug marketing practices.

During its first year HAI produced a critique of the International Federation of Pharmaceutical Manufacturers' Associations' International Code of Marketing Practices. HAI sees the industry voluntary code as a conspicuously unconvincing attempt to put its own house in order and forestall WHO controls. [89] In May 1982 HAI played an active role in lobbying at the World Health Assembly and prepared a special briefing pack focussing on the key issues confronting delegates to the Assembly. HAI's views were extensively reported in the press and the resolution on the Action Programme on Essential Drugs which the Assembly adopted gives HAI an added incentive to increase its worldwide membership and build up its campaigning strength on the international scene. [90]

INTERNATIONAL FEDERATION OF PHARMACEUTICAL MANUFACTURERS ASSOCIATIONS (IFPMA)

The IFPMA represents pharmaceutical manufacturers associations in 47 countries, over half of them in developing countries. Its Secretariat is based in Zurich. IFPMA was founded in 1968 to improve contact between national and industry associations, and participate in discussion in areas such as health legislation. One of IFPMA's declared objectives is "to promote and support continuous development throughout the pharmaceutical industry of ethical principles and practices voluntarily agreed on". [91]

IFPMA's public pronouncements on Third World policy issues have shown industry's ability to move with the consensus of medical and world opinion. For example, in 1977 IFPMA's initial reaction to the WHO Selection of Essential Drugs

16 Samples

16.1 Except when provided for identification or demonstration purposes, samples should only be supplied in response to a signed request from a doctor; such requests, except in respect of products controlled under the Misuse of Drugs Act, may not be accepted on a pre-printed card or form which incorporates more than the company name and address. The form must be handed by a representative to the doctor who should then add all other details.

Wherever practicable, an individual sample should not represent more than four days treatment for a single patient. When samples are provided to assist doctors in the recognition or identification of a product, or to demonstrate the use of a particular apparatus or equipment, only the minimum quantity necessary for this purpose should be supplied.

16.2 Where samples of products restricted by law to supply on prescription are distributed by a representative, the sample must be handed direct to the doctor or given to a person authorised to receive the sample on his behalf. A similar practice must be adopted for products which it would be unsafe to use except under medical supervision.

16.3 Samples of products restricted by law to supply on prescription, which are made available to representatives for distribution, should be strictly limited in quantity and an adequate system of accountability should be established.

16.4 Samples sent by post must be packed so as to be reasonably secure against the package being open by young children.

16.5 Distribution of samples in hospitals should comply with individual hospital regulations, if any.

V. Samples

Samples may be supplied to the medical and allied professions to familiarize them with the products, to enable them to gain experience with the product in their practice, or upon request.

Codes of Practice on samples. Left, the voluntary code of the Association of British Pharmaceutical Industries; right, from the Code of the IFPMA.

179

was decidedly hostile. An industry statement described the WHO initiative as "ill-advised and counter-productive". IFPMA did not mince its words in declaring that industry was "strongly opposed to the concept of a generally applied and restrictive essential list". According to IFPMA, if essential drug lists were taken up by governments they would "result in substandard rather than improved medical care and might well reduce health standards already attained". [92] But in 1979 IFPMA gave its qualified approval to the concept of limited lists for developing countries. This retraction of its earlier position followed after IFPMA received assurances from WHO that there had never been any suggestion that a single list should be universally applied, or that the WHO model list would not be updated to include useful new drugs as they came on to the market. [93]

Despite its initial opposition IFPMA has since taken an active interest in the WHO Action Programme on Essential Drugs and negotiated with WHO on behalf of its members. IFPMA continues to stress that "to focus attention on prices without giving proper attention to quality is a disservice to developing countries". [94] It has offered 3-6 months' training courses in drug quality control to trainees from developing countries on behalf of its members. To date only six candidates have been trained, one more is being trained and nine more traineeships are under discussion. [95] These places have not been taken up with the alacrity that industry expected, which may reflect reluctance on the part of some developing countries to have their officials develop a prediliction for the products of the brand-name producers.

THE IFPMA CODE

The IFPMA International Code of Pharmaceutical Manufacturing Practice includes some very positive statements on the "Obligations of Industry" in the preamble, which is almost as long as the code itself. [96] But the code is so loosely worded that there is a real danger it may only serve to legitimise existing unacceptable standards of promotion in developing countries. For example, this is the case even with such reasonable-sounding statements as: "Particular care should be taken that essential information as to pharmaceutical products' safety, contra-indications and side effects or toxic hazards is appropriately and consistently communicated *subject to the legal, regulatory and medical practices of each nation"*. (our emphasis) [97] This loads responsibility onto Third World governments, rather than manufacturers, to take measures to ensure that there is always a full disclosure of information.

A further illustration of the weakness of the IFPMA code is the short paragraph on samples, reproduced on p.179 alongside the corresponding section from the Association of British Pharmaceutical Industries (ABPI) Voluntary Code. Reservations about the IFPMA code were expressed even by some IFPMA members. The Swedish manufacturers association, LIF stated: "The code is unclear, unstructured and does not go far enough". [98] It is weakest in the area of monitoring and enforcement which is limited to industry personnel acting as "judges in their own cause". [99]

180

One commentator writing in the US industry newsletter *Pharmaceutical Executive* describes the IFPMA code as having been introduced to forestall "a coming WHO effort to impose unacceptable controls over all pharmaceutical commerce in the Third World". [100] He comments, "The code pledges industry to provide high quality products, to base its claims on valid scientific evidence regarding indications and conditions for use, to provide full scientific information with scrupulous regard for truth in all matters (including contra-indications and toxicity), and to use complete candour in dealing with government health officials, physicians, nurses, other health providers and the public. To some, this may sound like a pledge in favour of motherhood and against cancer. But the real political question is whether the code will be adequate to defeat the forces against private enterprise within WHO. " [101]

According to Catherine Stenzl, coordinator of the International Research Group for Drug Legislation and Programs, drug industry lobbyists are in a good position to block unwelcome moves towards controls on marketing within the United Nations system. She quotes a private communication from a Member of the European Parliament stating that "the pharmaceutical industry have a committee of six operating in Geneva whose sole job is to infiltrate every international institution to prevent mandatory legislation against the ... activities of multinationals". [102]

Unlike the Health Action International lobby on behalf of poor consumers, industry's views are directly represented in WHO proceedings. The IFPMA was officially accredited with NGO-status within WHO in 1971. According to Catherine Stenzl, this decision was "taken against the recommendations of the competent commission". [103]

DRUG MANUFACTURERS

The fact that the IFPMA Code was drafted at all is indicative that the drug industry is sensitive to its reputation. Manufacturers are acutely aware that reports of unethical marketing practices in the Third World have attracted criticism worldwide. They realise that sales performance in the more lucrative rich world markets may be conditioned by how they are seen to discharge their social responsibilities in the poor world. [104]

Manufacturers are increasingly conscious of the need to improve their Third World "image". For example, in May 1981 Ciba-Geigy held a special 3-day seminar on Third World policies attended by senior staff from their Basle headquarters and worldwide subsidiaries, and several UN officials. On the first day of the seminar participants were assigned the task of analysing "the problems and criticisms faced by the pharmaceutical industry and Ciba-Geigy in the Third World". [105] Executives taking part in Working Group One were asked to hold a brainstorming session to identify "whatever criticisms, attacks, or reproaches against the pharmaceutical industry and Ciba-Geigy" came to mind. Their next task was to discuss "who is mainly voicing them" and the "additional arguments these critics are using", the purpose of the session being to "try to develop ideas and strategies for dealing with arguments of this kind". [106]

181

NEW STRATEGIES

Ciba-Geigy certainly adopts a more open style than many manufacturers in acknowledging the need for a special Third World policy and in making clear what this is. A recent article in *Business International* refers to Ciba as "The first known major drug company to establish a specific corporate policy acknowledging an ethical responsibility to meet the 'special needs' of developing countries". [107] Ciba set up a new subsidiary company, Servipharm Limited, in 1977 - the very year that the first WHO selection of essential *generic* drugs was produced. Servipharm markets a range of its own brands of generic drugs ('branded generics') - many of them included in the WHO selection. [108]

Ciba-Geigy and other manufacturers that have diversified into producing branded generics have clearly not been motivated solely by a sense of corporate responsibility to the world's poor. As the Director of the British Office of Health Economics explains, "Many western research-based companies have seen the *economic* logic of supplying certain basic medicines to the less developed countries at lower prices than would be economic in relation to the more affluent nations". [109] (our emphasis)

Moreover, Ciba-Geigy has not been slow to make contingency plans to protect its profitable research base. Its Third World policy document states: "In cases where, for reasons of economy, it is impossible to include original Ciba-Geigy preparations (ie brand-name products) in these national lists, Ciba-Geigy Pharma will try to secure the necessary financing (eg via the World Bank, developmental aid organisations, etc) by taking the initiative itself." [110]

The issue of how to respond to the perceived threat to their market power from large-scale, low-priced generic production concerns all the research-based technology-intensive manufacturers. A book published in 1982 identifies over a dozen "defensive", "offensive" and "anticipatory" strategies open to the market leaders to safeguard their speciality medicines still under patent. [111]

The strength and weakness of the WHO model list of essential drugs - the fact that it is open to interpretation - makes it possible for the research-based manufacturers to try to persuade Third World regulatory authorities to include some of their latest patented products. As many as 63 of the drugs included in the WHO list are given as "examples of this therapeutic category" and health authorities are advised to "choose [the] cheapest effective drug product acceptable". [112] This leaves the door wide open for manufacturers of antibacterials, antidiarrhoeals, psychotherapeutic and other drugs to argue the special case for purchasing their more expensive but 'better' patented products which may offer few signifcant advantages over far cheaper, older drugs.

Some commentators see the strategy of diversification into branded generics pursued by some of the leading manufacturers as a very mixed blessing for the world's poor. They fear that the biggest companies, with the advantages of large economies of scale in production and advertising will undercut any smaller

182

producers. If competition in the generics market were eliminated in this way, industry could revert to its highly concentrated structure and prices might rise. In the words of UNCTAD, "an agreed price floor could emerge even for generics". [113] Furthermore, future rapid obsolescence in production technology could reinforce the Third World's dependence as a captive market.

The leading companies cannot be expected to relinquish their market power voluntarily. Consequently it would be unfair to dismiss any policy move to supply the Third World market with branded generics solely on the grounds that this might enable leading companies to undercut local industry. Manufacturers that move into generics production are at least offering Third World buyers an alternative to expensive brand-name products. It is then vital for Third World buyers to ensure that they do not become over-dependent on monopoly suppliers of branded generics.

POSITIVE RESPONSES TO THIRD WORLD NEEDS

We have already seen that through the IFPMA, industry has offered to supply essential drugs for public health service use in poor countries under 'special' conditions - although the precise advantages are not entirely clear. By May 1982, 42 manufacturers had contacted IFPMA expressing interest in supplying developing countries with a total of 230 drugs - 130 of them included in the WHO Selection of Essential Drugs. [114]

Just one illustration of industry's public expression of concern for the needs of developing countries is the statement that IFPMA made to the 1979 World Health Assembly that they wished "to put firmly on record that the pharmaceuticals industry entirely shares the WHO's concern in its objective of improving health care and in particular improving the access of drugs, vaccines and sera of the poorer developing countries". IFPMA also advised delegates that "As a particular illustration of this concern ... a number of companies in our industry have volunteered to place certain drugs used in communicable disease control at the disposal of the WHO under special conditions". [115]

The Belgian company, Janssen, echoes other manufacturers in demonstrating its awareness of the problems of drug supply in developing countries: "Unfortunately, we ascertain far too often that the drugs we found and developed after years of research, do not always reach the people who are most in need of them. It is often very difficult to reach the rural populations in developing countries. But the biggest problem for people who have to do with a strict minimum of existence remains ... the *price* of the drug. Therefore Janssen Pharmaceutica has contacted the WHO and proposed to supply mebendazole at a very low price for the use of worm eradication programmes." [116]

Some leading manufacturers have also been actively involved in providing consultancy services to advise on improvements in national drug policies and the logistics of supply. A recent example is the *Burundi Pilot Project* which is the result of collaboration between the Ministry of Health of Burundi, WHO, and Roche, Ciba-Geigy and Sandoz. [117]

183

We have already discussed industry's contribution to research into developing new drugs to treat tropical diseases. Some of this research is being carried out in developing countries, as in the case of four laboratories set up by the Wellcome Trust with profits made by Wellcome's manufacturing companies. [118]

Manufacturers have shown that they are open to persuasion and have cooperated with Third World governments in voluntarily agreeing to withdraw potentially harmful products. For example, Glaxo's subsidiary in Bangladesh agreed to withdraw its combined penicillin and streptomycin products, sold under the brand name Seclomycin. [119]. Meanwhile, some years ago Fisons (Bangladesh) Ltd was asked by the health authorities to produce fewer tonics and more life-saving drugs. In response, local managers claim that the company has been exploring the possibility of producing more speciality drugs to treat TB, cancer, hypertension and diabetes under licence from other manufacturers. [120] In India, Glaxo is responding positively to the Government's desire for foreign companies to produce more bulk drugs as opposed to formulations. Already, 15 drugs and intermediates are manufactured locally from the basic stages and Glaxo plans to expand basic drug production to include a further nine drugs to treat intestinal worms, diarrhoea and dysentery, heart disease, allergies and arthritis. [121]

Many industry spokesmen readily acknowledge that it makes sense for Third World governments to have limited drug selections for the public health services. But they resist the idea of a limited selection being applied to the private market. In response to our suggestion that manufacturers should only market essential drugs in poor countries, a senior executive of Ciba-Geigy expressed the view that ''This is a difficult question because of the needs of the prosperous minority in contrast to the bulk who are often very poor. I think the local health departments have to determine basic needs and draw up their version of the WHO 200 drugs list. I don't think one can suspend the normal basis of commerce except by government decree in a Communist type society, and many Third World countries do not want this.'' [122]

ADDRESSING THE CRITICS, NOT THE CRITICISMS

In listing six ''lessons'' to be learnt from the Anti Infant Formula Campaign (which led to the adoption of a code of marketing practice) a recent article in *Business International* urges manufacturers to ''address the issue, not the critics''. [123] Nonetheless, industry representatives have shown a marked tendency to devote their energies to accusing their critics of political extremism rather than focussing on the criticims they make.

For example, according to Lewis Engman, President of the US Pharmaceutical Manufacturers Association, ''The ultimate concern of at least some of the people behind the campaign for a WHO pharmaceutical marketing code is not the health of the Third World consumers. The ultimate concern is economic change in the direction of state control, and ultimately state ownership of private concerns. As such the code movement is part and parcel of the movement toward a new

184

economic order, a movement which touches health care only incidentally, a movement which has as its real goal the redistribution of wealth worldwide and the seizure - by political force if necessary - of economic power by those with no respect for the profit incentive and the rights of private property on which our society is based." [124]

Similarly a few manufacturers have responded to OXFAM's enquiries about their Third World policies and marketing practices by suggesting that these issues are not of legitimate concern to a charity. For example, the Group Public Relations Manager of Glaxo writes that "there must be considerable concern that your activities as reflected in your letter to us, seem totally out of keeping with the charitable objectives of OXFAM and more in keeping with those of a politically oriented pressure group". [125]

WE'VE PRODUCED THE GOODS...

Industry representatives often stress that manufacturers are doing all that can reasonably be expected of them for the Third World and that the onus must fall on governments to introduce new drug policies to ensure that the poor get the drugs they need. The Director of the British industry-funded Office of Health Economics has stated that "... the pharmaceutical firms have produced the goods. It is up to the developing countries to introduce the primary health care schemes which can make proper use of them - as China alone, so far, seems to have done." [126]

There is a great deal of truth in this statement as far as it goes. China, Mozambique, Sri Lanka and other developing countries that have succeeded in making the best use of limited resources to cater to the needs of the majority have done so because they have had the political resolve to introduce effective primary health care cover and comprehensive drug policies. But many developing countries have faced concerted opposition to their attempts to introduce new drug policies, not least from the drug industry itself. In the major drug-producing nations the degree of control on prices, promotion and production varies considerably. Manufacturers often complain that controls are too strict, but they rarely challenge the right of rich world governments to protect their citizens through some measure of control.

INDUSTRY OPPOSITION IN SRI LANKA

In an article entitled "National drug policies - more state intervention or less?", a senior executive of the US-based transnational Pfizer argues forcefully against state intervention and cites the "unfavourable results of introducing centralised drug procurement" in Sri Lanka. He makes no mention of the substantial savings that were achieved, but he does draw attention to the "acute shortages of certain important drugs" that followed the introduction of the new policies. [127]

It would however appear that some of the more critical drug shortgages experienced in Sri Lanka may have been aggravated by concerted opposition to the new policies from foreign manufacturers, and from Pfizer in particular. An account of the problems that arose has been provided by Dr. Sanjaya Lall of the Oxford Institute of Economics and Statistics and the late Professor Bibile of the University of Sri Lanka and former Chairman of the State Pharmaceutical Corporation. [128]

In 1973 the Government of Mrs Bandaranaike announced its new "34 Drug Programme" under which the State Pharmaceuticals Corporation (SPC) would centralise procurement of the chemical intermediates needed for local formulation of 34 drugs. A central aim of the new policy was to cut down on the high transfer prices manufacturers were paying for imported raw materials. [129]

From the outset the US Pharmaceutical Manufacturers Association were resolute in their opposition to the new policy. On 10 May 1973 their President, Joseph Stetler, wrote a six-page letter to Mrs Bandaranaike raising detailed objections to the new policy. Mr Stetler stated: "These actions, if implemented, would effectively destroy operations of the modern research-based pharmaceutical industry in Sri Lanka by removing all business incentives and internationally respected property rights. By so doing, the plan would call into question the Government's attitude toward *any future private investment in the country.*" [130] (our emphasis)

Lall and Bibile claim that: "A widespread ... campaign of denigrating low-cost supplies was launched. And a second source of opposition, the private practitioners, were drawn into the campaign. Reports were made of drugs being ineffective, substandard or toxic, but little hard evidence was produced." [131]

According to Lall and Bibile seven small local producers responded favourably to the new programme but all five foreign subsidiaries initially showed resistance. Glaxo was the first to accept the programme in principle; Pfizer the last. In Pfizer's case at least this agreement was a different matter from practical cooperation in implementing the policy. Lall and Bibile quote the then Managing Director of the SPC: ".... the SPC made an urgent appeal to Pfizer to make tetracycline capsules required in the cholera epidemic (in 1974) and offered quality tested raw materials and capsules." [132] Pfizer was asked to use raw materials purchased by SPC from a reputable supplier - the leading West German manufacturer, Hoechst. Lall and Bibile attribute Pfizer's reluctance to agree to this arrangement to the fact that they had been importing tetracycline from their parent company at almost five times more than Hoechst's price. [133] According to the Managing Director of the SPC, the outcome of the resulting delay during the cholera epidemic was "that the Hoechst tetracycline lay unused in SPC stores and Pfizer equipment lay idle, while capsules had to be airlifted to the country at enormous expense". [134]

Subsequently, the SPC and the Ministry of Industries recommended that Pfizer should be nationalised to ensure its compliance with the new policy. But powerful bargaining counters were brought into play. According to Lall and Bibile, "The reaction of the US was swift, and as it turns out, decisive in preventing such a measure. The US Ambassador personally intervened with the Prime Minister in the matter, and .... we can only speculate as to the nature of his intervention .... The Chairman of the SPC was ordered to 'continue negotiating' with Pfizer; no further disciplinary action was taken." [135]

186

When we asked Pfizer to comment on Lall and Bibile's article, they strongly defended their actions and stressed that "the facts of the case to which you refer are substantially different from what we have recorded". Their reply, from Dr. Hodin, Pfizer's Director of Public Affairs, concentrates on their role during the cholera epidemic when tetracycline was urgently needed. Dr. Hodin's account accepts that there was a delay. (Pfizer Sri Lanka was notified of the cholera emergency on 7 November 1974. On 23 December they made a firm quote to supply tetracycline. Discussion between Pfizer and the SPC continued into January 1975 - some months after the outbreak of the epidemic.) But Pfizer maintain that the SPC was to blame for the delay because they failed to clarify whether the tetracycline should be "supplied in capsules or tablets, sugar coated or not" and to stipulate the size and packaging. [136] Pfizer also say that they offered the SPC a specially reduced price because of the emergency, and subsequently reduced it further as SPC had received a lower quote. Pfizer conclude that the incident "indicates the inability of that state agency [the SPC] to cope adequately with the health needs of the Sri Lankan people," and emphasise that "we acted quickly, persisted in our efforts to help, and were responsible, with reference to price and other matters of detail that developed in this situation." [137]

The Sri Lankan experience also demonstrates the wholly negative way in which bold new policies are often portrayed. Pfizer sent us a heavily critical study of UNCTAD's 1977 report evaluating the SPC policies. [138] This "critical study" gives the impression that the whole purpose of setting up the SPC was to expand trade with Eastern Europe and China. It concludes: "Though the objectives were good, the practical implementation of changing sources from traditional to non-traditional suppliers did not bring any significant financial saving or provide the consumer with drugs of acceptable quality at a reasonable price. " [139] In fact the study misrepresents both the UNCTAD report and the original purpose behind the setting up of the SPC which was to obtain drugs from the *cheapest* source not to buy more drugs from Eastern Europe. [140] We have already seen that the savings achieved by the SPC policies have led to Sri Lanka's being singled out by WHO as an example for other countries to follow. [141] In the words of one analyst there were "dark spots" in the "success story" but instances of substandard imports were in fact few and far between. [142]

THE BANGLADESH LOBBY

Throughout this study we have focused a great deal on problems with the use and marketing of drugs in Bangladesh, which up until May 1982 the Bangladesh health authorities had failed to resolve. Thus, it is only fair that we should conclude by looking at the obstacles that health officials have encountered in recent years in attempting to implement policy changes.

In the early 1970s, attempts were made to improve the supply of essential drugs available to the health services by buying generics on worldwide competitive tender. These imports were centralised through bulk purchasing by the Trading

Corporation of Bangladesh (TCB). Increasingly orders were placed with Eastern European manufacturers - particularly in Hungary - because they quoted good prices. But the new policy ran into difficulties when doubts were raised about the quality of the Eastern European drugs, despite the fact that the drug control authorities were satisfied that they had undergone adequate quality control. [143]

Pressure was brought to bear for an official investigation into the increasing volume of imports from Eastern Europe to establish whether any political motive was involved. At the time the TCB was handling 40% of the national requirement for finished drugs and there were plans to expand its centralised procurement operations. In the event the commission of inquiry failed to establish any political motivation behind the imports from Hungary. Nonetheless, the TCB's share of imports was scaled down to 10%. [144]

Existing drug legislation in Bangladesh is based on the Drugs Act of 1940, which was described in a recent Expert Committee Report as "grossly inadequate". [145] Consequently, according to the Expert Committee: "Much of the unethical practices in manufacture and trade is possible because of the weakness of existing legislation ... There is no provision in the Drugs Act for the control of prices of pharmaceutical raw materials or finished products." [146]

Drug Administration officials have lacked the necessary legal powers to bring quick prosecutions and impose meaningful penalties even in cases of serious malpractice. Thus they have been seriously hampered in dealing with some of the worst abuses such as the case of a local company found to have been filling vials with tap water and selling them as distilled water for injections - a practice that can kill. Similarly, they could do little to control the black market in stolen drugs which we witnessed in operation in September 1980. A stallholder in Mitford market in the capital was selling tetracycline powder from a huge barrel stolen somewhere in transit. The yellow powder was tipped into paper sacks and whatever fell to the ground in the process was simply scooped back off the dirty floor.

The maximum penalty for offences of this nature has been a £14 fine and three years' imprisonment. There could be a delay of up to three years in bringing prosecutions through the courts. Drug Administration officials have long been critically aware of the need to tighten up legislation to safeguard health. They have put a great deal of effort into studying drug legislation in Britain, the United States, India and the WHO Model Drug Law, as a basis for new Bangladeshi drug laws. But when they tried to put their plans into action, they were obstructed. In 1978, a powerful lobby proved successful in blocking tougher legislation. Within months a new Health Minister replaced the man who had sanctioned the proposed new legislation. A committee was subsequently appointed to set about the task of redrafting the new drug laws. More attention was to be paid to local manufacturers' distaste for government controls. [147]

Local manufacturers have brought pressure to bear to block further controls proposed by the Health Ministry by lobbying the Ministries of Industries and Commerce. One recent example of this lobbying activity is a petition sent by the

Bangladesh Aushad Shilpa Samity (the Association of Pharmaceutical Industries) to the Deputy Prime Minister in charge of the Ministry of Industries in June 1981. The petition was sent in the name of individual member companies, including 25 of the largest nationally-owned manufacturers and all the foreign-controlled producers. [148] The covering letter dated 22 June 1981 stressed that the issues raised in the petition (on drug registration, production and price controls) were all inter-linked and the Association stated that "none of the issues is separable for solution in isolation, nor for any compromise solution". [149]

Despite the fact that 80% of the population has no ready access even to life-saving drugs, the manufacturers stress the export potential that would be blighted "unless our stand on the important matters is accepted in totality and policies are accordingly formulated for immediate implementation". [150] The manufacturers stated their opposition to tougher registration controls, including any attempt to regulate which drugs are marketed or produced locally on criteria of relevance to public health needs. The industry's 'stand' opposed any interference from the health authorities. "What manufacturers will produce and sell should best be left to the investors or their authorised representatives. Attempts should not be made to disrupt the laws of demand and supply through government dictum." [151]

The manufacturers stated that "price control should be abolished" and that they did "not feel that there is any *economic* justification in such control". [152] (our emphasis) An accompanying copy of a petition sent to the Minister of Commerce on 26 August 1980 repeated five times that not only did price control not benefit consumers, but that it was positively harmful to them. [153] No mention was made of any possible social and humanitarian criteria behind price controls. Government attempts to monitor and control transfer prices of raw materials were also resisted: "Drugs Administration should not assume the role of import regulatory body concerned with the approval of source, price and quality." [154]

Some of the manufacturers' arguments to support their 'stand' on registration policies would certainly cut no ice with regulatory agencies on their home markets. For example, they opposed any attempt by the Drugs Administration to withdraw licenses for drugs considered non-essential arguing that "Vitamins, enzymes, tonics etc. are manufactured because doctors prescribe them; these are essential because patients need them." Furthermore "All products which are prescibed by doctors are essential. Arbitrary criteria of essentiality should not be imposed. When the government is the buyer then it is free to choose the products needed; the doctors should have the same freedom to choose products..." [155] But governments in developed countries have been in no doubt for some decades that they need to control doctors' prescribing 'freedom' in the interests of the public as a whole.

The Bangladesh manufacturers also stated that any product registered for sale in developed countries "with stringent registration procedures" should automatically be licensed for sale provided it passes the necessary quality tests. This argument would carry little weight in Britain, as would the Association's insistence the registration of products should only be cancelled on the grounds

189

that they are found to be harmful or carry an "unacceptable level of risk". [156] In developed countries governments retain the right to withdraw registration from drugs on other criteria such as lack of proof of efficiency. In Britain drugs must also be licensed for each indication - a far cry from the blanket approval advocated in the Bangladesh manufacturers' stand.

The substance of this lobby directly contradicts many of the key policy measures that the UN agencies have urged developing countries to adopt to serve the interests of the majority of their people. However European and US parent companies that we have consulted fully endorse the stand taken by their Bangladesh subsidiaries. For example, the chairman of ICI Pharmaceuticals Division comments, "I cannot accept your assertion that the stand taken by the (Bangladesh) Association 'shows disregard for the social implications and the health needs of the mass of the poor in Bangladesh'. The substance of the Association's complaint is that retail prices are fixed by the government in an apparently arbitrary manner rather than according to a displayed and rational formula. As a consequence, of this manufacturers are not able to earn a return on their investment which will permit an adequate surplus for reinvestment and expansion of their business." [157] Other parent companies also critisise "arbitrary price fixing" in Bangladesh. None that we approached has responded to the critical issue of the social implications of their opposition to Government attempts to cut down on wasteful and unnecessary drugs.

*   *   *   *   *

BRAVE NEW POLICIES

This report might have ended here. The situation up to June 1982 gave little cause for optimism for the poor in Bangladesh and many other developing countries. Given the political and economic constraints, health authorities seemed unlikely to press ahead with the comprehensive new drug policies urgently needed to improve the supply of essential drugs.

However, recent events in Bangladesh mean that we can end with a positive and encouraging postscript. On 12 June 1982 the Chief Martial Law Administrator passed a Drugs (Control) Ordinance - the first step in implementing a radically new national drug policy designed to give priority to the production of 150 essential drugs. Under this ordinance the registration of over 1,700 unnecessary, harmful and otherwise undesirable drugs has been suspended. [158]

The Bangladesh Government acted on the recommendations of its specially appointed an eight-person Expert Committee which drafted the new national drug policy and carried out a major review of over 4,000 products licensed for sale in the country. Bearing in mind the country's priority needs, the Expert Committee identified 16 categories of non-essential or otherwise problematic drugs to provide

190

a guideline for assessing which formulations should be withdrawn or modified. [159] These criteria have been described as "admirable" and as combining "sound therapeutics with an attitude of commonsense economics" by other experts outside Bangladesh. [160]

The different categories recommended for withdrawal include tonics and enzyme mixtures; liquid multivitamin preparations (with the exception of a few for paediatric use); cough medicines, throat lozenges and gripe water; and combinations of antibiotics, corticosteroids and other drugs. Most combination drugs are to be withdrawn when single-ingredient drugs offer acceptable (often cheaper and safer) alternatives. [161] Drugs that can carry unacceptable risks particularly to children - such as liquid tetracyclines and anabolic steroids - have also been banned. In future no prescription drugs will be licensed unless they are formulations listed in the British Pharmaceutical Codex. [162]

The Expert Committee recommended that a National Formulary should be drawn up not later than 1983 to include only drugs considered essential to health needs. In the meantime national firms will be permitted to continue production of some non-essential drugs but subsidiaries of foreign companies must stop manufacture of simple over-the-counter products such as multivitamins, tonics and antacids. Instead, they will be offered incentives to import the necessary technology and know-how to formulate sophisticated essential drugs and produce bulk drugs. Foreign companies with no factory of their own will no longer be allowed to license other manufacturers to produce their brands locally if equivalent or similar products are already being manufactured in local factories. [163]

Other important aspects of the new policies include plans to strengthen the Drugs Administration department and the announcement of heavy penalties to control both unlicensed drug sales and the manufacture of spurious and sub-standard drugs. These controls will also apply to Unani, Ayurvedic and homeopathic drugs. The Expert Committee has recommended that generic names should be introduced and the Government has announced controls on prices of finished drugs and selected raw materials imported to produce essential drugs. [164]

These new policies have generated a great deal of controversy both inside and outside Bangladesh. Local manufacturers whose current production will be disrupted by the new measures are concerned about the short-term negative impact on sales turnover. One foreign-controlled producer estimates that about half their sales turnover may be affected. [165] Some foreign and national companies that are critical of the new policies have called for them to be "reviewed by a broader multi-disciplined forum". [166]

Under the Martial Law Ordinance 240 products were to have been withdrawn immediately and the remainder by the end of 1982. Local manufacturers expressed concern at the short timescale for products to be removed from the market because raw materials had already been ordered and paid for. Leading foreign and national producers that signed an "Appeal to the Martial Law Authority", stressed that previously they had been given a minimum notice period of two years to withdraw a drug "when it was found to be harmful by well-established drug monitoring systems". [167] Already, the original ruling on the timescale has been modified. There is now to be a phased withdrawal of different categories of drugs over a period of 3, 6 and 9 months. [168]

Opposition to the new policies in the local press recalls past experience in implying that there is a political bias behind the new policies. For example, the Expert Committee has been attacked for failing to consult industry and meeting "behind iron curtains". [169] The association representing leading manufacturers is reported to have warned that "if" the new policies are implemented local production will fall by "up to 80%"; there will be drug shortages and drug factories will be forced to close, "making thousands jobless". [170] According to one press report: "The treatment prescribed by the Expert Committee reminds one of the classic phrase, 'the operation was a success but the patient died'. In this case, unfortunately the patient is not the Pharmaceutical industry alone, but the whole economic structure of the country..." [171]

The opposition aroused suggests that the health authorities are unlikely to be successful in implementing the new policies unless they can count on the cooperation of the country's doctors and leading manufacturers. It is thus critical that short-term considerations should not be allowed to cloud the long-term goals behind the new policies. Manufacturers now have the option of expanding production to cater for the increasing demand for essential drugs.

HEALTHY PROFITS?

Can industry afford to adjust its priorities to suit the pressing needs of developing countries like Bangladesh? How significant is the Third World market to them?

One company's assessment of prospects in Bangladesh certainly indicates that there is room for concessions. "The market for pharmaceutical products is growing very fast in Bangladesh. Turnover in 1979 increased by more than 100% and business prospects shall be good for 1980 ... Most of the local as well as foreign firms having factories, are increasing their production capacity, modernising factories and introducing new products. Government is providing them with all sorts of assistance." [172]

The Third World as a whole is alrendy a significant market for major drug producers. In 1980 just over a third of Britain's total exports went to developing countries - though mainly to oil-rich countries like Nigeria and the Middle East. [173] But the potential is even greater. In the opinion of one company executive, "It is obvious that during the next 20 years drug therapy is going to be needed and will become available to a much greater extent in the Third World. Any pharmaceutical company should appreciate that perhaps 40% of its business will be in those areas by the year 2000." [174]

Balance sheets showing profits for single years and individual developing countries are misleading because the position of transnational companies can only be assessed on the basis of their worldwide operations. On these there is little doubt that the industry as a whole is doing well by comparison with other sectors of industry. In the words of a June 1982 *Financial Times Survey,* "The pharmaceutical industry has passed through the recession almost unscathed". Moreover, "the companies that originate and produce the world's key medicines have every reason to be confident about their current performance and prospects". [175]

The healthy financial state of drug manufacturers is further confirmed by a senior executive with 30 years working experience in the industry itself. "In pharmaceuticals there has been a tendency to resist all new regulations and to assume, yet again, that somehow, if only we could get through the next year then things will be 'back to normal'. The public stance of the industry has been to state categorically that if the regulations are not relaxed, then no new medicines will appear - or at least, so few as to force the industry to stop research and deny the public access to the new medicines to which it has a right. The financial results of the industry continue to be an embarrassing counter argument ..." [176]

The poor are not going to get the drugs they need unless Third World governments can count on widespread support in implementing what may be seen as unpopular controls on the free market. Governments of the major drug-producing nations have all voted in favour of WHO resolutions urging Third World governments to adopt the sort of policies that the Bangladesh Government has now resolved to introduce. The support of WHO, of rich world governments, and of professional and public opinion worldwide is now essential for the successful implementation of new health-centred drug policies throughout the Third World. This cooperation and understanding is vital to protect the health interests of millions of the world's poor.

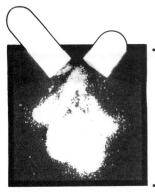

CHAPTER 11

HEALTH NOW
Action for Change

OXFAM has no intention of leaving this report to add to the cubic metres of analysis of the problems. It was written to highlight the distortions in drug marketing as they affect the world's poor and to show that there are positive solutions. But above all its purpose is to press for urgent action, and to demonstrate that meaningful changes are conditional on attitudes and actions in developed and developing countries.

An executive of one leading manufacturer gives his diagnosis of how changes can be made to happen: "Health care has to be a partnership between drug suppliers, governments and the medical profession, all acting in concert for the patients' benefit. It is difficult to achieve this because of problems with each side of the triangle. Provided dialogue takes place and there is understanding, tolerance and a general desire to be helpful on all sides, a great deal can be achieved, but it will nearly always be slow - too slow for many people." [1] Particularly, it must be added, for the Third World poor. But the triangle has also to be opened up to involve the *patients* - ordinary people as groups and individuals all have a crucial role to play in pressing for action.

What follows is a prescription for some of the more feasible changes that need to be made by governments, international and non-governmental organisations and manufacturers.

THIRD WORLD GOVERNMENTS

Political will is the key determinant of success. It is obviously unrealistic to expect manufacturers voluntarily to make either major changes in their current marketing practices or special concessions to the needs of the poor, in situations where governments are giving business interests priority over the health needs of their people.

The exact measures that governments need to implement will vary a great deal from one country to another depending, among other things, on what has already been achieved. But the crucial policy options identified by many governments and adopted by a few need to be acted on by all.

1. PREVENTION AND PRIMARY HEALTH CARE

Governments need to give preventive and primary health care services clear priority over costly hospital building projects and conventional cure-orientated medical training. A reallocation of health resources to benefit the poor majority has to be put into deeds as well as words.

2. COMPREHENSIVE NATIONAL DRUG POLICY

No country can solve the problems without a comprehensive national drug policy tailored to its specific needs. Key elements and important stages in implementing the policy include the following:

- Identification of priority health problems affecting the poor majority.
- Setting up a permanent multi-disciplinary team with the task of identifying which drugs are essential to the country's needs and to draw up a national formulary.
- Identification of the most vital drugs (to be given priority, for instance, in foreign exchange allocations and in setting up local production). More limited selections of drugs to be used by different categories of health workers also need to be drawn up.
- Rationalisation of the private market by withdrawing registration from non-essential, wasteful and 'problem' drugs not included in the national formulary.
- Making the use of generic names compulsory in prescribing, training, labelling etc.
- Ensuring that paramedics, doctors, nurses and other health workers all receive balanced drug information to suit their requirements, together with guidance on cost-effective treatments for different conditions. There should be a standard data sheet for each drug giving important information for both prescribers and patients.
- Establishment of an efficient public sector drug distribution system. This should have good communications from all units back to the centre on their requirements and any problems encountered with the quality of drugs or adverse reactions.
- Enforcement of controls on private drug distribution to prevent sales of prescription drugs by untrained and unlicensed drug sellers.
- Rationalisation of drug purchases for the public health services through bulk procurement on worldwide competitive tender, and progressive extension of this rationalisation to private sector imports.
- Setting up local (or where feasible regional) quality control laboratories.
- Regulating the type of drugs produced locally by private manufacturers so that they conform to national priorities. Self-reliance in local production of essential drugs needs to be encouraged with incentives to local manufacturers (both national and foreign) and export controls.
- Establishing public-sector production of esssential drugs.
- Adoption of comprehensive drug legislation covering areas such as price control, fair conditions on the transfer of drug technology, restricted patent protection and controls on marketing practices.
- Strict curbs on promotion should include banning sales representatives from visiting public health service doctors, and controlling the distribution of free samples, gifts and sales inducements to prescribers. Manufacturers' promotional leaflets and package inserts should be checked against information in data-sheets issued to doctors on the home market. Health authorities could levy a tax from companies on each sales representative they employ and this

195

revenue could be used to pay for the provision of independant drug information.
- Government departments responsible for administering and enforcing drug policies should be adequately staffed and financed and their rulings should be upheld by other ministries.

3. TRAINING

Governments will inevitably face opposition in implementing these drug policies unless they concentrate on winning over the country's doctors as firm allies. This can only be done if doctors and health workers understand what is at stake and what governments hope to achieve. The best approach is to influence the attitudes of health workers during training. Training should be refocussed and firmly rooted in social and economic realities so that, instead of being taught curative approaches to rich world diseases, Third World medical students learn their country's needs. During training doctors and paramedics should be encouraged to concentrate on prevention and appropriate non-drug treatments. All prescribers should also receive a firm grounding in the economics of drug prescribing and the critical need always to try the least expensive first-line treatment first. All health workers should be sent manuals with advice on standard treatments for common health problems. Efforts can also be made to influence the prescribing habits of practising doctors by encouraging them to take part in refresher courses, and sending them regular circulars on cost- effective prescribing.

4. HEALTH EDUCATION

Health authorities can use schools, the health services, community organisations and the mass media to put over basic health education and challenge people's dependence on drugs. For example, the message needs to be put across that it makes more sense to spend money on a diet of nutritious local foods than to buy imported vitamins. Health educators could usefully learn from commercial advertisers to put their message across in a lively and compelling way.

RICH WORLD GOVERNMENTS

Governments of developing countries are far more likely to succeed in implementing new drug policies if they can count on the goodwill and active support of rich world governments, particularly those of the major drug producing nations.

1. Rich world governments should increase their financial support to UN programmes that are designed to cater for the needs of developing countries, especially important initiatives such as the WHO Action Programme on Essential Drugs.

2. Having voted unanimously in support of the May 1982 resolution urging that the WHO Action Programme on Essential Drugs be implemented "in its entirety", rich world governments should make sure that it is. In particular they should not try to obstruct WHO from acting on mandates *they* have already given it such as the need to start work on the development of an international code of drug marketing practices.

3. The British and other major drug producers should actively support European initiatives to improve cooperation between the regulatory agencies of developed and developing countries. They should, for example, back the proposals of

the Nordic countries to assist developing countries with drug evaluations and improving their access to useful drug information.

4. The British and other Governments should set up their own investigation of drug policies and the Third World to identify which measures that they could take would be most helpful to health authorities in developing countries. A Government study could usefully focus on a possible tightening up of export controls and a contrasting opening up of access to information on drug exports. For example, as a first step to make it possible to evaluate the impact of existing export policies on developing countries, the Government could set up a register giving details of individual drug exports. This register should be open to public scrutiny, and could be compiled from information readily available to manufacturers, and other exporters.

Another important question for a Government investigation would be how best to assist Third World regulatory authorities by improving their access to expert evaluations of drugs. For instance, it would be particularly helpful for the British Government to make available copies of Licence Applications submitted for the Committee on Safety Medicines; to review the recommendations of the DHSS Medicines Division Professional Secretariat, and in some cases the deliberations of the Committee on Safety of Medicines itself.

5. Britain and other major drug producing countries should take a lead in getting new initiatives on drug exports and information policies morewidely adopted such as by all member states of the European Economic Community, OECD etc.

6. As part of a fundamental reappraisal of their development assistance, governments should review the *quality* of official health aid to ensure that it directly benefits the world's poor. Third World governments should not be tied to purchases of expensive pharmaceutical products or high-technology medical services. Instead, priority should be given to funding local projects that benefit poor communities - such as the training of paramedics.

7. Medical training paid for with official aid funds should include more priority for the training of medical and pharmaceutical civil servants from developing countries. For example more British aid funds could be allocated to DHSS courses to improve civil servants' skills in assessing drug submissions and clinical trials.

8. More needs to be done by governments of drug producing nations to promote the transfer of essential drug technology on terms favourable to the least developed countries.

INTERNATIONAL ORGANISATIONS

1. UN agencies should press ahead with their work programmes to assist developing countries in implementing comprehensive drug policies. But they should put more emphasis on 'marketing' policies such as the Selection of Essential Drugs and do more to ensure that their recommendations are translated into action.

2. The UN agencies should resolutely resist pressures to favour narrow rich-world interests and shift the balance so that 'international' policies really cater

for the needs of the majority of their members - the world's poorer nations.

3. WHO in particular should resist pressure to abandon its clear mandate to develop a UN-sponsored international code of drug marketing practices.

4. WHO should look for more allies in attempting to implement difficult programmes, both within the United Nations system and amongst non-governmental organisations. In the interests of balance, it would make sense to give official NGO-status to bodies such as Health Action International so that the needs of the world's poor are represented alongside those of industry.

NON-GOVERNMENTAL ORGANISATIONS

Non-governmental organisations are in a unique position to help set up a productive debate on solutions to the problems of drugs in developing countries.

1. NGOs should make use of their special access to information to publicise examples of constructive policy initiatives being undertaken in both developing and developed countries to provide an incentive to others to follow suit. They also have a duty to make the public aware of obstacles to changes that could benefit the poor.

2. They should take every opportunity to cooperate with other NGOs, international agencies, professional groups, trade unions, industry and governments in pursuing constructive solutions.

3. Aid agencies and other charities should stop giving 'aid' that is not wanted and only supply Third World countries and projects with drugs that they specifically request.

4. Aid agencies, including OXFAM, should continue to fund community health projects that encourage self-reliance, avoiding high-technology medical options wherever possible. More should be done to support grass-roots research into problems related to the use of drugs in poor communities and into creating awareness of positive alternatives to medicines. OXFAM and other agencies should continue to allocate funds to improving the supply of essential drugs.

MANUFACTURERS

We focus on the contribution that can be made by drug producers based in the rich world. Action is of course just as urgently needed on the part of smaller national producers in developing countries whose marketing practices are often far less scrupulous than the major transnational drug companies.

1. Manufacturers should do nothing to obstruct attempts by Third World governments to introduce new drug policies designed to safeguard and promote better health, even when these conflict with industry's immediate interests.

2. Manufacturers should be consistent in the standards they apply worldwide - irrespective of loose controls in developing countries. Marketing practices that would be unacceptable in Europe and North America should be seen as equally unacceptable in developing countries. Companies should abandon the tired old arguments that inconsistant standards are not 'illegal' because a Third World country's laws make them permissible. Instead, rich world manufacturers should take a lead in encouraging higher ethical standards in

promotional practices such as in disclosing full information and employing only suitably qualified sales representatives.

3. Companies should keep to their declared obligation of making sure that drugs "have full regard to the needs of public health" and demonstrate special social responsibility in poor countries by not encouraging demand for non-essential multivitamin tonics, cough and cold preparations and expensive and irrational combination drugs.

4. They should respect the purpose behind the WHO Selection of Essential Drugs and not pressurise public health officials into selecting unnecessarily expensive patented products when cheaper alternatives exist - sometimes in their own product range.

5. Parent companies should take a firm line in reminding their Third World subsidiaries of their social responsibilities, the need to maintain high standards and to comply with the wishes of government regulatory agencies.

6. Companies should cooperate wherever possible with the desire of developing countries to build up self-sufficiency through local production of essential drugs from basic stages.

7. As an immediate step, parent companies could review the product range of their subsidiaries and investigate the possibility of switching production to include more items on local essential drug lists (or on the WHO selection in the absence of a national list).

8. Companies could try to do more to ensure the safe and effective use of their products. They cannot afford to be complacent about labels that read prescription only in countries where drugs are sold in open air markets. A useful exercise would be for manufacturers (or their associations) to commission local research into how their products are actually used in developing countries to try to identify specific measures that *they* could take to counteract misuse.

* * * * *

These are OXFAM's suggestions for making more of the benefits of modern medicines available to the world's poor and counteracting harmful marketing practices. They are only a starting point. Others involved in the process of pushing for change will want to add to and improve on these proposals.

The changes we have suggested need different timescales, but they have one thing in common - the need to start work on them now. The longer action is delayed, the more the poor will suffer.

NOTES & REFERENCES

Some general notes on the terms and conventions used in this book.

THE POOR

It is difficult to measure poverty and the numbers affected by it. The World Bank estimates that about 800 million people are living in what it calls "absolute poverty", and probably as many again are only a little better off. The majority live in rural areas, and the greatest concentration is in South and East Asia.

THE THIRD WORLD

There is no satisfactory way of describing the group of countries which contain a high proportion of poor people. In this book the term 'Third World' is used as a shorthand which does at least reflect (through the use of the word 'world') the diversity of countries it encompasses. The Third World includes about a hundred countries containing some 3,000 million people.

THE RESEARCHERS

The research for this book was carried out by full-time OXFAM staff - principally the author, but with assistance from colleagues in the Third World and in Oxford. The researchers are referred to as 'we' in the text.

SOURCES

As well as books, articles and official documents, a large number of experts have been consulted in the course of the research and their letters provide a number of the sources quoted in the references. The term 'personal communication' refers to a letter from the person quoted. The phrase 'in interview with' means that no written record exists - but that the points made in the interview have afterwards been referred back to the person interviewed.

Some of the sources quoted are OXFAM files. Anyone wishing to see any of the files referred to should write to the Overseas Director, OXFAM, 274 Banbury Road, Oxford OX2 7DZ.

OXFAM SUPPORT

OXFAM seldom provides 100% of the cost of a scheme - so where projects are described as 'OXFAM-supported' or 'OXFAM-funded', it should be remembered that most of the cost is usually paid for by the local people and/or other aid agencies.

CURRENCIES

The sterling equivalent of local currencies is given in brackets in some cases. The exchange rate used is either that in force on the date in question, or, where the date is a year, the average of end-of-month exchange rates for that year, unless otherwise specified.

COMPANIES

Companies are referred to in the text by their short names - eg 'Glaxo' rather than the full name, 'Glaxo Holdings p.l.c.'

OXFAM's dialogue with the pharmaceuticals manufacturers continued after this report was completed. It has not been possible to take into account in the text all the points made after June 1982.

MEDICINES

The words drugs, medicines and pharmaceuticals are used interchangeably throughout the book.

CHAPTER 1

1   Figures derived from:
    -   Harford Thomas (ed), *A Picture of Poverty,* the 1979 OXFAM Report, OXFAM, Oxford, 1979.
        Life expectancy at birth in developing countries: 1935-39: 32 years 1965-70: 49 years
    -   World Bank, *World Development Report 1980,* Washington DC, 1980. (Low income countries, life expectancy at birth 1978 average 50 years - 1978)

2   -   *OXFAM Field Directors' Handbook,* Guidelines and Information for assessing projects, revised February 1980, pp.3-2, 3-3.
    -   Indian Council of Social Science Research (ICSSR) and Indian Council of Medical Research (ICMR) *Health for All - an alternative strategy,* Report of a study group set up jointly by ICMR/ICSSR, Indian Institute of Education, Pune, 1981, p.5.

3   Dr. Tony Klouda, "Prevention is more expensive than cure, a Review of Health Problems for Tanzania 1971-81", February 1982. (mimeo)

4   WHO, *Drug Policies Including Traditional Medicines in the Context of Primary Health Care,* Report and Background Documentation of the Technical Discussions held during the 32nd Session of the WHO Regional Committee for SE Asia Regional Office, New Delhi, November 1979, Table 1, p.28.

5   -   *OXFAM Field Directors' Handbook,* op. cit., p.22-1.
    -   ICSSR/ICMR Report, op.cit., p.5.
    -   Klouda, 1982, op.cit.

6   *OXFAM Field Directors' Handbook,* op.cit., p.26-1.

7   UNIDO, *Global Study of the Pharmaceutical Industry,* prepared by the Secretariat of UNIDO for the First Consultation meeting on the pharmaceutical industry, Lisbon, 1-5 December 1980, (ID/WG-33116) 22 October 1980, p.8.

8   Dr. David Morley, Professor of Tropical Child Health, Institute of Child Health, University of London, "Severe Measles: A Barometer of Childhood Nutrition". (mimeo)

9   Yemen General Grain Corporation, Ministry of Supply and Ministry of Health with the assistance of the US Department of Health and Human Services, Public Health Service, Centre for Disease Control and USAID, *Yemen Arab Republic National Nutrition Survey,* November 1980. Definition of anaemia: 11.0 g/dl for pregnant women and below 12.0 g/dl for all other women, lactating and non-lactating.

10 Prof. G. Peters, *Rapport Mission au Mozambique du 8 au 19 octobre 1980,* Institut de Pharmacologie de l'Universite de Lausanne, 26 March 1981, p.5.

11 Abram S. Benenson (ed), *Control of Communicable Diseases in Man,* twelfth edition, an official report of the American Public Health Association, 1975.

12 Dr. K.M.S. Aziz of the International Centre for Diarrhoeal Disease Research Bangladesh, in interview with the author, October 1980.

13 -   Government of the People's Republic of Bangladesh Ministry of Health and Population Control, Health Information Unit, *Bangladesh Health Profile 1977,* 1978.
    -   ICSSR/ICMR, op.cit., p.7.

14   -   UNCTAD, *Technology policies in the pharmaceutical sector in the United Republic of Tanzania,* United Nations, 1980, p.5.
      -    UNCTAD, *Technology policies in the pharmaceutical sector in Nepal,* United Nations, 1980, p.6.

15   ICSSR/ICMR, op.cit., p.7.

16   Dr. M. Fernex, "Im Teufelskreis von Krankheit und Armut", Roche Magazin No. 4, August 1978 (translated into English by Roche as "Roche and its fight against tropical diseases").

17   USAID *Environmental Impact Statement on the AID Pest Management Programme,* Washington DC, 1977, Vol.2, p.173.

18   -   L. Goodwin, P.O. Williams and D.W. Fitzsimons, "The Present State of Tropical Medicine in the United Kingdom", *Transactions of the Royal Society of Tropical Medicine and Hygiene,* Vol.75, Supplement 1981.
      -    Fernex, op.cit.

19   WHO, *Tropical Diseases,* Geneva (undated), pp.10-11.

20   W. J. Van Zijl, "Studies in Diarrhoeal Diseases in Seven Countries", *Bulletin of the World Health Organisation* 35 (Geneva, 1966) pp.249-261.

21   -   Klouda, 1982, op.cit.
      -    ICSSR/ICMR, op.cit., p.18.

22   Black Committee Report, *Inequalities in Health,* HMSO, 1980.

23   ICSSR/ICMR, op.cit., p.18.

24   Ibid., p.6.

25   *OXFAM Field Directors' Handbook,* op.cit., pp.3-2,3-3.

26   Klouda, 1982, op.cit.

27   *OXFAM Field Directors' Handbook,* op.cit., p.22-2.

28   Dr. Lesley Bacon, Medical Officer, University Hospital, Legon, Ghana, "Ghana - medical care amid economic problems", *Journal of the Royal College of General Practitioners,* July 1980. p.434.

29   O. Jakobsen, "Economic and geographical factors influencing child malnutrition, a study from the Southern Highlands, Tanzania", *BRALUP Paper No. 52,* University of Dar es Salaam, 1978.

30   Klouda, 1982, op.cit., p.9.

31   *OXFAM Field Directors' Handbook,* op. cit., p.3-2.

32   Ibid., pp.3-3, 22-2.

33   Ibid., p.24-2.

34   *World Development Report 1980,* op. cit.

35   ICSSR/ICMR, op.cit., p.7.

36   *Bangladesh Health Profile 1977,* op.cit.

37   Catholic Institute of International Relations, "Yemen Country Analysis", p. 40. (mimeo)

38   For example, female illiteracy in North Yemen recorded as 97.6%, Yemen Arab Republic Ministry of Health, *Annual Statistical Report,* 1979. p.3. Also, on unequal distribution of food: "As a result of the existing eating habits the best food is reserved for the adults, especially the men, and the children are thus deprived of necessary proteins." Sjaak van der Geest, "The Efficiency of Inefficiency: Medicine Distribution in South-Cameroon", paper presented at the Seventh International Conference on Social Science and Medicine, Noordwijkerhout, 22-26 June 1981. (mimeo)

39   D. B. Jelliffe, MD, FRCP and E.F.P. Jelliffe, MPH, FRSH, "Breast- feeding: A Necessity for Child Health in the Tropics", *Tropical Doctor,* July 1980.

40   Tanzanian Food and Nutrition Council, *Food and Nutrition Policy for Tanzania for 1st Tanzania Nutrition Conference,* Report No. 483 by TFNC, September 1980.

41   Klouda, "Prevention is more expensive than cure", July 1981. (draft)

42   ICSSR/ICMR, op.cit., p.6.

43   Smallpox vaccinations were introduced by Jenner in 1796 and well established during the nineteenth century (*British Medical Journal,* 1896).

44   -   Thomas McKeown, *The Role of Medicine,* Blackwell, Oxford 1979.
      -    Lesley Doyal with Imogen Pennel, *The Political Economy of Health,* Pluto Press, 1979, pp.56-57.

45   Office of Health Economics, *Medicines: 50 Years of Progress 1930-1980,* London, 1980.

46   Dr. John Yudkin, "Drugs, Drug Companies and the underdevelopment of health", paper presented at the Conference on Technology Transfer to the Third World, 10-12 January 1982 at Gonoshasthaya Pharmaceuticals Limited, Bangladesh.

47   Dr. J.R. Vane, "Drugs and the Third World", *Africa Health,* Volume I No. 7, April 1979.

48   The complexities of cost-benefit evaluation are discussed by Dr W.A.M. Cutting, "Cost-Benefit Evaluations of Vaccination Programmes", *The Lancet,* 20 September 1980, pp.634-636.

49   "BCG - Bad News from India", *Lancet* 12 January 1980.

50   Tony Klouda, personal communication, 11 September 1981.

51   -   *Control of Communicable Diseases in Man,* op.cit., pp. 312-314.
      -    Maurice King, Felicity King, Soebagio Martodipoero, *Primary Child Care: Book one,* a manual for health workers, Oxford University Press, 1978
      -    Bo Balldin, Richard Hart, Rolf Huenges, Zier Versluys, Child Health and Community Medical Depts, Kilimanjaro Christian Medical Centre, *Child Health,* a manual for Medical Assistants and other rural health workers, Africa Medical and Research Foundation, 1975, p.16.2.

52   Ibid.

53   ICSSR/ICMR, op.cit., p.54. (conversion rate from Rupees taken as £1 / Rupees 18)

54   Ibid., p.176: "The total output of the industry increased a hundredfold from Rs.100 million in 1947 to Rs.10,500 million in 1978-79 (at current prices). This was due to expanded production, especially of an ever-increasing number of sophisticated drugs and rising prices. The index of production rose from 64 in 1960 to 165 in 1979 (1970/100). The drug industry has enjoyed a higher man-average profitability so that investment therein has increased substantially from Rs.240 million in 1952 to Rs.4,5000 million in 1977." (i.e. approx. £250 million)

55   -   ICSSR/ICMR, op.cit., pp. 5 and 19.
      -    Kamala J. Jaya Rao, of National Institute of Nutrition, Hyderabad, "Kerala: a Health Yardstick for India", *Medico Friend Circle Bulletin*, October 1980.
      -    World Bank, *The Effects of Education on Health*, World Bank Staff Working Paper No.405, July 1980.

56   *OXFAM Field Directors' Handbook*, op. cit., Section 3.

57   "Alma-Ata Declaration", reproduced in *World Health Forum*, 2(1), 1981, pp. 5-22.

58   Ibid.

59   WHO, *National Policies and Practices in regard to medicinal products; and related international problems*, background document for reference use at technical discussions, Thirty-First World Health Assembly, A31/Technical Discussions/I, 6 March 1978, p.5.

60   World Health Organisation, *The selection of essential drugs*. Report of a WHO Expert Committee, Technical Report Series 615, WHO, Geneva 1977, and update Technical Report Series 641, WHO, Geneva 1979.

61   Ibid.

62   Dr. Mahler, Director General WHO: "But for the villager and urban slum-dweller great miracles can be achieved with fewer than 30 well-chosen drugs." ("The meaning of 'health for all by the year 2000 ' " *World Health Forum*, vol. 2, No. 1, 1981, p.17.)

63   United Nations Centre on Transnational Corporations (UNCTC), *Transnational Corporations and the Pharmaceutical Industry*, UN, New York, 1979, p.84.

64   *WHO* (A31/Technical Discussions/1) 1978, op. cit., p.5.

CHAPTER 2

1   Government of the People's Republic of Bangladesh Ministry of Health and Population Control, *Bangladesh Health Profile 1977,* Table 11a, p.105.

2   For example, *in Bangladesh*
     -    An estimated 325,000 active TB cases (aged over 10) receive no treatment.
     -    At least 90,000 under fives die each year of pneumonia.
     -    An estimated 136,000 under fives die of tetanus (mortality 8.6 per 1000).
     -    A WHO survey records the incidence of neonatal tetanus at 23.9 per 1000, with a case fatality rate of 93.5%.
     -    An estimated 32 million children under 15 need worm treatment. (Source: *Bangladesh Health Profile 1977,* op.cit.)

In Tanzania
- An estimated 130,000 leprosy cases not treated.
- An estimated 36,000 TB cases untreated.
- Hookworm affects up to 5 million. (Source: Dr Tony Klouda "Prevention is more expensive than cure, a Review of Health Problems for Tanzania 1971-1981," February 1982. (mimeo)

3   Consumption by sales value from M. P. Tifienbacher, director Fabwerke- Hoechst, Table I(i) and (iii) supplementary to paper published in the Proceedings of the US Institute of Medicine (National Academy of Sciences) Conference, *Pharmaceuticals for Developing Countries,* Washington, January 1979. Figures for the world pharmaceutical market in 1976 (manufacturers' price) The 19 industrialized: Australia, Austria, Belgium, Canada, Denmark, Finland, France, W. Germany, Ireland, Italy, Japan, Netherlands, New Zealand, Norway, South Africa, Sweden, Switzerland, UK and USA. The low income countries: Afghanistan, Bangladesh, Benin, Bhutan, Burundi, Burma, Kampuchea, Central African Empire, Chad, Ethiopia, Guinea, Haiti, India, Kenya, Lao PDR, Lesotho, Madagascar, Malawi, Mali, Mozambique, Nepal, Niger, Pakistan, Rwanda, Sierra Leone, Somalia, Sri Lanka, Tanzania, Uganda, Upper Volta, Vietnam, Yemen Arab Republic, Zaire.

4   - WHO, "National Policies and Practices in regard to Medicinal Products: and Related International Problems", Background Document A31/Technical Discussions/I, 6 March 1978, p.9 "... in economic terms the developed countries account for more than 80% of the world pharmaceutical consumption and the developing countries for less than 20%."
    - UNIDO, *Global Study of the Pharmaceutical Industry* (ID/WG.331/6) 22 October 1980, p.29, gives developing country consumption in 1978 as 17.55%. Pharmaceutical consumption in China equals 5.2% of total market (Tables 15-18).
    - David Taylor, *Medicines, Health and the Poor World,* Office of Health Economics, London 1982, p.30. World medicine consumption 1980 manufacturers' prices) was $76,000 million and 20% of sales were in developing countries.

5   Dr. V. Fattorusso, "Essential Drugs for the Third World", *World Health,* May 1981, p.3. Average drug consumption per head is considerably higher in some newly industrializing countries, particularly in Latin America: eg. Brazil $12 and Mexico $11.6 (1976) (UNIDO, op.cit., p.116). In Britain drug consumption per head in 1979 was $76 (retail prices) (*SCRIP,* World Pharmaceutical Newsletter, No. 621, p.4) and £19.55 (manufacturers' prices) for total UK market of £1,056 million (Association of British Pharmaceutical Industry - ABPI). But Britain ranks low amongst other developed countries, as W. Germany Japan, France, Sweden, Switzerland, USA and others have significantly higher average drug consumption. (UNIDO, 1980, op.cit., p.117.)

6   - UNIDO, 1980, op.cit., p.14.
    - Bangladesh Government report to WHO, "Drug Policy and Management in Bangladesh" (Country Information Paper), for Inter-Country Consultative Meeting on Drug Policies and Management, 13-16 October 1980, New Delhi, (WHO/SEA/DPM/Conslt. meeting 1/7). Drug market for 1979 US $70 million - (at trade prices). "The per capita consumption of drugs (allopathics) is about US $0.82, with a coverage of not more than 28% of the people."

7   See Chapter 9, "National and International Solutions".

8   - World Bank, Country Study *Yemen Arab Republic,* Development of a Traditional Economy, Washington DC, January 1979. Table 5:3, "Government Expenditures", 1967/7, p.245.
    - *Bangladesh Health Profile 1977,* op.cit., Table 5.2, "Central Government Current Expenditure".

9   Klouda, op. cit., p.12.

10 Bangladesh Government health budget 1978/9. Taka 350 million (£9.72 million) (£1/ 36 Taka). British NHS spending 1978/9 £8,850 million. NHS spending 1981/2 £11,000 million, of which £1,000 million on drugs (DHSS Press Office).

11   Tanzania Ministry of Health, *Evaluation of the Health Sector 1979,* October 1980.

12   Klouda, op.cit., p.15.

13   Ibid. p.17.

14   Government of People's Republic of Bangladesh, Planning Commission *The Second Five Year Plan (Draft)* 1980-5, Chapter XVII, "Health and Population Control".

15   *Bangladesh Health Profile 1977,* op.cit., p.69.

16   Suzanne Williams, OXFAM Field Director, Manaus, in interview with the author, September 1981.

17   Dr. Halfdan Mahler, "The meaning of 'health for all by the year 2000' ", *World Health Forum,* Vol.2, No.1, 1981, p.15.

18   Dr. K.M.S. Aziz, International Centre for Diarrhoeal Research, Bangladesh, in interview with the author, 8 October, 1980.
      5 year MBBS course consists of 2770 hours teaching, of which 940 hours (anatomy, embriology, histology); 780 hours (physiology, biochemistry); 10 hours (elementary bacteriology and pathology); 150 pharmacology (no *clinical* pharmacology); 40 forensic medicine; 25 clinical subjects; 180 medicine, including clinical medicine, paediatrics, skin and venereal disease and therapeutics.

19   Interview with Dr. Nelson Senise, "Os males da medicina", *Veja,* 23 April, 1980.

20   *Bangladesh Health Profile 1977,* op.cit.

21   Dianna Melrose, *The Great Health Robbery,* OXFAM, Oxford, 1981, p.10.

22   Mahler, op.cit, p.10: "Over three-quarters of the world's migrant doctors can be found in just five countries - Australia, Canada, W. Germany, the UK and the USA."

23   *Bangladesh Health Profile 1977,* op.cit., p.73.

24   Professor P.F. D'Arcy, Head of Department of Pharmacy, Queen's University of Belfast, Pharmacy in the Third World: a Cause for Concern, *Pharmacy International,* (FIP Sector), June 1980.

25   Figures given by WHO are contradictory:

(a)   The WHO Drug Policies and Management Unit Paper on the trend of essential drug prices in developing countries (1980) (mimeo), "General Principles Section", p.3 gives the figures as 15-20% of health budgets spent on drugs in developed countries, and 40-60% in developing countries.

(b)   The WHO Background Document, " *National Policies and Practices in Regard to Medicinal Products; and related international problems* " (A31/Technical Discussion/1), March 1978, gives expenditure on pharmaceuticals as 10-20% of health expenditure in developed countries, and "as high as 50% in developing countries."

(c)   But, drugs expenditure is shown to be under 30% in Burma, India, Indonesia and Sri Lanka in WHO, *Drug Policies Including Traditional Medicines in the context of Primary Health Care,* Report and Background Documentation of the Technical Discussions held during the 32nd session of the WHO Regional Committee for S.E. Asia, September 1979. Published WHO, Regional Office for S.E. Asia, November 1979, Table 1, p.28.

26   WHO, *Drug Policy and Management in Bangladesh,* op cit.

27   Tanzania Ministry of Health, *Evaluation of the Health Sector 1979,* op.cit.

28   Dr. Ann Hoskins, British Organisation for Community Development, "Discussion Paper from Basic Health Services Drug Committee on the problems of drugs in the Yemen Arab Republic", May 1981. (mimeo)

29   Letter from Pharmacist Barry Cohen, Pharmacy Department, Holy Rosary Hospital, Emekuku, IMO State, Nigeria to Ritchie Cogan, BBC, London, 23 July, 1979.

30   Sjaak van der Geest of the Anthropological-Sociological Centre, University of Amsterdam, "The Efficiency of Inefficiency: Medicine Distribution in South-Cameroon", paper presented at the Seventh International Conference on Social Science and Medicine, Noordwijkerhout, 22-26 June 1981. (mimeo)

31   Mark Bowden, Director, Save the Children Fund, Bangladesh, in interview with the author, 18 September, 1980, and others.

32   "KK exposes drug theft", *Zambia Daily Mail,* 3 May, 1980.

33   Prof. I.C. Tiwari, Dr S.C. Mohapatra and Dr S.D. Gaur, Department of Preventive and Social Medicine, Institute of Medical Sciences, Banaras Hindu University, "Drug Needs and Availability for Primary Health Care in a Rural Community in India", paper presented at Primary Health Care Symposium, 13-16 April 1982 at the Liverpool School of Tropical Medicine.

34   Ibid.

35   Oscar Gish and Loretta Lee Feller, School of Public Health, University of Michigan, *Planning Pharmaceuticals for Primary Health Care: the Supply and Utilization of Drugs in the Third World,* American Public Health Association International Health Programs, Monograph Series No. 2, 1979.

36   -   Dr. Balasubramanian, UNCTAD, quoted in *Provisional Summary Record of the Sixth Meeting Committee A,* Thirty-Fifth World Health Assembly, WHO Document A35/A/SR6, 11 May 1982, p.3.

      -    Dr. Humayun K.M.A. Hye, Director Drugs Administration Bangladesh, *Information on the Drug Sector in Bangladesh in the Context of Primary Health Care,* Bangladesh, May 1979.

      -    Dr. J Albably, Director Yemen Government Supreme Board of Drug Control, in interview with David Green of Oxfam and James Firebrace, Coordinator, British Volunteer Programme, August 1980.

      -    UNCTAD, *Technology Policies in the Pharmaceutical Sector in Nepal,* a study prepared by the UNCTAD Secretariat in co-operation with Dr. P.N. Suwal, U.N. 1980.

37   -   UK figures from *SCRIP,* No. 621, August 31, 1981.

      -    UN Commission on Transnational Corporations (UNCTC), *Transnational Corporations in the pharmaceutical industry of developing countries,* Report of the Secretariat E/C.10/85, UN Economic and Social Council, 15 July 1981, p.22.

38   *Drug Policies including Traditional Medicine in the Context of Primary Health Care,* op.cit.

39   *Bangladesh Health Profile 1977,* op.cit., p.75.

40   A. Giovanni, *A Questao dos Remedios no Brasil,* Polis, Sao Paulo, 1980, quoted by Mike Muller, *The Health of Nations, A North-South Investigation,* Faber & Faber, London, 1982, p.111.

41   Ann Ferguson, Department of Anthropology, Michigan State University, "The Role of Pharmaceuticals in the Process of Medicalization in Asuncion, El Salvador", paper delivered at the 1980 American Anthropological Association meetings held in Washington DC, December 2-7. (mimeo)

42   Ann Ferguson, "The effects of source of supply of medications on health care services dispensed in pharmacies in a Salvadoran town", paper presented at the Central States Anthropology Society 56th Annual Meeting, Ann Arbor, Michigan 9-12 April 1980. (mimeo)

43   van der Geest, op.cit., p.13.

CHAPTER 3

1   Dr. A. R. Phadke, "The Drug Industry - an analysis", *In Search of Diagnosis*, Ashvin J. Patel (ed), Medico Friend Circle, Vadodara, 1977. p.81.

2   *IFPMA Code of Pharmaceutical Marketing Practices,* March 1981 (draft) "Obligations of the Industry", pp.1-2.

3   George Teeling-Smith, Director, Office of Health Economics, quoted in *New Internationalist,* No. 50, April 1977, p.13.

4   -   United Nations Commission on Transnational Corporations (UNCTC), "Studies on the Effects of the Operations and Practices of Transnational Corporations", *Transnational corporations in the pharmaceutical industry of developing countries,* Report of the Secretariat, 15 July 1981, United Nations Economic and Social Council (E/C.10/85).
     -    United Nations Industrial Development Organisation (UNIDO), *Global Study of the Pharmaceutical Industry,* for First Consultation Meeting on the Pharmaceutical Industry Lisbon, Portugal, 1-5 December 1980, (ID/WG.331/6).

5   Ibid. Exports from Eastern European and other centrally-planned economies: 9.8% of world total (1977) and exports from all developing countries: 3.8% of total. Table 29)

6   United Nations Conference on Trade and Development (UNCTAD), *Technology policies and planning for the pharmaceutical sector in the developing countries,* study prepared by the UNCTAD secretariat in cooperation with Dr Nitya Anand. United Nations, 1980, (TD/B/C.6/56) p.20.

7   Ibid., pp.20-24. Besides production of synthetic drugs, biologicals such as insulin can be produced from slaughter-house wastes and others from plant extracts without very advanced technology.

8   Ibid.

9   UNIDO, 1980, op.cit., p.35.

10   -   UNCTC, *Transnational Corporations and the Pharmaceutical Industry,* United Nations, New York, 1979, (ST/CTC/9) (Table 25)
     -    UNCTC 1981, op.cit.
     -    WHO Country Information Paper for Inter-Country Consultative Meeting on Drug Policies and Management, New Delhi, 13-16 October 1980 (ICP DPM 001) *Drug Policy and Management in Bangladesh* (SEA/DPM/Conslt. Meet.1/7)

11   UNCTC, 1979, op.cit.

12   Indian Council of Social Science Research (ICSSR) and Indian Council of Medical Research (ICMR), *Health for all, an alternative strategy,* 1981.

13   -   UNCTC, 15 July 1981, op.cit.
     -    UNCTC summary draft report of 9 February 1981 with case studies on Argentina, Brazil, Colombia, Costa Rica, Egypt, India, Kenya, Malaysia, Mexico, Sierra Leone, Thailand.

14   Ibid.

15   UNCTC, 1979, op.cit., p.22.

16   OECD, *An Industry like no Other - The Pharmaceutical Industry as seen by the OECD,* (Summary of the report entitled "Multinational Enterprises, Governments and Technology; the Pharmaceutical Industry" by M. L. Burstall, J. H. Dunning and A. Lake, OECD, Paris 1981), Pharma Information Ciba-Geigy, Roche, Sandoz, Basle, February 1982, Table 11.

     There are only 3 British manufacturers in the top 25: Glaxo, Beecham and ICI. A league table (at 31 December 1980) on just prescription drugs includes Wellcome ranked No.21 (with ICI and Beecham at 22 and 23) and Fisons at 57. (*SCRIP* No. 653 & 654, 21 & 24 December 1981, p.19.)

17   UNCTC, 1979, op.cit., Table 14, pp.125-6.
      Concentration on *overall* sales is low in the drug industry compared to other high-technology manufacturing industries, eg. car production, in which the largest company had about 25% of the market in 1977. (UNIDO, 1980, op.cit. pp.55-6.)

18   UNCTC, 1979, op.cit., p.3.

19   Ibid.

20   For 18 Western industrialized contries this positive trade balance was $2,445.1 million and for just two Eastern European countries $170.2 million in 1977. (Unpublished data from UNCTAD.)

21   David Taylor, Office of Health Economics, *Medicines, Health and the Poor World,* OHE, London, 1982, p.30 (includes Western and Eastern bloc countries).

22   David Piachaud, London School of Economic, "Medicines and the Third World", 1979. (mimeo)

23   -   WHO, Background paper for the 33rd World Health Assembly, *NIEO and Health,* Annex 3 "Drug Policies and Essential Drugs: a casestudy", WHO, Geneva, May 1981.
      -    Piachaud 1979, op.cit.

24   Dr. Oliver Munyaradzi, Minister of Health, text of speech delivered at the meeting of Chief Pharmacists of the Africa Region in Harare, 26 April 1982, Department of Information, Press statement 358/82/DC.

25   WHO, May 1980, op. cit.

26   Prof. G. Peters, Rapport *Mission au Mozambique du 8 au 19 octobre 1980,* Universite de Lausanne, 26 March 1981.

27   WHO, *The Selection of Essential Drugs,* Second report of the WHO Expert Committee, Technical Report Series 641, Geneva, 1979.

28   See for example: Sidney Wolfe, Christopher Coley and, the Health Research Group founded by Ralph Nader, *Pills That Don't Work - Prescription Drugs That Lack Evidence of Effectiveness,* Farrar Stras Giroux New York, 1981.

29   Prof. Wilfred Lionel and Dr. Andrew Herxheimer, "Coherent Policies on Drugs: Formulation and Implementation", in Blum, Herxheimer, Stenzl and Woodcock (ed), *Pharmaceuticals and Health Policy,* 1981, Croom Helm, London, 1981, p.240.

30   WHO Background Document on *National Policies and Practices in regard to medicinal products and related international problems,* (A/31/Technical Discussions/1) March 1978, para.4.3.

31   -   Dr. Mohammed Jafer Saeed, "The Other Face of Drug Companies" (translated from Arabic), p.5. (mimeo)
      -    Dr. Ann Hoskins, British Organisation for Community Development, "Discussion Paper from the Basic Health Services Drug Committee on the problems of drugs in Yemen", 1981, p.3.

32   Ibid.

33   UNCTAD, *Technology policies in the pharmaceutical sector in the Philippines,* study prepared by Mr Esteban Bautista and Mr Wilfredo Clemente in co-operation with the UNCTAD Secretariat, (UNCTAD/TT/36), United Nations, 1980, p.25.

34   UNCTAD, *Case studies in the transfer of technology: Pharmaceutical Policies in Sri Lanka,* study prepared by Dr Senaka Bibile in co- operation with UNCTAD Secretariat, (TD/B.C.6/21), United Nations, 27 June 1977, pp.30 and 3.

35   UNCTAD, *Technology policies in the pharmaceutical sector in Nepal,* study prepared by the UNCTAD Secretariat in co-operation with Dr. P. N. Suwal, (UNCTAD/TT/34), United Nations, 1980, pp.15-16.

36   -   Dr G. J. Ebrahim, "The Problems of Undernutrition" in R. J. Jarrett (ed.) *Nutrition and Disease,* Croom Helm London, 1979.
     -   *British National Formulary 1981,* op. cit., p.225.

37   -   Dr. Mario Victor de Assis Pacheco, *A Mafia dos Remedios,* Brazil, 1978, pp.98-103.
     -   *British National Formulary* 1981, op. cit., pp.226 and 238-9.

38   Ibid., p.225.

39   Ibid., p.238.

40   -   Assis Pacheco, op. cit., pp.98-103.
     -   ABPI *Data Sheet Compendium 1979-80,* ABPI 1979, p.369.

41   BNF 1981, op. cit., p.226.

42   Dr. Carol Barker, "Pharmaceuticals Policy", unpublished draft, undated. (The maximum profit allowed was set at a fixed percentage of the CIF price.)

43   ICSSR/ICMR, *Health for All - An Alternative Strategy,* Report of a study group set up jointly by the ICSSR and ICMR, Indian Institute of Education, Pune 1981, p.178.

44   Ibid.

45   Ibid., p.7. (Also figure of 12 million leprosy sufferers from Goodwin, Williams, Fitzsimons, "Introduction" - "The Present State of Tropical Medicine in the United Kingdom", *Transactions of the Royal Society of Tropical Medicine and Hygiene,* Vol.75, Supplement 1981, p.3.)

46   UNCTAD, *Case studies in the transfer of technology the pharmaceutical industry in India,* study prepared by the Jawarharlal Nehru University and the Indian Council of Scientific and Industrial Research, United Nations, 1977, pp.4-7, Table 19 (p.38) and Table 20 (pp.40-41).

47   Ibid., p.39.

48   -   ICSSR/ICMR, op.cit.
     -   UNCTAD, 1977, op. cit.
     -   Hathi Report, *Report of the Committee on Drug and Pharmaceutical Industry,* Ministry of Petroleum & Chemicals, Government of India, April 1975.

49   Hathi, op.cit., p.95.

50   The April 1979 Drugs (Prices Control) Order attempted to keep down the prices of essential drugs by fixing lower price mark-ups for more essential items. In practice this has encouraged production of less essential drugs with higher profit margins. (Mukarram Bhagat *Aspects of the Drug Industry in India,* Centre for Education and Documentation, Bombay, February 1982, pp.90-95.)

51   Arnold Worlock, Group Marketing Director, The Wellcome Foundation Limited, personal communication, 28 May 1982.

52   Ibid. The policy of licensed capacity is intended to restrict production of non-essential drugs. In practice, many companies have been producing far in excess of their licensed capacities without action being taken, but the dapsone case has parallels. Alembic Chemical was required to export its unlicensed over-production of penicillin - a much-needed drug. The Indian public sector pioneered bulk drug production in the country and almost all its output is of important bulk drugs, but they have a poor record for reaching production targets, idle capacities and heavy financial losses. (Bhagat, op.cit.)

53   Bhagat, op.cit., p.116.

54   Expert Committee Report, *Evaluation of Registered/Licensed Products and Draft National Drug Policy,* Dacca, Bangladesh, 11 May 1982, p.92.

211

Chapter 3

THE 8 LEADING COMPANIES

1. Pfizer Laboratories Ltd. US subsidiary.
2. Glaxo (Bangladesh) Ltd. British subsidiary.
3. Fisons (Bangladesh) Ltd. British subsidiary.
4. Bangladesh Pharmaceutical Industry Ltd. Joint venture company of (BPI) Bangladesh Chemical Industries Corporation and May and Baker (UK) Ltd.
5. Hoechst Pharmaceuticals Co. Ltd. W. German subsidary.
6. Squibb of Bangladesh Ltd. US subsidiary.
7. Organon (Bangladesh) Ltd. Dutch subsidiary.
8. ICI Bangladesh Manufacturers Ltd. British subsidiary.

FOREIGN CONTROL

For example: *Glaxo:* Glaxo Holdings controls 70% of the equity and the Government 30%. Glaxo had 4 members on the Board to 3 Government representatives. (Information from Glaxo (Bangladesh) 1980). *ICI:* the British parent company also holds 70% of the equity. *Fisons:* The Bangladesh Government holds 51% of the equity shares, but Fisons holds 51% of controlling shares and has 3 representatives on the board to the Government's 2. *BPI:* May & Baker U.K. holds 60% of the equity; and is solely responsible for the management of the company under a management contract.

There are 25 medium-sized national companies which manufacture a further 15% of products and 133 small companies that account for the remaining 10% - these produce only simple liquid formulations.

55   Dr. H.K.M.A. Hye, then Director Drug Administration, personal communication, 7 May 1981. The Government tender is restricted to the local market for all items produced locally: "Procurement is by generic name but we have the constraint that the local market is dominated (80-85%) by large brand name producers and their subsidiaries. Drugs manufactured locally cannot be imported, even if cheaper foreign sources are available."

56   Dr. Hye in interview with the author, Delhi, 20 October 1980.

57   -   "Merck in Bangladesh Marketing Plan 1980 (-1982)", December 1979. Market Estimates 1978: Taka 805 million 1981: 1,440 million 1982: 1,728 million. (p.5 - "There is a fast growing market in Bangladesh (24%/1978).")

        -    Sales 1977 Taka 800 million ("Country Information Paper - Bangladesh" *Drug Polcies Including Traditional Medicines in the Context of Primary Health Care,* WHO Regional Office for S.E. Asia New Delhi, November 1979.)

        -    Drug expenditure 1981 estimated at 1,500 million taka (Expert Committee Report, Bangladesh, 11 May 1982, op. cit. p.92.)

58   -   Ibid.
        -    Dr. Hye in interview with the author, 20 October 1980.

59   Expert Committee Report, Bangladesh, op. cit.

60   "Merck in Bangladesh Marketing Plan 1980 (-1982)", op. cit., p.10.

61   Bristol-Myers (Bangladesh) Ethical Pharmaceutical Market in 1977 (estimates from Marketing division). Total market 50 million dollars.

	% of market
(a) vitamins, haematinics, tonics	30
(b) antibiotics	20
(c) analgesics	10
(d) antacids	10
(e) tranquilizers, antidepressants, sedatives	8
(f) antidiarrhoeals & anti-dysentric	7
(g) anti TB	6
(h) others 9	Total 100%

One local marketing manager interviewed (September 1980) considered (a) an underestimate and the true figure nearer 40%, and (c) and (d) overestimates in terms of *value*, not volume. The Marketing Director of Squibb of Bangladesh Ltd. gives turnover in 1980 as vitamins and nutritionals - 31.8% and antacids - 12.8%.

62   Expert Committee, *Evaluation of Registered/Licensed Products and Draft National Drug Policy,* Dacca, 11 May 1982, p.92.

63   We understand from inquiries made by our Field staff in Bangladesh that these product lists were current at the beginning of 1982, but we have no written confirmation from either company of precisely which drugs are currently marketed in Bangladesh. See Appendices II and III. Also, WHO, 1979, op.cit.

64   See Chapter 5,

65   Antidiarrhoeals: *Fistrep* (combination of streptomycin sulphate and clioquinol) and *Enterfram* (liquid preparation of neomycin sulphate and kaolin). For dangers of clioquinol, see page and for appropriateness of antibiotics for use in diarrhoea (especially ''infantile diarrhoea'' recommended in Fisons (Bangladesh) Limited *Price List of Products,* 1 September 1978) · ''Antibiotic....preparations should be *avoided* for the treatment of diarrhoea   even when a bacterial cause is suspected..'' (BNF, 1981, op. cit., p.40, original emphasis.)

66   BNF, 1981, op. cit., pp.291 and 286.

67   Wolfe, Coley and the Health Research Group, *Pills that Don't Work,* Farrar Straus Girouz, New York, 1981, p.35.

68   Prof.M.D. Rawlins, Head Department of Pharmacological Sciences, University of Newcastle upon Tyne, personal communication, 8 February 1982.

69   Letter from Fisons (UK) to Prof. Rawlins, 21 February 1981.

70   Dr. John Yudkin, personal communication 25 November 1980. *''Digeplex:* No justification for using enmzymes in ' 'indigestion ' '. The indications would be malabsorption for pancreatic failure - which can indeed happen in long-standing malnutrition, but needs specific diagnosis before it's used. Also vitamin B complex deficiency is *not* a basic cause of digestive disorders.'' (original emphasis)

71   Dr. Martin Schweiger, personal communication, 13 July 1980.

72   Schweiger, ''A Comparison of Drugs Marketed by Two British Companies in the United Kingdom and Bangladesh'', 1979. (unpublished paper)

73   GLAXO UK: In our letter of 8 May 1981 to Glaxo's Group Consumer Products Co-ordinator we wrote: ''On medicines you will remember I was keen to have the names of colleagues on the Ethical Pharmaceuticals side with whom I might discuss issues such as the product range in Bangladesh and the feasibility of switching production to drugs more in line with health needs and the priorities of the Government in Bangladesh.'' We received no reply. We wrote a long letter raising specific and general queries on 20 January 1982, with follow-up telephone calls on 26 March, 13 and 26 April and letters on 27 April and 19 May. On 29 January 1982 J. Barr (Group Public Relations) wrote: ''This our letter of 20 January has been passed to this office for actioning and further contact will be made when the matters raised have been fully considered''. A further letter of 16 June 1982 from Glaxo's Public Relations Manager does not respond to our request for comments on the range of products sold in Bangladesh (or give details of their current product range), citing the fact that in 1981 we discussed these issues with Mr Barnett, Glaxo Group Consumer Products Coordinator. In fact our discussion then focussed mainly on sales of artificial baby milk and Mr. Barnett suggested the Bangladesh pharmaceutical product range would be more appropriately discussed with colleagues on the ethical pharmaceuticals side.

GLAXO (BANGLADESH): Mr. Zaman, Marketing Services Manager and Mr. Chowdhury, Marketing Director, were helpful when we interviewed them on 7 and 8 October 1980.

213

FISONS: Mr. Mohammad Nurul Islam, Marketing Manager of *Fisons (Bangladesh) Ltd.* was also most helpful when we talked to him on 26 September 1980. Our letter to the Divisional Chairman of *Fisons UK* Pharmaceuticals Division of 18 January 1982 unfortunately did not reach Fisons, a copy was sent on 24 March which cut down the time for them to contact their subsidiary. Fisons Deputy Chairman wrote on 27 April 1982 to say: "Naturally I am very concerned about your criticisms, implied or otherwise, relating to the activities of Fisons (Bangladesh) and consequently you will appreciate that I find it necessary to investigate your ''facts '' thoroughly before responding on relevant matters due course." We had no further comments by time of going to press.

74   Expert Committee report, 11 May 1982, op. cit. Of the 1742 locally manufactured products recommended for withdrawal only 174 are produced by the 8 foreign-controlled manufacturers.

75   Ibid., p.9. Verdivitone is referred to as "multivatimin combination with alcohol and glycerophosphate. A highly misused habit-forming drug which is dangerous in hepatic malaisis. Chronic wastage of country's resources ..." (p.10) Squibb of Bangladesh point out: "Verdivitone is purchased mainly by the more affluent sector of the community and at 11% per volume, has a lower alcohol content than other vitamin tonics made here. Alcohol is used to preserve the B complex vitamins which would otherwise degrade quickly ... ". They also cite "the large rural industry producing cheap (and dangerous) alcohol from palm, sugar and rice." (R. Bower, Managing Director, personal communication, 3 May 1982.)

76   Dr. C. G. Roepnack and Dr. R. W. Timmers, Hoechst Head Office, personal communication, 22 March 1982.

77   F. K. Ghuznavi, Chairman ICI Bangladesh Manufacturers Ltd., in interview with the author, 1 October 1980.

78   Dr. Martin Schweiger, "In Sickness or in Wealth," B.B.C. Radio 4 transcript of tape No. TLN34/230P849, transmitted 26 August 1979, p.15.

79   Mohammed Nurul Islam, Marketing Manager, Fisons (Bangladesh) Ltd., personal communication, 19 February 1981.

80   *IFPMA Code of Pharmaceutical Marketing Practices,* March 1981, op.cit.

81   Dr. Halfdan Mahler, "The meaning of ' health for all by the year 2000 ' ", *World Health Forum,* vol. 2 No. 1, 1981, p.18.

82   ICSSR/ICMR, 1981, op.cit.

83   Veena Shatrughna, "Drug prescription: Service to whom?", *Medico Friend Circle Bulletin,* India, 1978, quoted by Brudon, 1981.

84   Ibid.

85   Dr. E. Snell and Mr. Lee (APBI) in interview with the author, 25 March 1981.

86   Dr. H.K.A. Hye, ex-Director Drug Administration - Ministry of Health, Bangladesh, personal communication, 7 May 1981.

87   "Merck in Bangladesh, Marketing Plan 1980(-1982)", op. cit. The marketing claims made for Neurobion are discussed in more detail in Chapter 5.

88   Ibid., pp. 3, 6, 11.

89   Dr. Hye, personal communication, 10 August 1981.

90   Government of the People's Republic of Bangladesh, Directorate of Drugs Administration, "Import Figures of Finished Drugs for the Calendar Year 1980."

91   E. Merck have argued that: "The import of our products to Bangladesh does not cost the country a penny in foreign exchange. As long as the country has been in existence, we have been closely cooperating with the Government in the conclusion of barter agreements, under which Merck supplies laboratory chemicals, reagents, diagnostics, industrial chemicals and

pharmaceutical specialities. Against the supply of these items, we purchase from Bangladesh goods such as molasses, textiles, industrial gloves, wheat grain for animal feed, jute and jute goods, wet blue skin, tea, cutlery, for none of which it is easy to find a ready buyer. We can even claim that we provide aid to Bangladesh through our contacts with customers for these goods by supplying know-how to that country, for example in the manufacture of textiles and for the production of cutlery. We feel this should be mentioned in order to complete the picture of our activities in the country ..." (Drs. Mehrhof and Niederehe, E. Merck, personal communication, 29 March 1982.) But the former Director of Drug Administration questions how much the barter arrangement is really helping Bangladesh in exchanging mainly finished medicines (many of which are "non-essential") for commodities (like jute, jute goods, tea and hides) which are 'easily exportable items, and if sold in the open international market would fetch valuable hard foreign exchange." "The statement that import of E. Merck products does not cost us a penny in foreign exchange is mischievous." (Dr. H.K.M.A. Hye, personal communication, 20 April 1982.)

92   Government of the People's Republic of Bangladesh, "Import Figures of Pharmaceuticals Raw Materials for the calendar year 1980".

93   Hye, 10 August 1981, op. cit.

94   Expert Committee, Bangladesh, op. cit., p.92.

95   Ibid.

96   Pascale Brudon, "L'Industrie Pharmaceutique Suisse dans les Pays sous developpes", Memoire presente pour le diplome de recherche en etudes de developpement, Institut Universitaire d'Etudes de Developpement, Geneva, 1981. Of the 36: 13 are for psychiatric and neurological use; 7 cardiovasculars; 3 antibiotics; 2 anti-cancer drugs. (p.211)

97   Ibid.

98   Ibid., p.202.

99   Ibid., p.203. Sandoz has a similar vanilla-flavoured preparation Meritene amongst its best-selling products in Mexico (p.207).

100 Ibid., p.257.

101 See Chapter 10.

102 Information Research Limited, "Opportunities for Pharmaceuticals in the Developing world over the next Twenty Years", June 1980, p.7.

CHAPTER 4

1   Dr. Roderick Rainford, at a Regional Pharmaceutical meeting, quoted by Robina Khan, Office of the Director General for Economic Cooperation and Development of the United Nations, New York, (previously UN/UNDP APEC Programme on Pharmaceuticals in Guyana) in "Effects of Drug Colonialism in the Caribbean", 22 October 1980, p.1. (mimeo)

2   Pascale Brudon, "L'Industrie Pharmaceutique Suisse dans les Pays Sous Developpes", Memoire presente pour le diplome de recherche en etudes de developpement, Institut Universitaire d'Etudes de Developpement, Geneva, 1981, pp.256-257 and p.197.

3   Ibid., pp.192-197, pp.202-203 and p.260. Bactrim was the 11th top-selling drug on the Mexican market in 1978. 20 tablets of the same drug were available more cheaply from: Burroughs Wellcome (Septrin) at 92.70 pesos. Laboratorios Tegur de Mexico (Bactifor) at 71.80 pesos. Industria Farmaceutica Andromaco (Andoprim) at 68.55 pesos. Laboratorios Fustery (Polibatrim) at 66 pesos. The 4 top-selling drugs can all be obtained more cheaply as generics: Bristol-Myers Pentrexyl and Bayer's Binotal as ampicillin; Upjohn's Lincocin as lincomycin, and Pfizer's Terramicina as oxytetracycline.

4   Khan, op.cit.

5   UNCTAD, *Technology policies in the pharmaceutical sector in the Philippines,* study prepared by Mr. Esteban Bautista and Mr. Wilfredo Clemente, in co-operation with the UNCTAD Secretariat, (UNCTAD/TT/36) United Nations, 1980, pp.18-19.

6

PRODUCT/ MANUFACTURER	TRADE PRICE BANGLADESH	TRADE PRICE UK £	PERCENTAGE DIFFERENCE %
BEECHAM			
Amoxcil	Taka 212.50		
100x250 mg caps.	= £5.90	12.47	111
Orbenin	Taka 165.75		
100x250 mg caps.	= £4.60	14.80	221
Penbritin	Taka 718.25		
100x250 mg caps.	= £19.95	25.21	26
CIBA GEIGY			
Tofranil	Taka 149.36		
100x25 mg tabs.	= £4.14	3.25	-27
FISONS			
Genaspirin	Taka 21.25		
250x300 mg tabs.	= £0.59	97.50	65
Imferon	Taka 331.50		
100x2 ml amp.	= £9.20	41.58	413
GLAXO			
Betnelan	Taka 53.80		
100 tabs.	= £1.49	4.00	168
Betnesol-N	Taka 12.25		
5ml drops	= £0.34	0.74	117
Grisovin	Taka 218.00		
500x125 mg tabs.	= £6.05	11.85	95
Piriton	Taka 4.50		
50x4 mg tabs.	= £0.12	0.45	260
Ventolin	Taka 27.75		
100x2 mg tabs.	= £0.77	1.35	75
HOECHST			
Lasix	Taka 38.95		
25x2 ml amps.	= £1.08	6.46	498
ICI			
Atromid-S	Taka 51.00		
50x500 mg caps.	= £1.41	1.62	14
Avloclor	Taka 165.75		
500x250 mg tabs.	= £4.60	3.75	-22
Fulcin	Taka 55.25		
100x125 mg tabs.	= £1.53	1.90	24
Inderal	Taka 63.75		
250x10 mg tabs.	= £1.77	3.92	121
250x40 mg tabs.	Taka 174.25		
	= £4.84	9.21	90

Mysoline 100x250 mg tabs.	Taka 27.55 = £0.76	0.88	15
Synalar ointment 5gm	Taka 10.20 = £0.28	0.30	7
Synalar N ointment 5gm	Taka 10.63 = £0.29	0.31	6
PFIZER Terramycin 100x250 mg caps.	Taka 90.50 = £2.51	5.19	106
Terramycin SF 100x250 mg caps.	Taka 95.20 = £2.64	5.39	104
Vibramycin 10x100 mg caps.	Taka 39.50 = £1.09	5.48	402
Vibramycin Syrup 50mg/5ml/30ml	Taka 14.40 = £0.40	1.72	339

Sources:
UK *Chemists and Druggists Price List,* February 1980. Bangladesh manufacturers price lists valid February 1980, except Hoechst Bangladesh price list dated 1.8.80. (£1 = Taka 36)

7   Monthly income of rural Bangladeshi family taken as Tk.400 (approx. £11) Prices from: Fisons Bangladesh Ltd. Price list (1.9.78) and ICI Bangladesh Manufacturers Limited Price list (4.1.80) effective November 1981 and UK Chemist & Druggist Price List, November 1981. UK family net monthly income taken as £583.

8   Brudon, op.cit., p.255

9   WHO, "National Policies and Practices in Regard to Medicinal Products; and Related International Problems", *Background Document,* A/31/Technical Discussions/1, 6 March 1978. Industry sources also concede that market factors influence prices. For example, Ciba Geigy's internal write-up of a hearing held as part of a seminar on Third World policies: It took nearly 45 minutes of persistent questioning for the company to admit that the price at which drugs are sold from its Basle headquarters to other countries is influenced by market factors.

10   UNCTAD, *Case studies in transfer of technology: Pharmaceutical Policies in Sri Lanka,* (TD/B/C.6/21), United Nations, 27 June 1977. See also Chapter 9.

11   "Merck in Bangladesh Marketing Plan 1980 (-1982)", dated December 1979, forwarded to E. Merck West Germany by H.G.Brotz, Bangladesh Branch of Emedia Export Co., 22 January 1980, p.13

12   "Prices of drugs in the private sector were uncontrolled and manufacturers charged what the market would bear." UNCTAD Report *Pharmaceutical Policies in Sri Lanka,* 1977, op.cit., p.6. Also: "The only general conclusion that can be drawn on this issue is that TNCs have charged whatever national markets would bear, and the market power of the leading firms has enabled them to limit the sales of many important drugs to that part of the population which could afford the going price - a part of which,in many countries, is very small indeed." Oscar Gish & Loretta Lee Feller, *Planning Pharmaceuticals for Primary Health Care,* American Public Health Association International Health Programs Monograph Series No.2., 1979. p.25.

13   *British National Formulary,* 1981, Number 1.

14   500 tablets Valium (5mg) trade price: £6.56; 500 tablets diazepam (5mg) trade price: £3. From *Chemists & Druggist Price List,* December 1981.

15   "Wasted spending on brand names increases health costs by £25 million", *Daily Telegraph,* 27 November 1979.

16   Dr. Zafrullah Chowdhury, "Essential Drugs for the Poor: Myth and Reality in Bangladesh", paper presented at the Primary Health Care Symposium, Liverpool School of Tropical Medicine, 13-16 April 1982, p.11, Table 3. (mimeo)

17   UNCTAD, *Technology Policies in the Pharmaceutical Sector in the Philippines,* op.cit.

18   "..price competition remains the most important tool of success for generics producers." (Ciba Geigy Pharma, *Generics Policy* Divisional Policy Affairs Pharma Policy V1/81, Basle, 1981.)

19   D.W. McMullan, Director of Operations, Beecham Research International, personal communication, 22 March 1982.

20   Ciba Geigy Pharma, "Generics are a fact", April 1981.

21   The situation is one of 'oligopoly ': "The principal rule is that price competition except on very limited occasions, is an antisocial practice to be strictly avoided." R.J. Barnett and R.E. Muller, *Global Reach: The Power of the Multinational Corporations,* Simon and Schuster, New York, 1974. p.32.

22   *Financial Times Survey* on Pharmaceuticals, 2 June 1982.

23   Dr. Klaus von Grebmer, Pharma Policy staff, Ciba-Geigy Limited, *Pharmaceutical Prices: A Continental View,* Office of Health Economics, London, 1978, p.13.

24   Senator Edward Kennedy, keynote address Proceedings Institute of Medicine Conference on Pharmaceuticals for Developing Countries, National Academy of Science, Washington, January 1979.

25   Estimates for 1978. Personal communication from David Taylor, Deputy Director, Office of Health Economics: 23,000 licences of right granted when Committee on Safety of Medicines came into existence, to cover sales of existing products. Since 1972, 13,000 licences withdrawn. Following licences granted by CSM: 3,250 priority category 3,500 prescription only 2,500 generics 8,000 over-the -counter drugs 750 herbal 500 homeopathic.

26   -   Government of Guyana in cooperation with UNCTAD,UNDTCD,UNIDO,WHO, *Pharmaceuticals in the Developing World, Policies on Drugs, Trade and Production,* Volume 1, General Report; referring to UNDP project INT/009/A/01/99 "Economic and Technical Co-operation among developing countries in the pharmaceutical sector", June 1979.
       -    UNCTAD, Case Studies in the transfer of technology, *The Pharmaceutical Industry in India,* study prepared by the Jawaharlal Nehru University and the ICSIR, (TD/B/C.6/20 United Nations, 1977, p.34.
       -    UNCTAD, *Technology Policies in the pharmaceutical sector in Nepal,* study prepared by the UNCTAD secretariat in cooperation with Dr. P.N. Suwal (UNCTAD/TT/34), United Nations, 1980, p.16.

27   Brudon, op.cit., p.212.

28   UNCTC, *Transnational Corporations and the Pharmaceutical Industry* (ST/CTC/9) United Nations, New York 1979.

29   von Grebmer, op.cit., p.8.

30   Ibid., p.7.

31   See also: Dr. Sanjaya Lall, Institute of Economics and Statistics, Oxford University, "Emerging Trends and future prospects in the less developed countries", in George Teeling-Smith and Nicholas Wells (ed), *Medicines for the year 2000,* OHE, London, 1979, p.104.

32   von Grebmer, op.cit., p.7.

33   WHO, A31/Technical Discussions/I, op.cit.

34   Office of Health, Economics Briefing Paper, *Trends in European Health Spending,* No.14, May 1981, p.5.

35   Others may put the question differently. For example, D.W. McMullan of Beecham writes: "It is unlikely that the pricing of pharmaceuticals to Third World countries will ever be seen as fair to all interested parties. One must remember that, if the pharmaceutical industry is to flourish, it must make a profit. However, it is a matter of debate whether a patient for example in the UK or in Germany should subsidise the price of medicines to a patient in Bangladesh or Poland." (Personal communication, 22 March 1982.)

36   -   Dr. Michael W. Hodin, Director of Public Affairs Pfizer International Inc., personal communication, 17 March 1982.
      -    *Financial Times* Survey, op.cit.

37   -   Alex Lumbroso, Managing Director, Laboratories Mariceau SA, "The Introduction of New Drugs", in Blum, Herxheimer, Stenzl and Woodcock (ed), *Pharmaceuticals and Health Policy,* 1981, p.63.
      -    *International Herald Tribune,* May 25, 1981.
      -    More recently the *Financial Times* reports that Smith-Kline "almost trebled its sales between 1976 and last year." R & D spending in 1981 was 120 million dollars and operating profit that year 525.8 million dollars. (*F.T.* Survey, op.cit.)

38   *Financial Times* Survey, op.cit.

39   Drs. J.P. Griffin and G.E. Diggle, UK DHSS Medicines Divison, review of ten years licensing experience quoted in *SCRIP* No.633, 12 October 1981, p.2.

40   FDA Bureau of Drugs *New Drug Evaluation Project,* Briefing book, October 1979, Table IV-i, quoted by Brudon, 1981, op.cit., p.226. Similarly in France according to Lumbroso out of about 250 drugs in each year, "only 5 are innovations of any therapeutic interest". (Lumbroso in Blum, et al. (ed), 1981, op.cit., p.62.)

41   *SCRIP,* No. 633, op.cit.

42   David Taylor, Deputy Director Office of Health Economics, *Medicines Health and the Poor World,* OHE, London 1982, p.35.

43   Ibid.

44   Lesley Doyal with Imogen Pennell, *The Political Economy of Health,* Pluto Press 1979. p.269.

45   "Roche and its fight against tropical diseases", translation (by Roche) of article in *Roche Magazine,* No.4, August 1978.

46   Ibid.

47   Ibid.

48   -   Prof. G. Peters, Univeristy of Lausanne, "Rapport Mission au Mozambique", 1981, p8.
      -    Dr. Milton Silverman, University of California, personal communication, 10 August 1981.

49   -   Wellcome, *In Pursuit of Excellence,* One Hundred Year Book 1880- 1980, pp.49-58.
      -    R. Lassere, "The Swiss Pharmaceutical Industry and Tropical Diseases", Roche translation of article in *Therapeutische Umschau,* 36 (1979) Part 3, pp. 263-266.
      -    And "Practical Roche responses to the special needs of Developing Countries", attachment 6 to personal communication from S. Redfern, Roche Products Ltd., 13 April 1982.

50   Peter Cunliffe, President of the Association of the British Pharmaceutical Industry and Chairman of the Pharmaceutical Division of ICI Ltd., text of paper "Pharmaceuticals in the Third World", presented to the All- Party Parliamentary Group on the Pharmaceutical Industry at the House of Commons, 15 December 1981.

51   Dr. L. C. Goodwin, Director of Science at the Zoological Society of London quotes the Research Director of Wellcome, Dr. John Vane, as saying that in 1978 Wellcome spent "£250,000 on the chemotherapy of tropical diseases, out of a research and development budget of more than

£29 million - less than 1 percent..'' ('Pharmacy and World Health Organisation Special Programme', extracts from Dr. Goodwin's Harrison Memorial Lecture, *The Pharmaceutical Journal,* 21 October 1978.) According to Wellcome in 1982 "R & D expenditure in respect of disease control in the poor communitiies of the developing countries is in fact many times greater". (Dr.Arnold Worlock, The Wellcome Foundation Limited, personal communication, 28 May 1982.) According to Roche about 10% of total R & D effort "is directly orientated to the needs of developing countries". (S. Redfern, Pharmaceutical Division, Roche Products Limited, personal communication, 4 May 1982.)

52   Goodwin, op.cit.

53   Taylor, op.cit., p.35.

54   Andras November, *Les Medicaments et le Tiers Monde,* Geneva 1981, p.52.

55   -   Dr. Michael Hodin, Director of Public Affairs, Pfizer International Inc., personal communication, 17 March 1982.
       -    *Financial Times* Survey, op.cit.

56   Prof. George Teeling-Smith, Director Office of Health Economics, personal communication, 17 February 1982.

57   Ibid.

58   WHO unpublished draft paper on the Trend of Essential Drug Prices in Developing Countries, 1980, p.6. of "General Principles" section. "It is estimated that in 1980 the World Consumption of Pharmaceuticals will reach 42.533 million dollars and, if the trend of investing 8-10% of sales (as the industry states) in research and development continues, the estimated amount for this purpose to be charged to developing countries will be considerable. Theoretically, the contribution could be 813.6 million dollars - 10% of the total consumption."

59   Estimated at 90,000 million US dollars 1982. (*Financial Times* Survey, op.cit.)

60   Ciba-Geigy Pharma, *Generics Policy,* Divisional Policy Affairs, Pharma Policy V1/81, Basle, 1981.

61   Ibid.

62   Ibid.

63   Ciba-Geigy, "Generics are a Fact", op. cit.

64   -   Ciba-Geigy, *Generics Policy* 1981, op.cit., p.6.
       -    P. F. Lumley, Manager, Public Affairs, The Association of the British Pharmaceutical Industry, personal communication, 21 June 1982.

65   Office of Health Economics, *Brand Names in Prescribing,* September 1976.

66   UNIDO, *Global Study of the Pharmaceutical Industry,* prepared by the Secretariat of UNIDO (ID/WG.331/6), 22 October 1980.

67   -   Government of Guyana et al., op.cit.
       -    Also UNCTAD, *Technology Policies and planning for the pharmaceutical sector in the developing countries,* United Nations, 1980.

68   For example, Zambia (Martyn Young,OXFAM Field Director, Zambia, personal communication, 28 March 1980).

69   "Generics are a Fact", op.cit.

70   Dr. Gordon Fryers, Director of Strategic Affairs, Reckitt and Colman, "The balance of public interest", in *Medicines for the year 2000,* OHE, op.cit., p.124.

71   Government of Guyana et al., op.cit., p.6.

72   UNCTAD, *Trade marks and generic names of pharmaceuticals and consumer protection,* report by the UNCTAD Secretariat (TD/B/C.6/AC.5/4), 15 December 1981, p.13.

73   Aspirin, chlorpromazine, ferrous sulphate, piperazine, analgin (aspirin + phenacetin + caffe –ine + codeine phosphate).

74   Advertisement appeared, for example, in *Indian Express,* 29 December 1980, and *India Today,* 1-15 February 1981.

75   Theo Fergusson, Manager Quality Control Laboratory, Lesotho Dispensary Association, personal communication, 2 July 1980.

76   WHO, *NIEO and Health,* Annex 3 (unpublished draft paper), May 1980.

77   WHO, "Quality assurance of drugs in multi-source purchasing", p.22. (unpublished draft 1980)

78   R.K.Menda, President of the Indian Medical Association, "The ethics of the Drug Industry", *Business India,* 7-20 July 1980.

79   UNCTAD *Case Studies in Transfer of Technology: Pharmaceutical Products in Sri Lanka,* 1977, op.cit.

80   Bangladesh *Prescriber's Guide 79,* pp.19-20.

81   UNCTC, 1979, op.cit.

82   Pharmacist J.V. Tapster, letter to the *Daily Telegraph,* 13 December 1979.

83   UNCTAD, *Case Studies in the Transfer of Technology: Pharamceutical policies in Sri Lanka,* 1977, op.cit.

84   UNCTC, "Case Study on India", draft report on "Transnational Corporations in the pharmaceutical industry of developing countries", 9 February 1981.

85   WHO Regional Office for the Western Pacific, Reference Document for the Technical Presentation on "National Drug Policies and Management", (WPR/RC28/TP/1) 22 July 1977.

86   Dr. Hye, personal communication, 20 April 1982.

87   Hearing before the Subcommittee on Monopoly of the Select Committee on Small Business, US Senate, 93rd Congress, Second Session, on Present Status of Competition in the Pharmaceutical Industry. Evidence sub- mitted by the American Public Health Association supporting the report on antisubstitution laws (laws requiring a pharmacist not to substitute a generic equivalent for a product named in a prescription). Quoted by Gish and Feller, 1979, op.cit.

88   The *Daily Telegraph,* 3 December 1979, "Drug Factories make one product for sale at two prices". Subsequently the Chairman of one of the companies, Arthur H. Cox and Co., wrote to the *Telegraph* supporting the arguments (15 December). But the Chairman of Thomas Kerfoot and Co. Ltd. wrote retracting his earlier statement that they manufactured Valium and Indocid on behalf of the brand-name producers.

89   UNIDO, op.cit.

90   WHO, *National Policies and Practices in regard to medical products: and related international problems,* 1978, op.cit.

91   Von Grebmer, op.cit., p.18.

92   Barnet and Muller, op.cit.

93   The Monopolies Commission, Chlordiazepoxide and Diazepam - *A Report on the supply of Chlordiazepoxide and Diazepam,* HMSO, London 1973.

94   Dr. Hye in interview with the author, 20 October 1980.

95   CIF prices per Kg of tetracycline (period July 1979-June 1980):

K.D.H. Lab	Taka	444
Pfizer	Taka	800
Squibb	Taka	1,440

But Pfizer has also paid comparatively higher prices, e.g. Taka 1,280 for oxytetracycline (per Kg CIF) compared to Taka 610 paid by local manufacturer, Albert David.

96   R. Bower, Managing Director Squibb of Bangladesh Ltd., personal communication, 3 May 1982.

97   CIF prices per kg for trimethoprim: Square - Taka 1,700 ICI (for Wellcome) - Taka 9,000. Dr. Arnold Worlock, Group Marketing Director, The Wellcome Foundation Ltd., comments: "On the subject of your query relating to the sale of trimethoprim in Bangladesh, we are fully aware that trimethoprim may now be purchased from sources other than the Wellcome Foundation Ltd., at prices which are considerably lower than our own. Our price includes necessarily an R & D cost element which does not arise in the case of trimethoprim which is shipped by companies that have not had to sustain over many years, technical and marketing risks in the discovery and development of the product. (No doubt you know that the cost of discovering and developing a new pharmaceutical substance is now estimated at £35 million or more.) Our price includes of course the stamp of Wellcome's quality control, which may not be available in all the cheap imitations of brand-name products whose patents have run out." (Personal communication, 28 May 1982.)

98   Dr. Hye, whilst Director, Drug Administration Bangladesh, in interview with the author, Delhi, 20 October 1980. Wellcome were compelled to reduce the price of trimethoprim from Taka 9000 to Taka 7700 per kg. "after a lot of argument and a few long-distance phone calls". (Dr. Hye, personal communication, 20 April 1982) Septrin (cotrimoxazole BP) is a combination of trimethoprim (80mg) and sulphamethoxazole (400mg).

99   CIF prices per kg. for levamisole:
Opsonin   Taka   1,081
Square   Taka   2,422
I C I   Taka   5,400

100   Peter Cunliffe, ICI Pharmaceuticals Division, personal communication, 11 February 1982.

101   Ibid.

102   Dr. Hye, personal communication, 20 April 1982.

103   Dr. Hye in interview with the author, 20 October 1980.

104   Comparative prices during 1979/80 (all per kg CIF) for Metronidazole:
Chemist Lab   Taka   266
Square   Taka   775
B P I   Taka   1,395

May and Baker tell us they are supplying metronidazole to Bangladesh at a price as low as they can afford in relation to UK production costs which are not comparable with those of Eastern Europe or China. (Mr. Washburton and Mr. Walker, in interview with author, 5 July 1982.)

105   - Import prices per kg CIF:

B P I   Taka   648
Therapeutics   Taka   1,680
from Cyanamid

The Drug Administration released the first consignment of 38 kg with a severe warning and the company subsequently reduced its price to Taka 1,100. (Dr Hye, personal communication, 20 April 1982.)

- Cyanamid advise us that they no longer supply this raw material to Bangladesh, "therefore comment with respect to purchase requirements from Therapeutics are no longer relevant". (Mrs Barri M. Blauvelt, Area Manager Far East Medical Products, American Cyanamid Company, personal communication, 17 May 1982.)

106   Dr Hye, "Drug Policy and Management". (undated mimeo based on a report prepared earlier for WHO)

222

107   *Procurement and manufacture of drugs for use in primary health care in Bangladesh,* May 1979, report of the study team recruited by the World Bank for the Government of the People's Republic of Bangladesh. "The relatively very high costs of some medicines produced commercially in Bangladesh is striking." (p.12)

108   Ibid.

109   -   *SCRIP,* No. 674, 10 March 1982, p.1.
          -    Brand name products make up just over 90% of medicines prescribed by GPs in the UK (excluding hospital sales) (P. F. Lumley, ABPI, personal communication, 21 June 1982)

110   Office of Health Economics, *Health Care Research Expenditure,* Briefing No. 6, June 1978.

CHAPTER 5

1   ABPI, "Code of Practice for the Pharmaceutical Industry", Fifth Edition (December 1978), para.15.1, *Data Sheet Compendium 1979-80* 1979.

2   Including in 1980, Glaxo, Merck Sharp & Dohme, Nicholas, Reckitt & Colman and Wellcome (*MIMS Middle East,* Volume 11, Number 2, 1980).

3   Merck Sharp & Dohme advise us in 1982 "The Mohdar Corporation, as you mention, distributes our products; it does not, we are assured, hire a ' 'part-time ' ' salesman to promote (our) products. Rather, representation is made by Merck employees who are well trained and carefully supervised. Merck has a large, worldwide organisation and for a distributor to be the Company's surrogate with physicians would certainly be the exception rather than the rule. The Company, cannot however, always provide professional representation where it operates through distributors, as in Yemen. In all arrangements with distributors, an agreement to comply with Merck standards is an important stipulation of the contract. Merck field and headquarters executives know these distributors well and visit them periodically to have first-hand knowledge of their operations. The training given to Company representatives is intensive and detailed..." "No system that we know of is infallible, which is why we took immediate steps to investigate the situation suggested by your letter." (John Stuart, Executive Director Public Affairs, Merck, Sharp & Dohme, 18 March 1982.) At the time of going to press, we have no response from Glaxo to this case specifically raised with them by letter on 20 January 1982.

4   Andras November, *Les Medicaments et le Tiers Monde,* Collection Centre Europe Tiers-Monde, (ed) Pierre Mariel Favre, 1981, p.157.

5   ABPI, "Code of Practice for the Pharmaceutical Industry", op.cit., Introduction, para d.

6   UNCTC, *Transnational Corporations and the Pharmaceutical Industry,* (ST/CTC/9), United Nations, New York, 1979. p.47 Some estimates suggest that marketing costs may be higher than 20% and more or less equal to actual production costs:

     Production: 30%   Trades promotion   11%
                              Sales   10%
                              Advertising   8%

                              TOTAL   29%

     (Plus research 10%,general overheads 15%, profit 16%.) Figures quoted by Charles Levinson, Secretary General International Federation of Chemical and General Workers Unions, "The Multinational Pharmaceutical Industry". (mimeo)

7   Dorit Braun, "Pharmaceutical Transnationals in Colombia", Chapter 8 of unpublished PhD thesis 1980. Figures are based on the estimated marketing expenditure of foreign firms (including 3 national firms with small sales volume) and health budgets 1971-1974. Marketing costs as % of health budget ranged between 46% and 55%. Estimated marketing expenditure taken as 26% of sales on the basis of a 1970 study by AFIDRO (industry representative body) - verified for costs of 10 foreign companies 1972/3 by Braun.

8   Wilfred Lionel and Andrew Herxheimer, "Coherent Policies on Drugs: Formulation and Implementation", in Blum, Herxheimer, Stenzl and Woodcock (ed), *Pharmaceuticals and Health Policy,* International Research Group for Drug Legislation and Programs, Croom Helm, London 1981, p.247.

9   S. Bethoud, "Profil de prescription en Suisse romande et au Tessin: analyse de 2006 ordonnences medicales" in *Journal Suisse de Medicine,* 109, No. 3, 1979, pp. 1194-1200, quoted in November, op.cit., p.157.

10   Lionel and Herxheimer, op.cit.

11   Dr. Burley, Head of International Medical Liaison, Ciba-Geigy, personal communication, "Comments on your list of requests to companies" attached to letter of 21 May 1981.

12   ABPI, "Code of Practice for the Pharmaceutical Industry", op.cit., p.vii (3.3).

13   *ABPI News,* No. 177, October 1979.

14   Professor M. D. Rawlins, University of Newcastle and advisor to Committee on Safety of Medicines, in interview with the author, 31 March 1982.

15   Dr. U.K. Sheth, quoted by Shiranand Karkal (winner of Rajika Kripalani Young Journalist's award, doing internship Kem Hospital, Bombay) "Drugging the Indian", article in *Debonair,* October 1980.

16   "Merck in Bangladesh, Marketing Plan 1980(-1982)", dated December 1979 (forwarded to E. Merck, West Germany with letter from Merck Emedia Export Co. m.b.H. Bangladesh Branch of 22 January 1980) p.11.

17   Ibid., pp.11 and 17.

18   Ibid., p.11, and from p.8: "3.4 SEGMENTATION OF DOCTORS

	Total 1978	Important visited	Actually to be visited	Planned estimated 1980	Total
G P	7,500	3,800	2,000	2,500	8,000
Specialists	500	400	250	300	700
TOTAL	8,000	4,200	2,250	2,800	8,700
Students	3,000	-	-	-	3,500

Medical opinion: British."

19   Ibid., p.29. Average sales proceeds per man/per year: 1978 DM 145,000(and 1981: DM250). Average cost/per representative per month 1978 DM 550. Average cost per call DM 3.20.

20   Dr. J.S. Yudkin, MRCP, Senior Lecturer in Medicine, Faculty of Medicine, University of Dar-es-Salaam, "To Plan is to Choose" 1978, p.9. (mimeo)

21   -   Jasper Woodcock, Director, Institute for the Study of Drug Dependence, "Medicines - the Interested Parties" in Blum, et al., op. cit., p.31.
     -   Milton Silverman and Mia Lydecker, "The Promotion of Prescription Drugs and other Puzzles", in Ibid., p.86. Guatemala, Mexico and Brazil, ratio 1:3.
     -   Dr. J.S. Yudkin, "The Economics of Pharmaceutical supply in Tanzania". (undated mimeo)
     -   UNCTAD *Technology policies in the Pharmaceutical sector in Nepal,* (UNCTAD/TT/34), United Nations 1980, p.13. ("Altogether therefore, there are 70 full-time and about 70-80 part-time detailmen employed by the private sector to promote its products to approximately 400 doctors. The main activity of these representatives is to visit the doctors with samples and brochures. It is estimated that some doctors with a large private practice in Kathmandu are visited by an average of three to four detailmen daily. There is no Government control on promotional activity by drug companies.")

22   R.J. Ledogar, *Hungry for Profits,* US Food and Drug Multinationals in Latin America, IDOC/North America Inc., New York, 1975.

23   Rajendra Shaw, Centre for Development Communication, Hyderabad, letter to Jeff Alderson, OXFAM Field Director for S. India, 13 August 1981.

24   Hathi Committee, *Report of the Committee on Drugs and Pharmaceutical Industry,* Government of India, Ministry of Petroleum and Chemicals, April 1975, p.87.

25   Barry Cohen, Pharmacist, Holy Rosary Hospital, Emekuku, Nigeria, Letter to Richtie Coggan, BBC, London, 23 July 1979.

26   D.E. Frizel, Laboratory Technician, Bo Government Hospital, Sierra Leone, personal communication, 28 August 1980.

27   Dr. Paul Nicholson, Searle Research and Development (UK), personal communication, 25 March 1982: "Water absorption in the small intestine is linked to sodium absorption. There are several mechanisms by which sodium is absorbed, of which glucose-facilitated sodium transport is most important for successful rehydration by the oral route. The concentration of glucose in the oral solution is of fundamental importance in optimising sodium transport. Solutions with low concentrations of glucose provide inadequate supplies for transport processes. High concentrations may lead to a reverse of the desired effect. Nevertheless, some believe that glucose must be present in adequate quantities to have nutritional value also. In addition, although the glucose and sodium are absorbed in equimolar concentrations, many paediatricians have been concerned that the administration of too much sodium can lead to hypernatraemia in some infants."

CONCENTRATION OF 3 DIFFERENT PREPARATIONS:

	WHO	REHIDRAT	BNF
Sugar	111	188	200
Sodium	90	50	35
Potassium	20	20	20
Chlorine	80	50	37
Bicarbonate	30	20	18
(Nicholson)			

28   Ibid.

29   Maurice King, Felicity King, Soebagio Martodipoero, *Primary Child Care,* A Manual for health workers, Book One, Oxford Medical Publications, OUP, 1980, p.120.

30   Dr. Tim Lusty, OXFAM Medical Adviser, in interview with the author, April 1982. The UNICEF price for a sachet to make up 1 litre of the WHO solution is $0.07 a sachet (*UNIPAC catalogue/Price List* 1982,UN children's Fund Supply Division Package and Assembly Centre, Copenhagen.)

31   Noor Mohammed, Senior Field Organiser, E. Merck, in interview with the author, Rajshahi, 29 September 1980.

32   A.N.P. Speight, MRCP, "Cost effectiveness and drug therapy", *Tropical Doctor,* April 1975.

33   IFPMA, Statement to the 32nd World Health Assembly, Geneva, 7-25 May 1979, item 2.7.2 on the subject of the WHO Action Programme on Essential Drugs.

34   IFPMA, "The IFPMA code of Pharmaceutical Marketing Practice", March 1981 (amended March 1982).

35   WHO, *Prophylactic and Therapeutic Substances,* Report by the Director General, 28th World Health Assembly, WHO, (A 28/11), 3 April 1978.

36   Letter from Barry Cohen, op.cit.

37   Noor Mohammed, op. cit.

38   Drs. Mehrhof and Niederehe, E. Merck, Darmstadt, West Germany, personal communication, 29 March 1982.

39   "Merck in Bangladesh", op.cit., p.17.

40   Ibid., p.27.

41   Ibid., p.22.

42   M.D. Rawlins, Professor of Clinical Pharmacology, Head of Department of Pharmacological Sciences, University of Newcastle, personal communication, 17 September 1981.

43   Drs. Mehrhof and Niederehe, op. cit.

44   Dr. Milton Silverman, *The Drugging of the Americas,* Berkeley and Los Angeles, University of California Press, 1976.

45   Silverman and Lydecker, in Blum, et al., op.cit., p.86.

46   Ibid.

47   Ibid., p.85.

48   Dr. Milton Silverman, personal communication, 10 August 1981.

49   The anomalies are documented in Milton Silverman, Philip Lee and Mia Lydecker, *Prescriptions for Death - the Drugging of the Third World,* University of California, Berkeley, 1982.

50   S. Redfern, Roche Products Limited, Attachment 1 "Product Information Leaflets" with particular reference to Mogadon and Valium in Thailand, personal communication, 4 May 1982.

51   Ibid. The current Thai Valium leaflet now includes a "Tolerance " paragraph, and the following "Precautions ": "(1) It may cause abnormality to the blood cells, liver and kidneys. (2) It should not be used during the first trimester pregnancy. (3) It may cause drowsiness. While taking this medicine, the patient should not drive nor operate machinery. (4) While taking this medicine, avoid alcohol, or drink or medicine containing alcohol." And the following warning: "It may cause habituation and be hazardous. It must be used according to the physician's instructions."

52   -   ABPI, *Data Sheet Compendium 1979-80,* 1979 op.cit., p.362.
        -    G. Potter, Group Public Relations Manager, Glaxo, personal communication, 16 June 1982.

53   Ibid., p.356. We have no comments from Glaxo on why these leaflets were issued without precautions on use.

54   The *British National Formulary,* 1981 (Volume 1) lists the following cautions for use of the combined Oestrogen-progestogen pills: diabetes, hypertension, cardiac or renal disease, migraine, epilepsy, depression, asthma, multiple sclerosis, wearing of contact lenses, cigarette-smoking, obesity, and drug interactions. Contra-indications: thrombosis and history of thrombo-embolic disease, recurrent jaundice, chronic liver disease, sickle-cell anaemia, hyperlipidaemia, mammary or endrometrial carcinoma, severe migraine, undiagnosed vaginal bleeding. And side-effects: nausea, vomiting, headache, breast tenderness, changes in body weight, changes in libido, depression, chloasma, hypertension, impairment of liver function, benign hepatic tumours, reduced menstrual loss, 'spotting' in early cycles, amenorrhoea. (p.210).

55   Government of the People's Republic of Bangladesh, Ministry of Health and Population Control (Health Division) Drugs Administration, "Requirements for Registration of New

and Unintroduced Medicines'', (undated), collected September 1980. Also form for "Application for Approval of Recipe of Pharmaceutical Preparation''.

56   ABPI, 1979, op.cit., p.369. Also comment on Cytamen current indications in Bangladesh from Geoffrey Potter, Group Public Relations Manager, Glaxo, personal communication, 16 June 1982.

57   *British National Formulary,* 1981, op.cit., p.225.

58   A.H. Goodspeed, MB BS MRCS LRCP Dip.Pharm.Med, personal communication, 2 April 1981.

59   Professor M.D. Rawlins, op.cit.

60   Ibid.

61   Drs. Mehrhof and Niederehe, op. cit. p.3.

62   Ibid.

63   "Merck in Bangladesh'', op.cit., p.15: daily cost of treatment with Neurobion (actual prices 31/12/79) Taka 11.88.

64   ABPI, 1979, para 17.2.p.x.

65   Dr. J.Z. Galvez-Tan, Personal communication, 2 May 1980. (Promotion observed in Samer and Leyte provinces and documented February 1980.)

66   Ibid. (Promotion in the Davao-Cotabato area, documented April 1980).

67   Ibid.

68   Dr. J.Z. Galvez-Tan, "Medical Plants: an alternative to the rising costs of medicines''. (mimeo)

69   Dr. Satoto, Semarang, personal communication, 25 June 1980.

70   Dr. Humayun K.M. Hye, personal communication, 10 August 1981.

71   For instance, in Bangladesh senior doctors, some of them professors in the government medical colleges, are shareholders of Pfizer and ICI. ICI comment: "It is not ICI's policy to encourage doctors in Bangladesh or in any other country to become shareholders. It is probable that amongst the 700,000 shareholders of ICI loan and equity stock some will be members of the medical profession.'' (P. Cunliffe, Chairman, Pharmaceuticals Division, 11 February 1982.)

    PFIZER advise us: "... it is not Pfizer's policy to encourage persons to become shareholders. We do not believe that it is our function to render investment advice to doctors or any other segment of the public. The situation in Bangladesh resulted from Pfizer's application to the Government (then Pakistan) a number of years ago, for the opening of a manufacturing branch in East Pakistan. The Government, in an effort to encourage local investment, granted approval of the project conditional upon a certain portion of the equity being allotted to members of the medical profession in East Pakistan.'' (M. W. Hodin, Director of Public Affairs, Pfizer, personal communication, 17 March 1982.)

72   Dilip Thakore, "The Ethics of the Drug Industry'', *Business India,* 7-20 July 1980.

73   Dr Hassani, private doctor and director of Norwegian Save-the-Children Fund Clinic, Ibb, in interview with the author, September 1980.

74   Anthony Hall, OXFAM Field Director, Recife, Brazil, personal communication, 10 June 1980.

75   Anne Ferguson, Department of Anthropology, Michigan State University, "The effects of source of supply of medications on health care services dispensed in pharmacies in a Salvadoran town'', paper presented at the Central States Anthropology Society, 56th Annual Meetings held in Ann Arbor, Michigan, April 9-12, 1980. (mimeo)

76   Ibid.

77   Dr. John S. Yudkin, "The Economics of Pharmaceutical Supply in Tanzania", *International Journal of Health Services,* Volume 10, number 3, 1980, p.460. In April 1982, in response to our enquiry, a spokesman of A.H. Robbins in Richmond, Virginia, US, advised us by telephone that a company executive was due to visit Tanzania and would look into the matter. The *British National Formulary* (1981) commen?s on cough expectorants like *Robitussin* (guaiphenesin): "There is no evidence that any drug given by mouth has specific action in promoting expectoration of bronchial secretions by stimulation or augmentation of the cough reflex... There is thus no scientific basis for prescribing these arugs although a harmless expectorant mixture may have a useful role as a placebo." (p.93) Prof. Peter Parish puts it more forcefully: guaiphenesin etc. "are present in many cough medicines and from the point of view of effectiveness you may as well choose them by taste or colour." (*Medicines,* A Guide for Everybody, Penguin, 1981, p.103). Regarding *Dimotane* (containing 4 drugs including an antihistamine and expectorant and sympathomimetic) the BNF comments: "Combinations such as expectorant and cough supressant, sympathomimetic and sedative, and any or all of these with other types of drug such as antihistamines are to be *deprecated.* " (p.95 original emphasis)

78   For example in Britain the ABPI "Code of Practice for the Pharmaceutical Industry", op.cit., includes 5 paragraphs of guidelines and restrictions on the distribution of samples. Para.16.1 states: "Except when provided for indentification or demonstration purposes, samples should only be supplied in response to a signed request from a doctor...When samples are provided to assist doctors in the recognition or identification of a product...only the minimum quantity necessary for this purpose should be supplied."

79   Hathi Committee, op.cit.

80   Paul E. Jenkins, UNAIS, Sahel Region Upper Volta, personal communication, 1 December 1981 (OXFAM Project VOL 114).

81   For example, stock at Ahmed Alhadry's Sandileer, the local pharmacy in Al Jabin, included 10 free samples, including Upjohn's Erythromycin, Boehringer's Gynaecosid, Warner & Co's (UK) Sinutab Decongestant, Dumex's antidepressive Imiprex, Knoll's Osadrin and others from Italian manufacturers. (Check made on 22 June 1980 by members of the British Organisation for Community Development Health Team.)

82   Government of the Yemen Arab Republic, "Fourth Annual Report on the Activities of the Supreme Board for Medicines and Medical Equipment during 1979", (translated from the Arabic) and as reported in *The Lancet,* 4 July 1981. Whilst waiting to see the WHO representative in Sana'a, September 1980, we observed a member of staff being given a free sample of an Asthma spray for a sore throat.

83   Dr. John Yudkin, "To plan is to choose", 1979. (mimeo)

84   Dr. Ann Hoskins, British Organisation for Community Development, Discussion paper from the BHS Drug Committee on the problems of drugs in Yemen, May 1981.

85   Priscilla Annamanthodo, OXFAM, "Medicines in Upper Volta", research paper, Ouagadougòu, October 1980. (mimeo)

86   S. Redfern, Roche Products Ltd., attachment to personal communication, 4 May 1982.

87   Professor Nurul Islam, in interview with the author, 6 October 1980.

88   ABPI, 1979, op.cit. Organon products, p.730.

89   *British National Formulary,* 1981, op.cit., p.159.

90   Dr. Sultana Khanum, paediatrician, SCF Children's Nutrition Unit, Dacca, in interview with the author, 24 September 1980.

91   ICSSR/ICMR, *Health for All - An Alternative Strategy,* 1981, p.179.

92   UNCTAD, *Technology policies and planning for the pharmaceutical sector in the developing countries,* (TD/B/C.6/56) United Nations, 1980.

93   Dr. Hassani, private doctor and director of Norwegian SCF Clinic, Ibb, in interview with the author, September 1980.

94   Nurul Islam, op.cit.

CHAPTER 6

1   Dr. Sultana Khanum, paediatrician, SCF Children's Nutrition Unit, Dacca, in interview with the author, 24 September 1980.

2   Letter from Dr. Cliff David, CIIR doctor, at the Mother and Child Health Centre, Sana'a, to CIIR London office, (PM/140) undated.

3   David Werner, personal communication, 20 July 1981.

4   Anne Ferguson, Department of Anthropology, Michigan State University, "The Role of Pharmaceuticals in the process of medicalization in Asuncion, El Salvador", paper delivered at the 1980 American Anthropological Association Meetings held in Washington, DC, 2-7 December. (mimeo)

5   A. Giovanni, *A Questao dos Remedios no Brasil,* Polis, Sao Paulo, 1980, quoted by Mike Muller, *The Health of Nations,* A North-South Investigation, Faber and Faber, 1982, p.111.

6   David Werner, seminar for OXFAM staff, OXFAM House, Oxford, 8 September 1981.

7   Sjaak van der Geest, University of Amsterdam, "The Efficiency of Inefficiency: Medicine Distribution in South-Cameroon", paper presented at Seventh International Conference on Social Science and Medicine, Noordwijkerhout, 22-26 June 1981, p.7. (mimeo)

8   Britain-Nepal Medical Trust, Annual Report, 1976. OXFAM File, NP5.

9   Anne Ferguson, "The Effects of Source of Supply of Medications on Health Care Services dispensed in pharmacies in a Salvadoran town", paper presented at the Central States Anthropology Society 56th Annual Meeting held in Ann Arbor, Michigan, 9-12 April 1980, p.31. (mimeo)

10   E. J Fullager, Divisional Manager Sandoz Products Limited quoting Indian colleagues. "The FAO/WHO Expert Group 1962 surveyed the food supplies of various parts of the world and summarised that India had the lowest calcium consumption (347 mg per day). The National Insitutute of Nutrition in India carried out a survey of the dietary habits of Indians and they found that the average daily intake of calcium of Indian children is 300 mg or less (ICMR 1980). The report mentioned that high levels of calcium intake "are not easy to achieve in practice in countries where the dietary calcium is mostly obtained from cereal and other vegetables and only to a lesser extent from milk and milk products ' ". (Personal communication, 9 June 1982.) This does not mean that health depends on calcium-intakes as high as Europe and North America (930 mg France; 1116 mg USA; highest: 1329 mg Finland). On high consumption, less is absorbed. "On a dietary intake of 600 to 1000 mg a normal adult absorbs about half the ingested calcium and net absorption varies little over this range. When calcium intakes fall below 500 mg adaptive mechanisms increase the proportion which is absorbed. In severe calcium restriction the efficiency of absorption can reach up to 70 to 80%..." (Dr G. J. Ebrahim, "The Problems of Undernutrition", *Nutrition and Disease,* in R. J. Jarrett (ed), Croom Helm London, 1979, p.105.) 11 Fullager, op.cit.

12   Whole cow's milk representative values for nutrients (per 100g of edible portion): Calories: 64, Protein: 3.3, Fat 3.6, Carbohydrate 4.7, Iron 0.1, vitamin A potency approx. 150, Thiamine 0.04, Riboflavin 0.15, Nicotinamide 0.1, Ascorbic acid 1.0 (B.S. Platt, *Tables of representative values of foods commonly used in tropical countries,* Liverpool School of Tropical Medicine, reprinted 1982, pp.26-27.)

229

Chapter 6

13 - Platt, op.cit.
   - Ebrahim, op.cit.,p.105.
14 - Brudon, op.cit.
   - David Werner in interview with Adrian Moyes, OXFAM Public Affairs Unit, 30 June 1980.

15 Solomon Agnew, Central Planning Office, Ethiopia, "Drug Business and its implication on the Development of Health Services in Ethiopia", part I paper presented at Institute of Development Research Seminar on Strategies for Socialist Rural Transformation in Ethiopia, Nazreth, 27-29 October 1978, p.11. (mimeo)

16 *British National Formulary 1981,* Number 1, 1981, p.15.

17 Peter Parish, Professor of Clinical Pharmacy and Director of the Medicines Research Unit, Cardiff, *Medicines,* Penguin, Third Edition, 1981, p.18.

18 Sir John Butterfield, "The contribution of modern medicines", in George Teeling-Smith and Nicholas Wells (ed), *Medicines for the year 2000,* Office of Health Economics, London, 1979, p.30.

19 Milton Silverman and Mia Lydecker, "The Promotion of Prescription Drugs and other puzzles", *Pharmaceuticals and Health Policy,* Blum, Herxheimer, Stenzl and Woodcock (ed), 1981, p.85.

20 Pascale Brudon, "L'Industrie Pharmaceutique Suisse dans les Pays Sous - developpes", Memoire presente pour le diplome de recherche en etudes de developpement, Institut Universitaire d'Etudes de Developpement, Geneva, 1981, p.192.

21 Ferguson, April 1980, op.cit., p.8.

22 - Cee-NU *British National Formulary 1981* op.cit., pp.213-214.
   - *SCRIP* No. 639 (2 November 1981) p.11 and No. 670 (24 February 1982) p.9.

23 Purchased Cee-NU 4 October 1980. Black market price of 2 capsules Taka 350 (£9.72) - This is only one of many prescription drugs that can be bought on the black market.

24 For example: "Widely divergent views and requirements of regulatory authorities often make it impossible to maintain our international standard and therefore, when starting to compare product information in different countries it is inevitable that deviations are noted ... Unfortunately again, there are as far as medical standards are concerned, in many instances no strict criteria as a result of transcultural differences .." (Dr T. Vossenaar, Organon, personal communication, 23 April 1982.)

25 For example a conversation between participants at the Mario Negri Institute in Milan in June 1981 revealed the very different thinking over painkillers in Europe. In Britain aspirin and paracetamol, are sold over the counter, but phenacetin and dipyrone have been removed from the market. But dipyrone is widely used in W. Germany. Italy considers the risks of kidney damage from phenacetin as less of a problem than the dangers of overdose of paracetamol.

26 WHO, *Treatment and Prevention of Dehydration in Diarrhoeal Disease* (A Guide for use at the Primary Level), WHO, Geneva, 1976.

27 King, King and Martodipoero, *Primary Child Care,* A manual for health workers, Oxford University Press, 1978, p.129.

28 Ibid.

29 Both Ciba-Geigy and Searle agree there is a problem. Dr. Burley, *Ciba-Geigy:* "You are almost certainly right about the unconsidered use of clioquinol in children, particularly young children where diarrhoea needs to be treated with fluid replacement and proper food. I will look into exactly what we say about the use of clioquinol in young children now. " (Personal communication, 23 February 1982.) But Ciba's package insert (dated 21 December 1981), forwarded by Dr. Burley on 12 March 1982, contains *no warning* about the importance of oral rehydration in treating children. Package inserts for *Searle's* Lomotil purchased in Egypt

in 1982 contain no warnings about oral rehydration. But Dr. Nicolson of G. D. Searle writes: "We have agreed that the importance of replenishng fluid and salts in the treatment of diarrhoea particularly in children is something which should be further emphasised in our literature (advertising, package inserts, etc.) It is true that the problem of dehydration in the context of diarrhoea may not be fully appreciated by physicians in private or public health practice. While we may help in the educational process by providing responsible information, the problem is one which must be tackled fundamentally in professional medical education on a worldwide basis." (Personal communication, 25 March 1982.)

30   ABPI, *Data Sheet Compendium, 1979-80,* p.936.

31   "Lomotil for Diarrhoea in Children", *The Medical Letter,* (25, 1975) p.104, quoted by Charles Medawar and Barbara Freese, *Drug Diplomacy,* Social Audit Ltd, 1982, pp.12-13.

32   S. M. Uthman, "Some complications of Diphenozylate Hydrochloride with Atropine", *Lebanese Medical Journal,* 27.5, 1974, pp.521-2, quoted by Medawar and Freese, 1982, op.cit., pp.12-13.

33   G. Upunda, J. Yudkin and G. Brown, *Therapeutic Guidelines,* (A Manual to assist in the rational purchase and prescription of drugs), African Medical and Research Foundation (AMREF), Nairobi, 1980, p.96, quoted in ibid.

34   "Lomotil for Diarrhoea in Children", in *The Medical Letter,* 25, 1975, p.104, quoted in ibid.

35   M. E. Drake and M. E. Drake Jr., "Lomotil Intoxication in Pediatric Patients", *J. Med. Soc. New Jersey,* June 1974, pp.501-2, quoted in ibid.

36   Ibid., p.8.

37   ABPI, *Data Sheet Compendium 1979-80,* p.936.

38   Medawar and Freese, op.cit., p.16.

39   -   *British National Formulary 1981,* No. 1, op. cit., p.40.
     -   WHO, 1976, op. cit.

40   *SCRIP,* No 630, 30 September, 1981, p.11.

41   AMREF, 1980, quoted by Medawar and Freese, op. cit., pp.12-13 Worldwide Sales of Lomotil in 1981 totalled $31.2 million (*SCRIP* 684, 14 April 1982).

42   Medawar and Freese, op.cit.

43   "You have raised the question of communicating information to the illiterate. This problem we presume, is not one which confronts only Searle or the pharmaceutical industry. Your practical suggestions will be welcomed and considered." (Dr. Nicholson, Searle Research and Development (UK), personal communication, 25 March 1982.)

44   Dr. Olle Hansson, "Is Entero-Vioform a killer drug?", *New Scientist,* 23 November 1978.

45   -   Parish, op. cit., p.137.
     -   Hansson, op. cit.

46   ICADIS News, No 1, Information Centre Against Drug-Induced Sufferings, Japan, November 1981.

47   -   Hansson, op. cit.
     -   Prof. Rawlins of Committee of Safety of Medicines, in interview with the author, 31 March 1982.

48   -   *British National Formulary 1981.* Unigreg's Unidiarea (125 mg clioqunol and 200 mg neomycin sulphate).
     -   UK *MIMS,* February 1980.

49   WHO, *Drug Information Bulletin,* WHO, Geneva, January-March 1978.

50   -   Dr. D. M. Burley, Head of International Medical Liaison, Ciba-Geigy, Horsham, England, personal communication 4 February 1982.

Chapter 6

- Silverman, Lee and Lydecker, *Prescriptions for Death, The Drugging of the Third World,* University of California Press, 1982, pp.44-58.

51   Dr. D. M. Burley, personal communication, 21 May 1981.

52   - Dr Sayeed Hyder (ed), *The Prescriber's Guide, '79,* June 1979. Dose: Adults 1-2 tablets thrice daily (250 mg clioquinol x 6 / 1500 mg daily x 7 / 10.5 gms.)
      - "An investigation by Professor Tadao Tsubaki established that 96 per cent of the SMON patients in the sample had taken oxyquinoline. He also found that neurological symptoms generally began to appear when a total dose of 10 to 50 grammes had been reached, and that the time span between the taking of oxyquinoline and the beginning of neurological symptoms was 50 days at a daily dose of 600 mg and 30 days at a daily dose of 1200 mg oxyquinoline, that a larger dose tended to produce a more severe patho-logical picture." (Hansson, op.cit.)

53   - *The Lancet,* Editorial 28 May 1977:.. "the companies deny that the neurological damage from clioquinol is a serious risk outside Japan. This denial is unconvincing because cases of clioquinol damage have been observed outside Japan, and identical abnormalities of the nervous system have been reproduced in animals."
      - *The Lancet,* 2 September 1978: "A quiet change in the indications is not enough. Drug regulatory authorities, manufacturers and distributors ... should now emphasise to the public that these drugs should no longer be used for ... non-specific diarrhoeas." (From: Social Audit leaflet on clioquinol: "Bad information means Bad Medicine..", 1981.)

54   Mr A. Wahid, Managing Director of Fisons Bangladesh quoted in "Crisis in the Drug Industry", *Robbar,* 1 June 1980, Dacca - cited by Dr. Zafrullah Chowdhury, "Essential Drugs for the Poor: Myth and Reality in Bangladesh", paper presented at the Primary Health Care Symposium, Liverpool School of Tropical Medicine, 13-16 April 1982. (mimeo)

55   Prof. G. Peters, University of Lausanne, "Information and Education about Drugs", in Blum et al. (ed), op.cit., pp.105-106.

56   Mohammed Nurul Alam, Marketing Manager, Fisons (Bangladesh) Limited, in interview with the author, 26 September 1980.

57   Ferguson, 2-7 December 1980, op. cit., p.9.

58   Ibid., pp. 15-16.

59   *British National Formulary,* 1981, op.cit., p.201.

60   H. R. Gribbin, S.G. Flavell Matts, "Mode of Action and Use of Anabolic Steroids", *The British Journal of Clinical Practice,* Vol. 30 No. 1, January 1976, pp.3-9.

61   Ibid.

62   Parish, op.cit., p.201.

63   *British National Formulary* 1981, op.cit., p.201.

64   Gribbin, Flavell Matts, op.cit., p.9.

65   Text of advertisement distributed in Bangladesh.

66   Dr. Martin Schweiger, Rangpur Dinajpur Rehabilitation Service, personal communication, 28 September 1980.

67   Organon (Bangladesh) Limited, *Therapeutic Index,* undated.

68   ABPI 1979, op.cit., p.730.

69   Dr. R.J. Bloemen, Organon, personal communication, 21 December 1981.

70   "Organon Product Safeguards" re: Orabolin tablets and drops. The revised therapeutic index has not been received at the time of going to press, June 1982. Four months after Organon advised us of their intention to revise the entry for Orabolin, we were informed: "The entry

in the Therapeutic Index should be corrected, including incorporation of side-effects and contra-indications. As soon as this has been printed I will send you a copy." (Dr. T. Vossenaar, Organon, personal communication, 23 April 1982.)

71   ABPI, 1979, op.cit., p.1013.

72   *British National Formulary 1981,* op.cit., p.201.

73   P. W. Cunliffe, Chairman Pharmaceuticals Division, ICI, personal communication, 11 February 1982.

74   Dr. D. M. Burley, Ciba-Geigy, personal communication, 1 April 1982.

75   -   Ciba-Geigy statement on aminophenazone (amidopyrine) *SCRIP* No. 666, 10 February 1982, p.14.
        -    Dr. D. M. Burley, Ciba-Geigy, personal communication, 4 February 1982.
        -    Silverman, Lee and Lydecker, op.cit., p.60.

76   -   Dr. Burley, personal communication 4 February 1982.
        -    Dr. G. R. Venning, "Validity of anecdotal reports of suspected adverse drug reactions: the problem of false alarms", *British Medical Journal,* Volume 284, 23 January 1982,. p.250.

77   -   The withdrawal of amidopyrine was recommended "because of its ability to form carcinogenic nitrosamines either spontaneously or by interaction with nitrites in food", P. Epstein and J. S. Yudkin, letter to *The Lancet,* 13 August, 1978.
        -    *SCRIP* No. 666, op.cit.
        -    Burley, personal communication 4 February 1982, op.cit.

78   -   Ibid.
        -    Brudon, op.cit., p.236.

79   J. S. Yudkin, letter to *The Lancet,* 14 November 1981, p.1114.

80   Entry for Cibalgin (with aminophenazone) *MIMS Middle East,* Volume 11, Number 2, 1980, p.57.

81   Brudon, op.cit., p.236.

82   Dr. Burley, personal communication, 4 February 1982.

83   -   Ibid.
        -    *SCRIP* No. 666, op. cit.

84   *The Lancet,* 14 November 1981, op.cit.

85   Brudon, op.cit., p.236.

86   *The Lancet,* 14 November 1981, op. cit.

87   -   Ibid.
        -    Personal communication from Stephen de Winter of Belbo Film Productions.

88   Dr. Burley, personal communication, 4 February 1982.

89   "Special Report", *The Hindu,* 6 January 1981.

90   Ibid.

91   *The Lancet,* 2 August 1980, op. cit.

92   Dr. Burley, Ciba-Geigy, personal communication, 12 March 1982. Ciba have stressed that "It is not right to infer that amidopyrine has been dumped in the Third World. On the contrary far more has been sold in the developed world ..." (Burley, personal communication, 4 February 1982, op. cit.)

93   C. M. Huguley, "Agranulocytosis induced by dipyrone, a hazardous antipyretic and analgesic", JAMA 189; 1964, pp.938-941, quoted by J. S. Yudkin," The Economics of Pharmaceutical Supply in Tanzania", *International Journal of Health Services,* Volume 10, Number 3, 1980, pp.455-477.

94 Yudkin, 1980, op. cit. Of course manufacturers do not agree: "Novalgin (dipyrone) is still an irreplaceable analgesic having a wide therapeutic profile encompasing excellent analgesic, spasmolytic, antiinflammatory and antipyretic activity". (Dr R. W. Timmers and Dr C. G. Roepnack, Hoechst, West Germany, personal communication, 22 March 1982.)

95 - "Drugs for Human use containing Dipyrone", *Federal Register,* 1976, quoted in WHO *Drug Information Bulletin,* January-March 1977.
   - *Martindale:* "Its (dipyrone) use is justified only in serious or life-threatening situations where no alternative antipyretic is available or suitable." (p.191)

96 In early 1982 an expert advisory committee proposed that pyrazolone products such as dipyrone should be placed under prescription only regulations. This was subsequently altered to apply to injectables only. (*SCRIP* No. 679, 29 March 1982.) 70 manufacturers and 162 products are affected by the new proposals. Decisions on a further 1,000 plus combination products are awaited (*SCRIP* No. 685, 19 April 1982). Hoechst objection: "The authorities justify these measures by saying that there are grounds for believing that ... metamizole (dipyrone) can cause agranulocytosis and shock. We have repeatedly pointed out that the available data do not in any way justify measures as severe as those the BGA is now requiring. Reliable figures on the - much overestimated - frequency of the adverse reactions will be available next year from the Boston study on agranulocytosis and aplastic anaemia." (*SCRIP* No. 689, 3 May 1982.) Also Timmers and Roepnack, personal communication 22, March 1982, op.cit.

97 Dr. K. Balasubramanian, UNCTAD, "Drug Policies in Third World Countries", paper presented at the International NGO Seminar on Pharmaceuticals, Geneva, 27-29 May 1981.

98 Brudon, op.cit., pp.195-6.

99 Hoechst have sent us the product inserts for Novalgin (for Bangladesh) which contain a warning in red in *English:* "The drug may cause fatal agranulocytosis." From our research drug-sellers had no idea of any safety warnings. 'Agranulocytosis' meant nothing to most.

100 Dr. H.K.M. Hye, while Director Drugs Administration, personal communication, 10 August 1981. Novalgin and other dipyrones are included in the drugs recommended for withdrawal in the 1982 Expert Committee Report: "Evaluation of Registered/Licensed Products and Draft National Drug Policy, May 11, 1982", Dacca, Bangladesh.

101 Priscilla Annamanthodo, OXFAM, "Medicines in Upper Volta", Ouagadougou, 1980. (mimeo)

102 Dr. Tony Klouda, OXFAM Medical Adviser Tanzania, personal communication, 11 September, 1981.

103 - Dr. Hassani, private practitioner and director of Norwegian SCF clinic, Ibb, in inteview with the author, September 1980.
   - Dr. Ann Hoskins, British Organisation for Community Development, discussion paper from the BHS Drug Committee on the problems of drugs in Yemen, May 1981, p.10.

104 Dr. Ann Hoskins, op. cit., p.10.

105 Institute of Development Studies Health Group, *Health Needs and Health Services in Rural Ghana,* Volumes 1 and 2, IDS in collaboration with ISSER, University of Ghana; NHPU, Ministry of Health, Government of Ghana and Department of Community Health, Korle Bu; IDS, Brighton, June 1978.

106 Ibid.

107 - Mohammed Nurul Islam, Fisons (Bangladesh) Marketing Manager, in interview with the author, 26 September 1980.
   - Dr. H.K.M. Hye, personal communication, 10 August 1981.

108 Dr. Mira Shiva, Voluntary Health Association of India, personal communication, 24 August 1981.

109 Dr. Martin Schweiger, "In Sickness or in Wealth", BBC Radio 4, transcript of programme transmitted 26 June 1979.

110 - UNCTAD, *Technology policies in the pharmaceutical sector in Nepal,* 1980, op. cit., p.169.
     - Similarly tonic preparations containing isoniazid and vitamins are on sale in the Philippines - David Werner, in interview with the author, 8 September, 1981.

111 *British National Formulary 1981,* op.cit., pp. 38 and 40.

112 - Sumycin (tetracycline oral suspension) purchased on 28 September 1980 at drug store in Baragharia village, Rajshahi.
     - In Britain tetracycline is contraindicated in pregnancy and for children under twelve. (*British National Formulary 1981,* op.cit., p.159.)
     - "Tetracyclines may cause a yellow to brown discolouration of the teeth in the developing foetus or child..." (ABPI 1979, op.cit., p.467.)

113 The Managing Director of Squibb of Bangladesh Limited writes: "I am puzzled as to why you have singled out Sumycin Syrup as being sold over the counter when most pharmaceuticals in Bangladesh can be purchased in this manner. We in Squibb share your concern about this practice, but regrettably there is little we can do about it .. I would welcome your letting me have the name and address of the dealer you allege recommends Sumycin for young children suffering from diarrhoea in order that we can investigate. *We never have promoted this product for the treatment of diarrhoea.* "(R. Bower, Squibb, personal communication, 3 May 1982.) *Mr. Bower makes no comment on the lack of any warnings on the Sumycin pack or bottle,* but writes: "Since you raise the question of product information in general, I take the opportunity of informing you that Squibb worldwide policy is to place all product facts before doctors. Bangladesh is no exception." (op.cit.)

114 *Prescriber's Guide 79,* op.cit., p.17.

115 *British National Formulary 1981,* op. cit., p.164.

116 Bruce K. Berger, Public Relations Associate, The Upjohn Company, personal communication, 19 March 1982.

117 Brudon, op.cit., p.197. Upjohn comment: "Lincocin sells well in Mexico. But it also sells well in Japan, Italy and other countries. And it sells well because it is an effective, life-saving antibiotic, not because of the magnitude of promotion in any particular country." (Berger, 1982, op.cit.)

118 Package insert for Rivomycin Strepto, manufactured by Rivopharm Laboratories, Manno, Switzerland, purchased in Ibb, North Yemen, September 1980.

119 - *Martindale,* p.1107.
     - *British National Formulary 1981,* op. cit.: "chloramphenicol is a potent, potentially toxic, broad-spectrum antibiotic which should be reserved for the treatment of life-threatening infections..."

120 Dr. E. Tagman and Dr. S. Balluz, Rivopharm SA, Manno, Switzerland, personal communication, 11 February 1982.

121 Drs Tagman and Balluz, personal communications 8 April 1982 and 17 May 1982. Rivomycin Strepto is no longer licensed for sale in Switzerland. Rivopharm comment: "We still consider chloramphenicol and dihydrostretomycin a useful combination in the treatment of intestinal infection with susceptible organisms; but it should only be given under medical supervision." (Personal communication, 17 May 1982, op. cit.)

122 Albert David (Bangladesh) Ltd, *Vademecum,* medical products list. (Current September 1980.

123 - Information from: David Newell, OXFAM Field Director, and Concern Volunteers, Dacca, Bangladesh;
     - Sue Becklerleg, Nutritionist, "Breastfeeding case studies in the town of Ibb". (mimeo

1980) Injections prescribed by the Nasser Hospital ;
Suzanne Williams, OXFAM Field Director, Manaus.

124 Norman S. Lane, WHO Pharmaceutical Services Adviser, Addis Ababa, "A National Drug
Policy: Why and How", (Ferdis Health Station, Hararge Province), November 1977. (mimeo)

125 Shamsud Doha, Pharmacist, Save the Children Fund, Dacca, in interview with the author,
9 October 1980.

126 Annamandthodo, op. cit.

127 Letter from a VSO worker at Institute of Medicine, Kathmandu to Ritchie Coggan, BBC,
London, 5 June 1979.

128 - Gaby Taylor, OXFAM Field Director, Zaire in interview with the author, 1980.
- Annamanthodo, op. cit.

129 - Dr. Abhay Bang, Medico Friend Circle, Gopuri, Wardha, personal communication,
September 1980.
- Bharat Dogra, researcher and journalist, personal communication December 1980,
quoting studies by Dr. K. B. Sharma, the Salmonella Centre at Lady Harding Medical
College, Delhi; Central Research Institute, Kesouli.

130 Prof. Philip Lee, Statement before the sub-committee on Monopoly, Small ?Business
Committee, United States Senate, 26 May, 1976.

131 Dr. C. E. Gordon-Smith, Dean of the London School of Hygiene and Tropical Medicine,
paper delivered at the US Institute of Medicine, National Academy of Sciences, Proceedings
Conference on Pharmaceuticals for Developing Countries, Washington, January 1979.

132 Lee, op. cit.

133 Mike Muller, *The Health of Nations; A North-South Investigation,* Faber and Faber, 1982,
pp.114-115.

CHAPTER 7

1 WHO, "WHO urges a blending of merits between Western and Traditional Medicine", *WHO
Features No. 46,* April 1979.

2 Dr. W. D. Sutherland, "A systems analysis of a rural primary health centre in India including
a study of the integration of indigenous practitioners into the primary health centre", dissertation
for Master of Community Health, Liverpool School of Tropical Medicine, 1978.

3 Ibid.

4 Mrs. Najma Sarwar, social researcher, carrying out survey of patients at SCF Children's
Nutrition Unit, Dacca, in interview with the author, 24 September 1980.

5 Priscilla Annamanthodo, OXFAM, "Medicines in Upper Volta", Ouagadougou, 1980. (mimeo)

6 WHO, op.cit.

7 Dr. H.K.M Hye, "Utilisation of Traditional Medicines in Primary Health Care". (undated
mimeo)

8 WHO, op.cit.

9 Dr. Aziz, International Centre for Diarrhoeal Disease Research, Dacca, in interview with the
author, 8 October 1980.

10 Dr. Tony Klouda, "Prevention is more expensive than cure", a Review of Tanzania's Problems
in Health, 1971-81, July 1981 draft, p.11.

11 WHO, op.cit.

12 Klouda, op.cit.

13   -   Mark Bowden, Director, Save the Children Fund, Bangladesh, in interview with the author, 18 September, 1980.
      -    Dr. Martin Schweiger, personal communication, 13 July 1981.

14   Dr. Dhruv Mankad, "Proposal for the Self-Reliant Alternatives to Western Medicine Project", 7 January 1981, OXFAM file, MAH.87.

15   Dr. Jaime Galvez-Tan, "Medicinal Plants: An alternative to the rising costs of medicines", May 1979. (mimeo)

16   -   Prof. K. N. Udupa, Banaras Hindu University, "The Role of Indian medicine in Primary Health Care", paper presented at the symposium on Primary Health Care, Liverpool School of Tropical Medicine, 13-16 April 1982. (mimeo)
      -    Dr. J. S. Yudkin, Whittington Hospital, in interview with the author, October 1981.

17   WHO, op. cit.

18   -   Neem / azadirachta indica-meliaceae. Dr. Hye, personal communication, 10 August, 1981.
      -    P. C. Roy Chaudhury, "Herbal Medicines for Common Ailments", *The Himachal.* - The International Organisation of Consumer Unions warns that neem oil has been identified as the cause of Reye syndrome, where there is an acute onset of damage to the liver, kidneys and brain. Symptoms of poisoning are observed within 2-4 hours of consuming 5-30mg of the oil (studies of the University of Malaya Hospital, Kuala Lumpur). (Personal communication from Foo Gaik Sim, Head of Information and Research, 5 August 1981.)

19   -   Peter Parish, *Medicines,* A Guide for Everybody, Penguin, 1981.
      -    Anil Agarwal, *Drugs and the Third World,* an Earthscan Publication, International Institute for Environment and Development, August 1978. -Digoxin and quinine are included in the WHO *Selection of Essential Drugs,* (Technical Report Series No. 641, Geneva 1979). Ephedrine and reserpine are included in the WHO Selection as "complementary" rather than "essential" drugs. ?

20   UNCTAD, *Case Studies in the transfer of technology: The Pharmaceutical Industry in India,* study prepared by the Jawaharlal Nehru University and the Indian Council of Scientific and Industrial Research, 1977.

21   Dr. H.K.M. Hye, in interview with the author, Delhi, 20 October 1980.

22   Galvez-Tan, op.cit.

23   Agarwal, op.cit.

24   Hye, "Utilisation of Traditional Medicines in Primary Health Care", op. cit., p.6.

25   Prof. Arnold Beckett, quoted in *SCRIP,* No. 628, 23 September 1981, p.13.

26   Hye, "Utilisation of Traditional Medicines in Primary Health Care", op.cit., p.5.

27   Ibid., p.4.

28   Agarwal, op.cit.

29   Hye, "Utilisation of Traditional Medicines in Primary Health Care", op.cit., p.6.

30   Sheila Hillier, lecturer London Hospital Medical College, in interview with the author, 25 April 1981.

31   WHO, *Drug Policies and Management Problems, Constraints and Strategies,* Report on the Inter-Country Consultative Meeting on Drug Policies and Management, New Delhi, 13-16 October 1980, (ICP DPM 001.00) WHO Regional Office for S.E. Asia.

32   Dr. Tcheknavorian-Asenbauer, Chief Pharmaceutical Industries Unit, UNIDO, in interview with the author, 27 May, 1981.

33   WHO, *Drug Policies and Management-Problems, Constraints and Strategies,* op.cit.

34   Agarwal, op.cit. "Some scientists believe that their knowledge may be more valuable than

that available in the Ayurvedic texts, as the tribal communities have lived in far greater dependence on nature.''

35   Dr. Pham Ngoc Thach, quoted by Agarwal, op.cit., p.58.

36   Galvez-Tan, op.cit.

37   - Sutherland, op.cit.
      - A.C. Alexander and M.K. Shivaswany, "Traditional Healers in the Region of Mysore'', *Social Sciences and Medicine,* Pergamon Press, 1971, volume 5, pp. 595-601.

38   Sutherland, 1978, op.cit. At the Chiraigaon and Harahua joint clinics (Uttar Pradesh) 200 questionnaires revealed that 70.2% of patients consulting the traditional healers were educated beyond primary school revel (against regional average for population with secondary education of 11.8%). By contrast 68% of patients seeing allopathic staff were either illiterate or had only primary school education. Most patients consulting the traditional healers were educated young men, many with psychosomatic complaints.

39   WHO, *National Policies and Practices in regard to Medicinal Products; and Related International Problems,* background document A/31/Technical Discussions/1, 6 March 1978, p.30.

40   Dr. D. B. Nugegoda, Department of Community Medicine University of Peradeniya, "Cooperation and Conflict between Allopathic and Ayurvedic Systems of Therapy in Sri Lanka'', paper delivered at the Primary Health Care Symposium, Liverpool School of Tropical Medicine, 13-16 April 1981. (mimeo)

41   Agarwal, op.cit, p.57.

42   OXFAM Project File, MAH 87.

43   - OXFAM Project File MAH 74.
      - Hugh Goyder, OXFAM Field Director, S. India, personal communication, 29 September 1981. (Homeopathy was started by Dr. Samuel Hahnemann in Saxony in the early nineteenth century, but spread to India where the system was culturally acceptable.)

44   Deoki Nardan et al., S. N. Medical College, Cegra, India quoted in *Message from Calcutta* (Highlights of the III International Congress of the World Federation of Public Health Associations and the XXV Annual Conference of the Indian Public Health Association "Primary Health Care: World Strategy'', 23-26 February 1981), Geneva and Washington, 1982, p.93.

45   - Jackie and Tim Lusty "Report on visit to Yemen Health Projects, CIIR and Concern'', 10-23 March 1980. (mimeo)
      - Oxfam Project write up, Yemen 15C, August 1980.
      - Dianna Melrose, *The Great Health Robbery,* OXFAM Public Affairs Unit, 1981.

46   Jackie and Tim Lusty, op.cit.

CHAPTER 8

1   Information on Gonoshasthaya Kendra based on research visit by the writer, September, 1980. Also:
      - OXFAM Project Write-up, "Bangladesh 20'', August 1978. (mimeo)
      - Gonoshasthaya Kendra "Progress Report'', No. 7, August 1980. (mimeo)
      - "Gonoshasthaya Pharmaceuticals'', Newsletter, undated (1981). (mimeo)
      - "The Paramedics of Savar: an experiment in community health in Bangladesh'', *Medico Friend Circle Bulletin,* 1 September 1980.
      - Dr. Abhay Bang "Learning from the Savar project'', *Medico Friend Circle Bulletin,* October 1980.

2   Dr. Zafrullah Chowdhury.

3   Gonoshasthaya Kendra, "Progress Report'', No. 7, op. cit.

238

4   Ibid.

5   Information on Gonoshasthaya Kendra Pharmaceuticals: as note (1). Also:
    -    Dr Zafrullah Chowdhury and Susanne Chowdhury, "Essential Drugs for the Poor: Myth and Reality in Bangladesh", paper delivered at the Primary Health Care Symposium, Liverpool School of Tropical Medicine, 13-16 April 1982. (mimeo)
    -    OXFAM Project Write-up BD 20c, "Gonoshasthaya Pharmaceuticals Ltd."
    -    NOVIB, Report on proposal to set up Gonoshasthaya Pharmaceuticals: "Gegevens over de te medefinancieren aktiviteiten", 21 August 1979.
    -    Dr. Zafrullah Chowdhury, letter to *The Lancet,* 7 November 1981.
    -    Barry Newman, *Wall Street Journal,* July 3 1981.
    -    David Newell, OXFAM Field Director, "1980-81 Bangladesh and Burma Annual Report". (mimeo)

6   "Gonoshasthaya Pharmaceuticals" Newsletter, op.cit., p.3.

7   Initial funding included:

NOVIB (Holland) US $	2.62m
Christian Aid	0.16m
Bangladesh Shilpa Bank] GK Trust and others	1.00m

    (Source Gonoshasthaya Pharmaceuticals Newsletter, op.cit.)

8   Dr. Zafrullah Chowdhury, in interview with author, April 1982.

9   "Gonoshasthaya Pharmaceuticals" Newsletter, op.cit., p.5.

10   Chowdhury and Chowdhury, 1982, op.cit., p.11.

11   Ibid., p.12

12   Ibid.

13   *In Touch,* VHSS Newsletter, 1980.

14   I.C. Tiwari, S.C.Mohapatra and S.D. Gaur, Department of Preventive and Social Medicine Banaras Hindu University, "Drug Needs and Availability for Primary Health Care in a Rural Community in India", paper presented at Primary Health Care Symposium, Liverpool School of Tropical Medicine, 13-16 April 1982, p.5.

15   VHAI, "Our concern about drugs", 1981, p.1. (mimeo)

16   Dr. Premchandran John of the Deenabandbu Medical Mission, in interview with David Bull of OXFAM, 14 September 1980.

17   VHAI, op.cit.

18   Selim Ahmed, VHSS, Dacca, in interview with the author, 24 September 1980.

19   -   Dr. Sathya Mala and S. Srinivasan of VHAI, in interview with the author, Delhi, 21 October 1981.
    -    S. Srinivasan, personal communication, 15 July, 1981.

20   -   UNCTAD, *Technology Policies and the Pharmaceutical sector in Nepal,* (UNCTAD/TT/34) United Nations 1980.
    -    Dr. Andrew Cassels, Medical Director Britain Nepal Medical Trust, "Drug Supply in Rural Nepal: The Bhojpur Drug Scheme". (mimeo (1982))
    -    OXFAM Project write-up "Nepal 5", March 1982. (mimeo)

21   -   "The Britain-Nepal Medical Trust Quarterly Report", Asoj-Mangsir 2037, mid-September to mid-December 1980.
    -    UNCTAD, 1980, op.cit., and Cassels, op.cit.

22   -   "The Britain Nepal Medical Trust Quarterly Report", op.cit.
    -    Dr. Don Patterson, "A Scheme for the purchase and distribution of drugs in a developing

country - Nepal'', paper delivered at Primary Health Care Symposium, Liverpool School of Tropical Medicine, 13-16 April 1982.

23   ''The Britain Nepal Medical Trust Quarterly Report'', op.cit.

24   Cassels, op. cit., p.10.

25   Ibid., p.9.

26   Ibid., pp.1-8.

27   Ibid., p.11.

28   David Werner, Director, Project Piaxtla, personal communication, 20 July 1981.

29   David Werner and Bill Bower, *Helping Health Workers Learn,* a book of methods, aids and ideas for instructors at the village level, Hesperian Foundation, Palo Alto, California, 1982, pp.27.14-27.18.

CHAPTER 9

1   Dr.V.Fattorusso, then Director of the Division of Prophylactic, Diagnostic and Therepeutic Substances, WHO, ''Essential Drugs for the Third World'', *World Health,* May 1981, WHO, p.5.

2   WHO, ''National Policies and Practices in Regard to Medicinal Products; and Related International Problems'', Background Document (A31/Technical Discussions/1)6 March 1978,p.5: ''In spite of the general recognition that medicinal products should be viewed as essential tools for health care and for the improvement of the quality of life, it is not uncommon to find that drug policies are mainly directed towards industrial and trade development and sometimes contradictory policies exist independently and are implemented in different sectors of the administration.''

3   -   David Taylor, *Medicines, Health and the Poor World,* Office of Health Economics, May 1982, pp.22-23.
       Dr.H.Mahler, ''The meaning of 'Health for all by the year 2000' '', *World Health Forum,* 2 (I), WHO, 1981, pp.5-22.

4   Fattorusso, op.cit., p.5.

5   For example, Jay J. Kingham, US Pharmaceutical Manufacturers Association, ''Preliminary Observations on UNCTC Draft Summary Report 'Transnational Corporations in the Pharmaceutical Industry of Developing Countries ' '', 23 February 1981,p.3.
     See also: Chapter 10.

6   Sjaak van der Geest, Anthropological-Sociological Centre, University of Amsterdam, ''The Efficiency of Inefficiency: Medicine Distribution in South-Cameroon'', paper presented at the Seventh International Conference on Social Science and Medicine, Noordwijkerhout, 22-26 June 1981,p.12.

7   WHO, ''Action Programme on Essential Drugs'', *Report by the Executive Board Ad Hoc Committee on Drugs Policies on behalf of the Executive Board,* (A35/7), Thirty-Fifth World Health Assembly, 1 April 1982.

8   David Werner, personal communication, 20 July 1981.

9   Adrian Moyes, Oxfam Public Affairs Unit, ''Don't Compare us with India'' - A visit to China, September 1980. (mimeo) The position of the communes may have changed with more recent political changes.

10   Sheila Hillier, London Hospital Medical College, talk given at Politics of Health Group meeting, London, 25 April 1981.

11   David G. Beynon, Pharmaceutical Supply Officer, Department of Health, Provincial Medical Store, Madang Province, personal communication, 4 July 1980.

240

12   -   Letter from Dr. Luise Parsons, Medical Officer, Immanuel Hospital, Enga Province, Papua New Guinea to Ritchie Cogan, BBC Producer, London, 7 June 1979.
      -   Letter from Dr. J. Moir, Medical Officer, rural health centre, Madang Province, Papua New Guinea to Ritchie Cogan, BBC, 11 July 1979.

13   -   Dr. Carol Barker, "Drugs Policy in Mozambique", paper delivered at the Primary Health Care Symposium, Liverpool School of Tropical Medicine, 13-16 April 1982. (mimeo)
      -   Dr. Carol Barker, "Pharmaceuticals Policy", draft of unpublished chapter, undated.

14   Ibid.

15   WHO, *The Selection of Essential Drugs,* Report of a WHO Expert Committee, Technical Report Series 615, WHO, Geneva, 1977.

16   UNCTAD, *Case Studies in transfer of technology: Pharmaceutical Policies in Sri Lanka,* study prepared by Dr. Senaka Bibile, Professor of Pharmacology University of Sri Lanka and Chairman of the State Pharmaceuticals Corporation, in cooperation with the UNCTAD Secretariat, (TD/B/C.6/21), United Nations, 27 June 1977,p.6.

17   -   WHO, 1982 (A35/7), op.cit., p 30.
      -   Barker, op.cit., p.1.

18   Barker, 1982, op.cit., p.3.

19   Pascale Brudon, "L'Industrie Pharmaceutique Suisse dans les pays Sous Developpes", (Memoire presente pour le diplome de recherche en etudes de developpement), Institut Universitaire D'Etudes de Developpment Geneva, 1981, p.209.

20   Dr. Braga quoted in *Provisional Summary Record of the Fifth Meeting of Committee A,* Thirty Fifth World Health Assembly (A35/A/SR/5) 10 May 1982, p.7.

21   -   United Nations Centre for Transnational Corporations (UNCTC) *Transnational Corporations and the Pharmaceutical Industry,* United Nations, New York, 1979, p.87.
      -   UNCTC, "Case Study on Brazil", draft report, 9 February 1981.

22   Ibid.

23   Government of Guyana, in collaboration with UNCTAD, UNDTCD, UNIDO, WHO, Pharmaceuticals in the Developing World, *Policies on Drugs, Trade and Production, Volume I General Report* (related to UNDP Project INT/009/A/01/99 "Economic and Technical Cooperation Among Developing Countries in the Pharmaceutical Sector"), June 1979, p.11 and p.77. Afghanistan passed its Generic Drug Law in 1976, before the political changes in 1980.

24   UNCTAD, 1977 (TD/B/C,6/21), op.cit.

25   Barker, 1982, op.cit.

26   - WHO, "Drug Policy and Management in Bangladesh", Country Information Paper for Inter-Consultative Meeting on Drug Policies and Management, (ICP/DPM/001) New Delhi, 13-16 October 1980.
      -   UNCTAD, 1977, (TD/B/C. 6/21) op.cit.
      -   Professor G. Peters, University of Lausanne, "Rapport Mission au Mozambique du 8 au 19 octobre 1980".

27   *Proposed Essential Drug List for Zimbabwe,* Ministry of Health, Harare, 1981.

28   -   Professor Wilfred Lionel (University of Colombo) and Dr. Andrew Herxheimer (Senior Lecturer in Clinical Pharmacology and Therapeutics, Charing Cross Hospital Medical School), "Coherent Policies on Drugs", in Blum, Herxheimer, Stenzl and Woodcock (ed), *Pharmaceuticals and Health Policy,* 1981, p.248.
      -   Peters, op.cit.
      -   Joseph Hanlon, "Are 300 drugs enough?" *New Scientist,* 7 September 1978.

29   Hathi Committee, *Report of the Committee on Drugs and Pharmaceuticals Industry,* Government of India, Ministry of Petroleum and Chemicals, April 1975, pp.252-254 and p.271.

30   UNCTC, "Case Study on India", draft report, 9 February 1981.

31   -   UNCTAD, 1977 (TD/B/C.6/21) op.cit.

        -    Professor S. R. Kottegoda, in interview with the writer, April 1982.

32   Government of Guyana et al., op.cit., p.77.

33   Ibid., p.78.

34   Letter from Dr. Luise Parsons to Ritchie Cogan, BBC, 7 June 1979.

35   Barker, 1982, op.cit.

36   Government of Guyana et al., op.cit., p.64.

37   UNCTAD, 1977 (TD/B/C.6/21) op.cit.

38   Ibid., p.25-26 and Annex IV.

39   Ibid., p.26.

40   With a change of Government in Sri Lanka in 1977, the private sector is again permitted to import drugs.(D.C.Jayasuriya, "Regulating the drug trade in the Third World", *World Health Forum,* Vol.2 (3), 1981, pp.423-426.)

41   -   UNCTC, *Transnational corporations in the Pharmaceutical Industry of Developing Countries,* Report of the Secretariat, United Nations Economic and Social Council (E/C.10/85) 15 July 1981, p.17.

        -    "Case Study on Costa Rica", UNCTC draft report, 9 February 1981.

42   Ibid.

43   Government of Guyana et al., June 1979, op.cit.

44   Dr. F. S. Antezana, Senior Scientist, WHO, personal communication, 30 April 1981.

45   UNCTAD, "Technology Policies in the Pharmaceutical Sector in Cuba", study prepared by the Medico-Pharmaceutical branch of the Ministry of Public Health, Cuba, for the UNCTAD secretariat, 1980.

46   Peters, op.cit.

47   Barker, draft chapter,op.cit., p.13.

48   Hathi Committee, April 1975, op.cit.

49   UNCTC, 15 July 1981, op.cit., p.30.

50   For example: *SCRIP* No.668, 17 February 1982, p.11. and *SCRIP* No.694, 19 May 1982, p.13.

51   Indian Council of Social Science Research (ICSSR) and Indian Medical Research Council (ICMR), *Health for All - an Alternative Strategy,* 1981, p.180.

52   Dr. H.K.M. Hye, whilst Director of Drug Administration, in interview with the author, Delhi, 20 October 1980.

53   Ibid.

54   -   WHO,(A35/7), 1 April 1982, op.cit., p.21.

        -    Stuart Kingma, Christian Medical Commission, talk at Primary Health Care Symposium, Liverpool School of Tropical Medicines, 13-16 April 1982.

55   Government of Guyana et al., op.cit., p.10.

56   UNCTAD, *Technology Policies in the Pharmaceutical sector in Cuba,* 1980, op.cit.

57   UNCTC, "Case Study on Egypt", draft report, 9 February 1981.

58   Ibid.

59   Ibid.

60   David Beynon, M.Pharm, Drug Cost Comparison, "Improving Pharmaceutical distribution to the rural areas", 21 February 1980. (mimeo)

61   Dr. Pham Ngoc Thach, First Health Minister of the Democratic Republic of Vietnam, quoted in *Health in the Third World: Studies from Vietnam,* Dr. Joan K. McMichael (ed.), Spokesman Books, 1976.

62   Anne Ferguson, "The effects of source of supply of medications on health care services dispensed in pharmacies in a Salvadoran town", 1980, p.8. (mimeo)

63   A limited list of products to be sold off prescription in grocers' shops was drawn up in August 1977. (Barker, op.cit.)

64   UNCTAD, *Technology Policies in the Pharmaceutical Sector in Cuba,* 1980, op.cit.

65   Ibid.

66   *SCRIP,* No. 689, 3 May 1982, p.11.

67   Yemen Arab Republic Ministry of Health, *Fourth Annual Report on the activities of the Supreme Board for Medicines and Medical Equipment,* 1979: "The majority of (import) authorisations have been given without their being presented to the Supreme Board." (translation from the Arabic).

68   Government of Guyana, et al., op.cit.

69   UNCTC, 15 July 1981, op.cit., p.14.

70   -   UNCTC, "Case Study of India", draft report 9 February 1981, op.cit.
     -   But controls have held the rise in the drug price index below the rate of other sectors of the chemical industry.

71   UNCTC, 15 July 1981, op.cit., p.16.

72   -   Study by Constantine Vaitsos quoted by R.J. Barnet and R.E. Muller, *Global Reach,* Jonathan Cape, London, 1975, p.158.
     -   Oscar Gish and Loretta Lee Feller, *Planning Pharmaceuticals for Primary Health Care,* American Public Health Association, International Health Program Monograph Series No.2, 1979.

73   UNCTC, 15 July 1981, op.cit., p.16.

74   UNCTAD, *Pharmaceutical Policies in Sri Lanka,* 1977, op.cit., p.26 and Annexe VIII.

75   Professor Lionel, Faculty of Medicine, Colombo, in interview with David Bull of OXFAM's Public Affairs Unit, 11 September 1980.

76   UNCTC, 15th July 1981, op.cit., p.16.

77   Peters, op.cit.

78   UNCTC, 15 July 1981, op.cit., p.21.

79   Ibid., p.23.

80   Professor Lionel, op.cit.

81   UNCTC, 15 July 1981, op.cit., p.23.

82   Comision Popular Nacional de Salud, Ministerio de Salud, Dimavi, *Jornadas Populares de Salud,* 1981.

83   Professor Carlos Mazargao, quoted by Joseph Hanlon, "Are 300 drugs enough?", *New Scientist,* 7 September 1978.

84   UNCTAD, *Pharmaceutical Policies in Sri Lanka,* 1977, op.cit., p.7.

85   WHO, "Country Information Paper-Sri Lanka", in *Drug Policies including Traditional Medicines in the context of Primary Health Care,* op.cit.

86   Dr. Mahler, *World Health Forum*, 2(1), 1981, op.cit., p.18.

87   Government of Guyana et al., op.cit., p.1 and annex 1.

88   *Provisional Summary Records* of the Fourth, Fifth and Sixth Sessions of Committee A on the Action Programme on Essential Drugs, 10/11 May 1982, WHO, (A35/A/SR/4-6) and the Resolution on the Action Programme on Essential Drugs adopted by the Thirty-Fifth World Health Assembly.

89   -   Government of Guyana et al., op.cit., pp.16-17.

      -    WHO (A35/7) April 1982, op.cit.

90   UNCTAD *Report and recommendations of the workshop on trade and technology policies in the pharmaceutical sector,* Abidjan, Ivory Coast, 12-23 October 1981, UN, 1982.

91   Dr. Oliver Munyaradzi, Minister of Health, text of speech delivered at the Zimbabwe meeting of Chief Pharmacists of the Africa Region, in Harare, 26 April 1982, (''Press Statement'' 358/82/DC) Department of Information, Zimbabwe.

CHAPTER 10

1   *North-South: A Programme for Survival,* the Brandt Report, Pan Books,1980.

2   World Health Organisation, United Nations Conference on Trade and Development, United Nations International Children's Emergency Fund. Other UN agencies involved in pharmaceuticals include: United Nations Development Programme (UNDP), United Nations Action Programme for Economic Co-operation (UNAPEC), United Centre for Transnational Corporations (UNCTC). Other international organisations such as the World Bank and Asian Development Bank are helping to fund drugs projects, for example setting up local production.

3   WHO Regular Budget 1980/1 Total: $477,135,300 United States $115,158,410) (24%) France 26,058,955) W.Germany 34,078,960) Italy 14,518,920) 51.9% of total budget. Japan 38,774,010) U.K. 19,106,305) Source: WHO, *Proposed Programme Budget* for the financial period 1982-1983 (PB/82-83), Geneva, 1980, pp.31-37

4   Dr.Mahler: ''How often do I still see you misusing its WHO's very limited financial resources by perpetuating fragmented projects, requesting fellowships that have very little relevance to your essential manpower needs, and asking for equipment and supplies of marginal utility!'' ''Review of the Report of the Director-General on the work of WHO in 1980'', Second Plenary Meeting, Thirty-Fourth World Health Assembly, Geneva, 4-22 May 1981, Verbatim Record of Plenary Meetings, (WHA34/1981/REC/2) Geneva 1981,p.19

5   Dr. J. F. Dunne, Chief of the Pharmaceuticals Unit, Division of Diagnostic, Therapeutic and Rehabilitative Technology collects information from member states on regulatory decisions taken (approving and banning drugs) and compiles these into *Drug Information Bulletins.* These are then circulated to health and regulatory authorities worldwide. Unfortunately as Dr.Dunne is almost a one-person department, these bulletins have been appearing only at 6-monthly intervals.

6   Dr. Mahler was appointed as DG in May 1973, and reappointed in May 1978, (his re-election is due in 1983). WHO, ''Prophylactic and Therapeutic Substances'', *Report by the Director-General,* Twenty-eighth World Health Assembly, (A28/11) 3 April 1975, p.1.

7   Ibid.,p.2.

8   Catherine Stenzl, Coordinator International Research Group for Drug Legislation and Programs, ''The Role of International Organisations in Medicines Policy'', in Blum, Herxheimer, Stenzl and Woodcock (ed) *Pharmaceuticals and Health Policy,* Croom Helm, London, 1981, p.223.

9 Dr. Balasubramanian, Technology Division, UNCTAD, *Provisional Summary Record of the Sixth Meeting,* Committee A discussion on Action Programme on Essential Drugs, Thirty-Fifth World Health Assembly (A35/A/SR/6) 11 May 1982, pp.2-3.

10 Mrs. Quintero, UNIDO, *Provisional Summary Record of the Fifth Meeting,* Committee A discussion on the Action Programme of Essential Drugs, Thirty-Fifth World Health Assembly (A35/A/SR/5) 10 May 1982, pp.2-4.

11 Stenzl, op.cit.,p.226 There has been discussion on expanding the Copenhagen operation and for WHO to cooperate with UNICEF in bulk-purchasing on behalf of Third World governments.

12 WHO, Action Programme on Essential Drugs, *Report by the Executive Board Ad Hoc Committee on Drug Policies on behalf of the Executive Board,* Thirty-Fifth World Health Assembly (A35/7) 1 April 1982.

13 Ibid.,Annex 1 "Relevant Health Assembly Resolutions" (WHA31.32)

14 WHO,(A35/7) 1 April 1982,op.cit.

15 Prof. Ofosu-Amaah, *Provisional Summary Record of the Fourth Meeting,* Committee A discussion on Action Programme on Essential Drugs, Thirty- Fifth World Health Assembly, (A35/A/SR/4) 10 May 1982,p.7.

16 Prof. Benhassine, WHO (A35/A/SR/5) 10 May 1982,op.cit.,p.15. Delegates expressing disatisfaction with slow progress included France, Netherlands, Mozambique, the Nordic countries and Bolivia. The West German delegate expressed concern that 4 years had passed since the adoption of resolution 31.32 with no detailed work plan.

17 WHO,(A35/7) 1 April 1982, p.5 Also Dr. Morck, Chairman of the Ad-Hoc Committee reported to delegates: "The Ad-Hoc Committee, at its most recent meeting, in March 1982, had anticipated that detailed information on the IFPMA offer would be available in time for it to be distributed to the Health Assembly...That was not the case...As the Director-General had said in January 'Due appreciation could be expressed only when the Health Assembly fully understood the extent of the offer and its effect in practical terms'." (WHO (A35/A/SR/4) 10 May 1982, op.cit., pp.2-3.

18 WHO Minute of Executive Board Meeting (Document EB69/SR/9), January 1982.

19 *SCRIP.* "WHO and Germans Pushing ahead with discussions on World Drug Scheme", 4 June 1977, p.7.

20 International Federation of Pharmaceutical Manufacturers Associations (IFPMA), "WHO Action Programme on Essential Drugs", Statement by Dr. Ernst Vischer, President of IFPMA, to Committee A, Thirty-Fifth World Health Assembly, 10 May 1982.

21 Ibid.

22 Dr.F.S. Antezana, Senior Scientist, Action Programme on Essential Drugs, WHO, Geneva, in interview with the author, 26 May 1981. Health Action International, "The WHO and the Pharmaceutical Industry". HAI briefing paper for the Thirty-Fifth World Health Assembly: "There was disagreement between WHO and the industry because industry... claimed that Rwanda's request resembled a 'straightforward tender' and that not all drugs requested were intended for primary health care. WHO felt that the industry's reasons for turning down the request from Rwanda were spurious.

"This episode has wider implications, since the WHO seemed unhappy about the industry's package approach, in which drugs were supplied only if technical services were provided as well. The Manager of the WHO's Action Programme on Essential Drugs, Dr. W. B. Wanandi, has been reported as saying that the WHO wanted the industry to quote separately for the supply of drugs and associated services - since 'the WHO's primary concern was the price of the actual drugs ' . (*SCRIP* No.592. 20 May 1981, p.13.) A third reason why the negotiations faltered is that WHO considered some of the industry's conditions to be unduly restrictive.

The industry's insistence on near-monopoly conditions suggested it was in effect bidding for preferential supply terms in exchange for technical cooperation.''

23   Dr. Braga, WHO (A35/A/SR/5) 10 May 1982, op.cit., p.7.

24   For example: Dr. Annandale (Samoa): "That dialogue between WHO and industry did not appear to have made much progress and the small developing countries could not afford to wait indefinitely.'' Mr. Rahman (Bangladesh) hoped that suitable mechanisms could be worked out without hampering progress towards self-reliance and without jeopardising the interests of individual developing countries as regards their own needs and choice.'' Also Dr. Quamina (Trinidad & Tobago), Prof. Benhassine (Algeria), Dr. Sikkel (Netherlands), Prof. Lacronique (France). But others like the West German delegate argued that the scheme would not inhibit local production because it was only a first step. WHO *Provisional Summary Records,* (A35/A/SR/4-5-6) op.cit. 25 'Catalyst ' expression used by Chilean and Cuban delegates, WHO (A35/A/SR4-5-6), op.cit.

26   Action Programme on Essential Drugs, text of Resolution adopted May 1982, Third Report of Committee A (A35/40) 14 May 1982. No specific mention is made of continuing dialogue with industry.

27   Dr. Borgono (Chile), WHO (A35/A/SR/5) 10 May 1982,op.cit.,p.2.

28   Text of Dr. Sikkel's intervention in Committee A. Also recorded in WHO (A35/A/SR/5) op.cit., pp.14-15.

29   WHO, *International Code of Marketing of Breast-Milk Substitutes,* Geneva, 1981.

30   -   WHO, "Draft resolution proposed by the delegations of Algeria, Bahrain, Congo, Greece, India, Kuwait, Mozambique, Norway, Qatar, Rwanda, Saudi Arabia and Sweden.'' (A35/A/)Conf.Paper No.2) Agenda Item 24, 11 May 1982.

      -    Text of resolution adopted in WHO Third Paper of Committee A (A35/40) op.cit.

31   Dr. J. Bryant, quoted in Minutes of 15th Executive Board Meeting EB 69/SR/15) 21 January 1981, p.6.

32   Prof. Hayes, quoted in *Provisional Summary Record,* Committee A (A35/A/SR/5) op.cit., p.10.

33   -   Dr. J. Bryant quoted in *SCRIP* No. 697, 31 May 1982. Also reported as saying "If the international industry can be seen to be addressing the criticisms of its marketing practices and cooperates in the essential drugs list, he believes a WHO marketing code could be held off''.

      -    Dr. C.E. Koop (US Surgeon General) "praised the assembly for having avoided divisive discussions of a WHO pharmaceutical code similar to the code on the marketing of breast milk substitutes...the United States believes it is inappropriate for the WHO to get involved in commercial marketing codes''. (From: "World Health Assembly Gives Impetus to WHO Programs'', EURG-1, Press Release, Geneva, 14 May 1982.)

34   In 1976 out of total OECD drug exports to developing countries four-fifths came from 5 countries: France (17.6%) West Germany (17.1%) USA (17%) UK (15.6%) and Switzerland (11.9%)

35   Office of Health Economics, George Teeling-Smith and Nicholas Wells (ed.) *Medicines for the Year 2000,* a Symposium held at the Royal College of Physicians, London, September 1978, 1979, p.89.

36   *The Medicines Act 1968,* Section 48, "Postponement of restrictions in relation to exports'', HMSO.

37   David A. Kay, *The International Regulation of Pharmaceutical Drugs,* A Report to the National Science Foundation on the application of International Regulatory Techniques to Scientific/Technical Problems, The American Society of International Law, 1976.

38 Statement of Hon. Michael D. Barnes, a Representative in Congress from the State of Maryland, Export of Hazardous Products, hearings before the Sub-Committee on International Economic Policy and Trade of the Committee on Foreign Affairs, House of Representatives, Ninety-sixth Congress, June 5, 12, and September 9 1980, US Government Printing Office, Washington, 1980, p.3.

39 In Britain, Member of Parliament Jack Ashley was told that detailed breakdowns of drug exports were not available and could only be collected at disproportionate cost.

40 Ralph Cox, Department of Health and Social Security, personal communication, 29 October, 1981.

41 Lord Wells-Pestell, Parliamentary Under-Secretary of State, Department of Health and Social Security, House of Lords, *Hansard,* 21 February 1979.

42 *Hansard,* 30 January 1979, column 1433.

43 "The Penang Declaration on the Export of Hazardous Substances and Facilities", signed by participants at the First International Consumer Testing Course in Penang, 29 October - 25 November 1980, para.1(a).

44 Ibid, para.1(b)(i).

45 Barnes, op.cit.

46 "Report to the President on the Review of US Hazardous Substances Export Policy and cover letter to US Trade Representative Brock from Secretaries Haig and Baldridge", 10 May 1982, *US Export Weekly* - Memorandum from S. Jacob Scherr, Natural Resources Defense Council, Inc., 24 June 1982.

47 Roland Moyle, DHSS, Replies to Parliamentary Questions, *Hansard,* 12 and 19 March 1979.

48 - Letter from Kenneth Clarke, Health Minister, to Sydney Chapman M.P., 6 April 1982.
    - Cox, personal communication, 29 October 1981, op.cit.

49 WHO, *Quality Control of Drugs,* A. Good Practices in Manufacture; B. Certification scheme for products moving in international commerce, Geneva, 1977.

50 WHO, (A35/7) 1 April 1982, op.cit., pp.3-4.

51 As (49) and (50).

52 As (49).

53 Cox, op.cit.,: "The United Kingdom for its part would certainly respond sympathetically and constructively to any approach from a reGulatory authority which sought additonal help."

54 Hakan Mandahl, Assistant Director, Department of Drugs, National Board of Health and Welfare, Uppsala, Sweden, in interview with the author, 15 April 1982.

55 "WHO Europe meeting turns down drug evaluation scheme," *SCRIP* No. 628, 23 September 1981, p.2.

56 Dr. Dukes, WHO (Europe) Regional Officer for Pharmaceuticals, at international drug regulation session of the US Food and Drug Law Institute, Washington, quoted in *SCRIP* No. 697, 31 May 1982, p.10.

57 *SCRIP* No. 628, op.cit.

58 Review in *SCRIP* No. 684, 14 April 1982, p.5. "Drug Problems in Nordic countries in the light of the control of psychopharmaceuticals". Regulatory authorities in developed countries face difficulties in finding independent experts to assess drugs because of "industry's penetration of the medical profession".

59 The EEC Council has rejected the concept of "need " (relative efficacy compared with marketed drugs) as registration criteria. (Gilles de Mourot, "The industry and the international regulatory environment" *EFTA Bulletin,* No. 3, Volume XXII, June/August 1981, p.2.)

Chapter 10

60   WHO, (A35/A/SR/5) op.cit., p.5. WHO, (A35/A/SR/4) p.6.

62   WHO (A35/7) 1 April 1982, op.cit.

63   Overseas Development Administration, *Statistics of UK Assistance in Developing Countries in 1980,* Table 9.

64   Cox, op.cit.

65   Ken Temple, Health and Population Division of Overseas Development Administration, personal communication, 11 February 1982. Total UK multilateral and bilateral health aid in 1980 was £109 million (12.7% of total aid). Mr. Temple gives a helpful break down: "We would not wish you to give importance to this figure since prominent within it are the food aid items, both multilateral and bilateral, which is on the borderline of health aid. But similarly the 4.4% figure reached by totalling amounts of direct health benefit gives a false impression, because it leaves out sizeable contributions to the International Development Association and European Development Fund (some of which must be devoted to health projects) as well as one-quarter of our bilateral aid. We guess that the true figure lies somewhere between 8% and 10%."

66   Department of Trade and Industry, statistics on UK exports of Medicinal and Pharmaceutical Products for 12 months ended December 1980. (Complete statistics for 1981 exports are not available.)

67   ODA, 1980 Statistics, op.cit., Table 5, p.20.

68   See for example Real Aid: a Strategy for Britain, the report of the UK Independent Committee on Aid (forthcoming).

69   Peggy Burton, SRN, *Cheaper by the Million,* H.E. Walter, Worthing, 1979.

70   Dr. James Burton, Medical Director ECHO, personal communication 25 August, 1981.

71   Burton, 25 August, 1981, op. cit.

72   Dr. Burton and Bill Davies is interview with the author, 5 August, 1980.

73   Burton, 25 August, 1981, op. cit.

74   Dr. H.K.M. Hye and Dr. Martin Schweiger, in interview with the author, during September/October 1980.

75   Dr. Tim Lusty, OXFAM's Medical Adviser, in interview with the author.

76   Priscilla Annamanthodo, OXFAM, "Medicines in Upper Volta", 1980. (mimeo)

77   -   Prof. P.F. D'Arcy, personal communication, 12 July 1981. - D'Arcy "Pharmacy in the Third World - A cause for concern 11" , *Pharmacy International,* June 1980.

78   Prof. G. Peters, "Information and Education about Drugs", in Blum, et.al., op.cit. p.99. Dr. Andrew Herxheimer, Editor of *Drug and Therapeutics Bulletin,* in various interviews with the author.

79   These publications include:

-    Malcolm Segall and Carol Barker, "Two papers on Pharmaceuticals in Developing Countries", *IDS Communication 119,* 1975.

-    Oscar Gish and Loretta Lee Feller, *Planning Pharmaceuticals for Primary Health Care,* Monograph Series, American Public Health Association, International Health Programs, 1979.

-    Dr. J. S. Yudkin, "The Economics of Pharmaceutical Supply in Tanzania", *International Journal of Health Services,* Volume 10, November 3, 1980.

-    Dr. J.S. Yudkin, "To Plan is to Choose", Dar es Salaam, 1978. (Mimeo).

-    The Haslemere Group, *Who Needs the Drug Companies?* a Haslemere Group, War on Want and Third World First publication, undated.

- Anil Agarwal, *Drugs and the Third World,* Earthscan, London, 1978.
- Dr. Tom Heller, *Poor Health, Rich Profits,* Spokesman Books, Nottingham, 1977.
- R.J. Ledogar, *Hungry for Profits,* IDOC, New York, 1975.
- And a series of studies and articles by Dr. Sanjaya Lall of the Oxford Institute of Economics and Statistics.
- Silverman, Lydecker, Lee, 1982, op.cit.
- Dr. Milton Silverman, *The Drugging of the Americas,* University of California Press, 1976.
- Milton Silverman and Philip Lee, *Pills, Profits and Politics, University of California Press, 1974.*

80   *The Alliance for the Prudent Use of Antibiotics (APUA), "Statement Regarding Worldwide Antibiotic Misuse", (APUA President, Prof. Stuart Levy, Department of Molecular Biology and Microbiology, Tufts University, Boston, USA.)*

81   *"Report of the International NGO Seminar on Pharmaceuticals", co-sponsored by IOCU and BUKO, Geneva, 27-29 May 1981.*

82   - *Charles Medawar, Insult or Injury?* Social Audit, 1979.
        - Charles Medawar, *Drug Disinformation,* Social Audit, 1980.
        - Charles Medawar and Barbara Freese, *Drug Diplomacy,* Social Audit, 1982.

83   See Chapter 6.

84   Medawar and Freese, 1982, op.cit.

85   "Summary of the President's Closing Remarks", 10th IOCU World Congress, The Hague, 22-26 June 1981 .

86   Khor Kok Peng, CAP Research Director, various interviews with the author during 1980/1.

87   "Forty-four Problem Drugs", a consumer action and resource kit on pharmaceuticals, IOCU, Penang, May 1981.

88   Linda Bolido, Depth News Asia Press Release, "Asian Nations Urged to set up Consumer Interpol", 19 December 1980.

89   HAI Booklet, "Not to be Taken. At least, not to be taken seriously", critique of IFPMA International Code of Pharmaceutial Marketing Practice, revised edition produced for the World Health Assembly, Geneva, May 1982.

90   Just one example of press coverage: "Maneouvring by Critics Upstages Drug Industry in World Health Forum", *Business International,* 28 May 1982. Also coverage in *Le Monde, SCRIP, Financial Times, Guardian, Herald Tribune,* German and Dutch press and Swiss, Dutch and US radio.

91   "IFPMA Structure and Activities", IFPMA, Zurich, 1981.

92   *SCRIP* No. 281.

93   IFPMA Statement to the Thirty-second World Health Assembly, Geneva, 7-25 May 1979.

94   Dr. Ernst Vischer, IFPMA President, Statement to Committee A, 35th World Health Assembly, May 1982, p.3.

95   Ibid.

96   IFPMA International Code of Pharmaceutical Marketing Practice, 1981 (amended March 1982).

97   Ibid.

98   *SCRIP,* No. 650, 9 December 1981.

99   HAI, 1982, op.cit.

Chapter 10

100 Dr. H. Schwartz, *Pharmaceutical Executive,* August 1981.

101 Ibid.

102 Catherine Stenzl, "The Role of International Organisations" in Blum, et al., op.cit., p.228.

103 Ibid, p.227.

104 For example Swedish doctors have taken part in a boycott of Ciba-Geigy products. Drug manufacturers could also be vulnerable to consumer boycotts because of their diversification from prescription drugs into over-the- counter medicines, cosmetics, toilet and household articles, food & drink products etc.

105 Dr. D. M. Burley, Head of International Medical Liaison, Ciba-Geigy, Horsham, personal communication, 21 May 1981.

106 Ciba-Geigy Pharma policy meeting, Ciba-Geigy Pharma and the Third World, Instructions - Working Group I - Research and Development, Medicine: "Criticisms faced by the Pharmaceutical Industry and Ciba-Geigy Pharma in the Third World".

107 *Business International,* 26 March 1982.

108 Dr. Burley, Ciba-Geigy, personal communication, 3 March 1982. Servipharm also offers consultancy services in seting up rural drug schemes and contributes training materials, such as copies of David Werner's *Where There is No Doctor.*

109 George Teeling-Smith, *ABPI News.*

110 Ciba-Geigy, *Pharma and the Third World,* p.204.

111 Barrie James, *The Marketing of Generic Drugs,* 1982, quoted in *SCRIP* No. 680, 31 March 1982, p.8.

112 WHO, *The Selection of Essential Drugs,* 1979.

113 UNCTAD, *Trade marks and generic names of pharmaceuticals and consumer protection,* report by the UNCTAD Secretariat, (TD/B/C.6/AC.5/4) 15 December 1981, p.21.

114 Vischer, IFPMA, May 1982, op.cit.

115 IFPMA, May 1979, op.cit.

116 Janssen Pharmaceutica, "The Worm Problem in the World".

117 WHO, *Action Programme on Essential Drugs. Burundi Pilot Project,* Ministry of Health of Burundi in collaboration with WHO/Interpharma, 30 April 1982.

118 *The Wellcome Trust,* pp.80-85.

119 S.Q.Zaman (Marketing Services Manager) and Mr. Chowdhury (Marketing Manager) of Glaxo (Bangladesh) Ltd.,in interview with the author,7/8 October 1980.

120 Mohammed Nurul Alam, Marketing Manager, Fisons (Bangladesh) Ltd., in interview with the author, 26 September 1980.

121 *The Illustrated Weekly of India,* 6 September 1981.

122 Dr. D. M. Burley, Ciba-Geigy, personal communication, 21 May 1981.

123 *Business International,* 5 February 1982, p.42.

124 Address to the PMA Public Relations Section annual meeting, excerpts reported in "Quotes of Notes" broadsheet "PMA President Engman on the Third World", PMA, 28 September 1981.

125 Geoffrey Potter, Glaxo, personal communication, 16 June 1982.

126 George Teeling-Smith, "Drug Companies and the Third World", *ABPI News, August 1976.*

127 *R. D. Douglas, Vice-President, Public Affairs, Pfizer Europe, "National drug policies - more state intervention or less?", World Medicine,* 28 July 1979.

128   Sanjaya Lall, (Institute of Economics and Statistics, Oxford University) and Senaka Bibile (University of Sri Lanka), "The Political Economy of Controlling Transnationals: the Pharamceutical Industry in Sri Lanka (1972-76)", in *World Development,* Vol.5. No.8. 677-697, Pergamon Press, 1977.

129   Ibid.,p.685.

130   Letter from C. Joseph Stetler, President Pharmaceutical Manufacturers Association to the Honorable Mrs. Sirimavo R.D. Bandaranaike, 10 May 1973.

131   Lall and Bibile, 1977 op.cit., p.685.

132   Ibid., p.686.

133   Ibid.

134   -   UNCTAD, case studies in transfer of technology: Pharmaceutical policies in Sri Lanka (TD/B/C.6/21), UN,1977, p.31.

       -    Ibid., note 26, p.696.

135   -   Anil Agarwal, Drugs and the Third World, Earthscan, London, 1978, p.38.

       -    Ibid., p.686.

136   Dr. Michael Hodin, Director of Public Affairs, Pfizer, personal communication, 17 March 1982.

137   Ibid.

138   Dr. Gladys Jayewardene, Chairman SPC (after the Bandaranaike Government was replaced by the Jayewardene Government), *A critical study of the purchases of the State Pharmaceuticals Corporation of Sri Lanka referred to in the UNCTAD Report 1977,* Rainbow Printers, Colombo, 21 September 1981. WHO was sent the critical study by the author asking them to publish it. WHO declined.

139   Ibid.

140   The reference to expanding trade with Eastern Europe and China comes from one sentence, (quoted out of context), of a 2-page article by S. A. Wickremansinghe and S. Bibile (who developed the new Sri Lankan drug policies). *British Medical Journal* 1971, 3, pp.757-758. Dr. Jayewardene's study is critical that the 1977 UNCTAD Report did not make it clear that most SPC purchases after the adoption of the new policies continued to be from traditional suppliers. But para. 109 and Table 3 of the UNCTAD Report make it clear that most drug imports in 1976 were still from developed market economies.

141   V.T. Herat Gunaratne, Director WHO Regional Office for South-East Asia, 'Bringing down drug costs: the Sri Lankan example', *World Health Forum,* 1 (1,2) WHO, 1980, pp.117-122.

142   D. C. Jayasuriya, Attorney-at-Law, "Regulating the drug trade in the Third World", *World Health Forum* 2(3), WHO, 1981, pp 423-426. It is also interesting to note that the SPC was criticised by the medical establishment and the press for buying tetracycline from the Polish company Polfa, as this was said to be sub-standard. But in 1980/1 - after liberalisation of drug import - Polfa tetracycline held over 80% of the market in Sri Lanka.

143   In view of our criticism in the previous section, it is only fair to Pfizer to emphasise that we have no firm evidence that they were actively involved in the Bangladesh lobby. It is intertesting to note that Dr. Hodin of Pfizer informs us that "the managing director of Pfizer Bangladesh is a man as interested in the progress and development of his country as he is in the success of his business. As such, he is quite active in Community and Country affairs in Bangladesh, including the Bangladesh Assocation of Pharmaceutical Industries.." (Dr. Hodin, personal communication, 17 March 1982). Jayasuriya, 1981, op.cit., p.423.

144   Dr. H. K. M. Hye and Dr. Jahangir, Director and Deputy Director, Drug Administration, Bangladesh, in interview with the author, September and October 1980.

145   Expert Committee *Report Evaluation of Registered/Licensed Products and Draft National Drug Policy,* 11 May 1982, p.93.

146   Ibid.

147   Dr. Hye, whilst Director of Drug Administration, in interview with the author, 20 October 1980.

148   Letter from Bangladesh Association of Pharmaceutical Industries to the Deputy Prime Minister in-charge at the Ministry of Industries, 22 June 1981.

149   Ibid.

150   Ibid.

151   "Association's Stand on Important Matters concerning Pharmaceutical Industry", p.2.

152   Ibid, p.3.

153   Letter from Bangladesh Association of Pharmaceutical Industries, to the Honourable State Minister for Commerce, 26 August 1981. Retail prices have been pegged for some years. We have seen in Chapter 4 that they have been described as ' 'strikingly '' high in relation to actual production costs. The Association's letter argues somewhat bizarrely that "the benefit of control, although intended for the consumer, hardly reaches them, because "intermediaries in the distribution channel... make unauthorised profits and black money." Whereas if price control were to be lifted "the average increase in the cost of medicines computed based on maximum retail price will increase by 12% to 15%. But, since the consumers are already paying higher prices for some of the products than the approved MRP, the real cost increase to the consumers will be about 5-7%." (Somehow, magically without price controls retailers will stop overcharging customers.) The letter also states: "Once our products are correctly priced in terms of their real value these will be available in adequate quantities and consumers will pay less than what they are currently paying." (Retailers and manufacturers in Bangladesh each accused the other of holding back supplies of drugs to make their sale more profitable when interviewed during our 1980 research trip.)

154   "Association's Stand on Important Matters concerning Pharmaceutical Industry", op.cit., p.3.

155   Ibid., p.1.

156   Ibid., p.2.

157   P.W. Cunliffe, Chairman Pharmaceuticals Division, ICI, personal communication, 11 February 1982. ICI is not amongst the offenders in selling a mass of tonics and other over-the-counter remedies.

158   Government of the People's Republic of Bangladesh Ministry of Law and Land Reforms, The Drugs Control Ordinance, 1982, Ordinance No. VIII of 1982.

159   Expert Committee Report, 11 May 1982, op.cit.

160   -   Letter from Prof. M. D. Rawlins, University of Newcastle to Prof. Nurul Islam, 20 July 1982.

         -    Letter from Dr. J. S. Yudkin, Consultant/Senior lecturer in General Medicine, Whittington Hospital to Prof. Nurul Islam, 18 July 1982.

         -    The criteria have also been praised by Dr. G. Tognoni, Head, Laboratory of Clinical Pharmacology, Instituto di Ricerche Farmacologiche Mario Negri, Milan (Temporary Adviser to WHO Expert Committee on the Selection of Essential Drugs (letter to Prof. Nurul Islam, 26 July 1982).

161   -   Expert Committee Report, 11 May 1982, op.cit.

         -    Wolfe, Coley, "Pills that Don't work", Health Research Group, Washington, 1981. British National Formulary, London, 1982.

162   -   Expert Committee Report, op.cit.

163   Ibid.

164   Ibid.

       -    The Drugs (Control) Ordinance, 1982.

165   K. Washbourn and B. Walker, May and Baker Ltd., in interview with the author, 5 July 1982.

166   "An Appeal to the Martial Law Authority" by members of the Bangladesh Anshad Shilpa Samity, *The New Nation*, 23 June 1982.

167   Ibid.

168   Dr. Z. Choudhury, personal communication, 24 June 1982.

169   *The Pulse*, 9 May 1982.

170   *The New Nation*, 10 June 1982.

171   *The Pulse*, 20 June 1982.

172   -   "Merck in Bangladesh, Marketing Plan 1980 (-1982)".

       -    Ciba-Geigy is planning to set up production in Bangladesh (Dr. Burley, personal communication, 1982).

173   Department of Trade and Industry, *Overseas Trade Statistics*. Nigeria was Britain's largest export market with sales worth over £64 million (compared to exports of over £20 million to the USA and £59 million to W. Germany).

174   Dr. Burley, Head of International Medical Liaison, Ciba-Geigy, personal communication, 21 May 1981.

175   -   *Financial Times*, 2 June 1982.

       -    In 1978 a British Minister of State drew attention to a report by the Economic Development Committee for the Chemicals Industry showing that the "innovative pharmaceutical industry as a whole remains one of the major growth sectors of the chemical industry as a whole." (Roland Moyle quoted in *Medicines for the year 2000*, OHE 1979, op.cit.)

176   Dr. Alan Hayes, Chairman, Plant Protection Division ICI, "What can the Agrochemical Industry Learn from the Pharmaceutical Industry?", Agrochemical Conference, Dolder Hotel, Zurich, September 1981.

CHAPTER 11

1.   Dr. Burley, Head of International Medical Liaison, Gba-Geigy, personal communication, 21 May 1981.

THE WHO SELECTION OF ESSENTIAL DRUGS, 1979

	MAIN LIST	COMPLEMENTARY DRUGS
1. ANAESTHETICS	ether,anaesthetic	
1.1 general anaesthetics	halothane	
nitrous oxide		
oxygen		
thiopental		
1.2 local anaesthetics	bupivacaine	
	lidocaine	
2. ANALGESICS, ANTIPYRETICS NONSTEROIDAL ANTI-INFLAMMATORY DRUGS USED TO TREAT GOUT	acetylsalicylic acid	colchicine
	allopurinol	probenecid
	ibuprofen	
	indometacin	
	paracetamol	
3. ANALGESICS, NARCOTICS AND NARCOTIC ANTAGONISTS	morphine	pethidine
	naloxone	
4. ANTIALLERGICS antihistamines	chlorphenamine	
5. ANTIDOTES		
5.1 general	charcoal, activated	
	ipecacuanha	
5.2 specific	atropine	methylthioninium
	deferoxamine	chloride
	dimercaprol	penicillamine
	sodium calcium edetate	
	sodium nitrite	
	sodium thiosulfate	
6. ANTIEPILEPTICS	diazepam	carbamazepine
	ethosuximide	valproic acid
	phenobarbital	
	phenytoin	
7. ANTIINFECTIVE DRUGS		
7.1 amoebicides	metronidazole	diloxanide
		emetine
		paromomycin
7.2 anthelmintic drugs	mebendazole	bephenium
	niclosamide	hydroxy-
	piperazine	naphthoate
	tiabendazole	

7.3 antibacterial drugs	ampicillin benzathine benzyl- penicillin benzylpenicillin chloramphenicol cloxacillin erythromycin gentamicin metronidazole phenoxymethylpenicillin salazosulfapyridine sulfadimidine sulfamethoxazole + trimethoprim tetracycline	amikacin doxycycline nitrofurantoin procaine benzyl- penicillin
7.4 antifilarial drugs	diethylcarbamazine suramin sodium	
7.5 antileprosy	dapsone	clofazimine rifampicin
7.6 antimalarials	chloroquine primaquine pyrimethamine quinine	sulfadoxime + pyrimethamine
7.7 antischistosomals	metrifonate niridazole oxamniquine	antimony sodium tartrate sodium stibocaptate
7.8 antitrypanosomals	melarsoprol nifurtimox pentamidine suramin sodium	
7.9 antituberculosis drugs	ethambutol isoniazid rifampicin streptomycin	
7.10 leishmaniacides	pentamidine sodium stibogluconate	
7.11 systemic antifungal drugs	amphotericin B griseofulvin nystatin	flucytosine
8. ANTIMIGRAINE DRUGS	ergotamine	

9. ANTINEOPLASTIC AND   azathioprine
    IMMUNOSUPPRESSIVE DRUGS   bleomycin
                                busulfan
                                calcium folinate
                                chlorambucil
                                cyclophosphamide
                                cytarabine
                                dexorubicin
                                flurouracil
                                methotrexate
                                procarbazine
                                vincristine

10. ANTIPARKINSONISM DRUGS   levodopa   levodopa +
                                trihexyphenidyl   carbidopa

11. DRUGS AFFECTING THE
    BLOOD

    11.1 antianaemia drugs   ferrous/salt   iron dextran
                                folic acid
                                hydroxocobalamin

    11.2 anticoagulants and   heparin
         antagonists   phytomenadione
                                protamine sulfate
                                warfarin

12. BLOOD PRODUCTS AND
    BLOOD SUBSTITUTES

    12.1 plasma substitute   dextran 70

    12.2 plasma fractions   albumin, human   antihaemophilic
         for specific uses   normal   fraction
                                                       fibrinogen
                                                       plasma protein
                                                       factor IX
                                                       complex
                                                       (coagulation
                                                       factors
                                                       II, VII, IX, X
                                                       concentrates)

13. CARDIOVASCULAR DRUGS

    13.1 antiaginal drugs   glyceryl trinitrate
                                isosorbide dinitrate
                                propranolol

13.2 antiarrhythmic drugs	lidocaine procainamide propranolol	quinidine
13.3 antihypertensive drugs	hydralazine hydrochlorothiazide propranolol sodium nitroprusside	methyldopa reserpine
13.4 cardiac glycosides	digoxin	digitoxin
13.5 drugs used in shock or anaphylaxis	dopamine epinephrine	isoprenaline

14. DERMATOLOGICAL DRUGS

14.1 antiinfective drugs	neomycin + bacitracin
14.2 antiinflammatory drugs	betamethasone hydrocortisone
14.3 astringents	aluminium acetate
14.4 fungicides	benzoic acid + salicyclic acid miconazole nystatin
14.5 keratoplastic agents	coal tar salicylic acid
14.6 scabicides and pediculicides	benzyl benzoate gamma benzene- hexachloride

15. DIAGNOSTIC AGENTS   edrophonium
                                tuberculin, purified
                                  protein derivative

15.1 ophthalmic	fluorescein
15.2 radiocontrast media	adipiodone meglumine barium sulfate iopanoic acid meglumine amidotrizoate sodium amidotrizoate

	MAIN LIST	COMPLEMENTARY DRUGS

16. DIURETICS

amiloride
furosemide
hydrochlorothiazide
mannitol

chlortalidone

17. GASTROINTESTINAL DRUGS

17.1 antacids

aluminium hydroxide
magnesium hydroxide

calcium
carbonate

17.2 antiemetics

promethazine

17.3 antihaemorrhoidals

local anaesthetic,
astringent and
antiinflammatory drug

17.4 antispasmodics

atropine

17.5 cathartics

senna

17.6.1 antidiarrhoeal

codeine

17.6.2 replacement solution

oral rehydration salts

18. HORMONES

18.1 adrenal hormones
and synthetic hydrocortisone
substitutes

dexamethasone

prednisolone

fludrocortisone

18.2 androgens

testosterone

18.3 estrogens

ethinylestradiol

18.4 insulins

compound insulin
zinc suspension
insulin injection

18.5 oral contraceptives

ethinylestradiol +
levonorgestrel
ethinylestradiol +
norethisterone

norethisterone

18.6 progestogens

norethisterone

18.7 thyroid hormones
and antagonists

levothyroxine
potassium iodide
propylthiouracil

18.8 ovulation inducer

clomifene

259

19. IMMUNOLOGICALS

19.1 sera and   anti-D immunoglobulin
      immunoglobulins   (human)
                                       antirabies hyperimmune
                                         serum
                                       antivenom serum
                                       diphtheria antitoxin
                                       immunoglobulin, human
                                         normal
                                       tetanus antitoxin

19.2 vaccines

19.2.1 for universal   BCG vaccine
       immunisation   diphtheria-pertussis-
                                       tetanus vaccine
                                     diphtheria-tetanus
                                       vaccine
                                     measles vaccine
                                     poliomyelitis vaccine
                                     smallpox vaccine
                                     tetanus vaccine

19.2.2 for specific groups   influenza vaccine
       of individuals   meningococcal vaccine
                                     rabies vaccine
                                     typhoid vaccine
                                     yellow fever vaccine

20. MUSCLE RELAXANTS AND   neostigmine   pyridostigmine
     CHOLINESTERASE INHIBITORS   suxamethonium
                                     tubocurarine

21. OPHTHALMOLOGICAL PREPARATIONS

21.1 antiinfective   silver nitrate
                                     sulfacetamide

21.2 antiinflammatory   hydrocortisone

21.3 local anaesthetics   tetracaine

21.4 miotics   pilocarpine

21.5 mydriatics   homatropine   epinephrine

21.6 systemic   acetazolamide

22. OXYTOCICS   ergometrine
                                     oxytocin

23.   PERITONEAL DIALYSIS   intraperitoneal dialysis
      SOLUTION   solution

24.   PSYCHOTHERAPEUTIC DRUGS   amitriptyline
                                   chlorpromazine
                                   diazepam
                                   fluphenazine
                                   haloperidol
                                   lithium carbonate

25.   DRUGS ACTING ON THE RESPIRATORY TRACT

      25.1 antiasthmatic drugs   aminophylline   beclometasone
                                   epinephrine   cromoglicic acid
                                   salbutamol   ephedrine

      25.2 antitussives   codeine

26.   SOLUTIONS COLLECTING WATER, ELECTROLYTE AND
      ACID-BASE DISTURBANCES

      26.1 oral   oral rehydration salts
                                     (for glucose-salt
                                     solution)
                                   potassium chloride

      26.2 parenteral   compound solution of
                                     sodium lactate
                                   glucose
                                   glucose with sodium
                                     chloride
                                   potassium chloride
                                   sodium bicarbonate
                                   sodium chloride
                                   water for injection

27.   SURGICAL DISINFECTANTS   chlorhexidine
                                   iodine

28.   VITAMINS AND MINERALS   ascorbic acid   calcium
                                   ergocalciferol   gluconate
                                   nicotinamide
                                   pyridoxine
                                   retinol
                                   riboflavin
                                   sodium fluoride
                                   thiamine

*Note: Spellings in this Appendix follow those given by WHO but do not always correspond to
accepted British spelling.*

APPENDIX II

GLAXO (BANGLADESH) LTD. PRODUCT RANGE.

PRODUCT	DESCRIPTION	FORMULA-TION ON UK MARKET	FORMULA-TION ON WHO LIST	PRODUCT RECOMMENDED FOR WITH-DRAWAL, BANGLADESH EXPERT COMMITTEE MAY 1982
ANTIBIOTICS				
1. CLINMYCIN Capsules	A broad spectrum antibiotic containing 250 mg oxytetracycline dihydrate in each capsule	No	No	No
2. CLINMYCIN Syrup	Pleasantly flavoured broad spectrum antibiotic syrup, containing 125 mg oxytetracycline calcium in each 5 ml	No	No	Yes
3. CRYSTAPEN Injection	Single dose injection containing 500,000 units of crystalline sodium salt of benzylpenicillin	Yes	Yes	No
3. CRYSTAPEN V Granules	A flavoured syrup produced by adding 5 spoons of boiled & cooled water (spoon provided). Each teaspoonful of syrup (5 ml) contains 125 mg phenoxymethyl penicillin	Yes	Yes	No
5. CRYSTAPEN V Tablets	Tablets containing phenoxymethyl penicillin 125 mg 250 mg	No Yes	No Yes	No No
6. GRISOVIN-FP Tablets	Each tablet contains 125 mg fine particles of griseofulvin	Yes	Yes	No
7. NEOBACRIN Ointment	Skin & eye ointment containing 5 mg neomycin and 500 units zinc bacitracin in each gram	No	Yes	No

262

PRODUCT	DESCRIPTION	FORMULA- TION ON UK MARKET	FORMULA- TION ON WHO LIST	PRODUCT RECOMMENDED FOR WITH- DRAWAL, BANGLADESH EXPERT COMMITTEE MAY 1982
8. SECLOPEN Injection	Single dose injection containing 300,000 units of procaine penicillin G and 100,000 units of benzylpenicillin	No	Yes	No
9. STREPTOMYCIN SULPHATE Injection	Single dose injection containing equivalent of 1 gram streptomycin sulphate	Yes	Yes	No

CORTICOSTEROIDS

10. BETNELAN Tablets	Each tablet contains 0.5 mg betamethasone	Yes	Yes	No
11. BETNESOL-N Eye Ointment	0.1% betamethasone disodium phosphate with 0.5% neomycin sulphate in a bland paraffin base	Yes	No	Yes
12. BETNESOL-N Eye, Ear & Nose Drops	0.1% betamethasone disodium phosphate with 0.5% neomycin sulphate	Yes	No	Yes
13. BETNOVATE-N Cream	0.1% betamethasone 17-valerate with 0.5% neomycin sulphate	Yes	No	Yes
14. BETNOVATE-N Ointment	0.1% betamethasone 17-valerate with 0.5% neomycin sulphate in a bland paraffin base	Yes	No	Yes

PHARMACEUTICALS

15. ADEXOLIN Liquid	Containing vitamin A 12,000 units and vitamin D 2,000 units per ml	Yes	No	Yes
16. ANCOLOXIN Tablets	Each tablet containing 25 mg meclozine hydro- chloride and 50 mg pyridoxine hydrochloride	Yes	No	No

263

PRODUCT	DESCRIPTION	FORMULA-TION ON UK MARKET	FORMULA-TION ON WHO LIST	PRODUCT RECOMMENDED FOR WITH-DRAWAL, BANGLADESH EXPERT COMMITTEE MAY 1982
17. BECADEX Drops	Multivitamin drops	No	No	Yes
18. BECADEX Syrup	Fruit-flavoured multivitamin	No	No	Yes
19. BECADEX Tablets	Sugar-coated multivitamin tablet	No	No	Yes
20. BERIN Injection	100 mg thiamine hydrochloride per ml (vitamin B1)	No	No	No
21. BERIN Tablets	100 mg thiamine hydrochloride per tablet (vitamin B1)	No	Yes	No
22. *CALCI-OSTELIN Injection		No	No	Yes
23. CALCI-OSTELIN + B12 Injection	0.5 mg colloidal calcium 5,000 units vitamin D and 50 mcg vitamin B12 per ml	No	No	Yes
24. CALCI-OSTELIN + B12	Syrup of calcium vitamin D and vitamin B12	No	No	Yes
25. CALDEFERRUM Tablets	Coated tablets containing iron, calcium and vitamin D	No	No	No
26. CELIN Flavoured Tablets	Orange-flavoured tablets containing 250 mg ascorbic acid (vitamin C)	No	No	No
27. CYTAMEN Injection	Injection of vitamin B12: 250 mcg per ml 1000 mcg per ml	Yes	No	No
28. CYTEXIN Liquid	Vitamin B-complex with vitamin B12	No	No	Yes
29. DEQUADIN Lozenges	Pleasantly flavoured lozenges each containing 0.25 mg dequalinium chloride	Yes	No	Yes

PRODUCT	DESCRIPTION	FORMULA-TION ON UK MARKET	FORMULA-TION ON WHO LIST	PRODUCT RECOMMENDED FOR WITH-DRAWAL, BANGLADESH EXPERT COMMITTEE MAY 1982
30. ERBOLIN Tablets	Each tablet contains 0.4 mg of the total alkaloids of ergot	No	No	No
31. FESOLATE Tablets	Sugar-coated tablets containing ferrous sulphate 200 mg, copper sulphate 2.5 mg and manganese sulphate 2.5 mg	No	No	No
32. GLAXOSE-D	Finely powdered dextrose monohydrate B.P. (98.9%) with vitamin D (250 units per oz) and calcium glycerophosphate	No	No	Yes
33. HALIBORANGE	Syrup of vitamin A, C. & D with concentrated orange juice	No (only tablets)	No	Yes
34. HELMACID	Pleasantly flavoured anthelmintic syrup con-taining in each teaspoonful (5 ml) equivalent of 600 mg piperazine hydrate	No	Yes (with-out flavour)	No
35. HELMACID with Senna	Chocolate-flavoured anthelmintic granules, containing in each 10 gms (4 teaspoons) piperazine phosphate 4 g and calcium sennosides equivalent to 1.5 g of powdered senna pod	No	No	No
36. KAOPEX-N Suspension	Suspension of light kaolin, pectin and neomycin	No	No	Yes
37. KAPILIN Tablets	Each tablet contains 10 mg acetomenaphthone	No	No	No

PRODUCT	DESCRIPTION	FORMULA-TION ON UK MARKET	FORMULA-TION ON WHO LIST	PRODUCT RECOMMENDED FOR WITH-DRAWAL, BANGLADESH EXPERT COMMITTEE MAY 1982
38. KAPILIN Ampoules	1 ml ampoules each containing 10 mg menaphthone sodium bisulphite	No	No	No
39. LAXENNA Tablets	Tablets containing activity of 600 mg senna pod	No	No	No
40. MINADEX Syrup	mineral vitamin tonic in orange-flavoured syrup	Yes	No	Yes
41. MYCIL Ointment	Anti-fungal ointment containing 0.5% chlorphenesin	Yes	No	No
42. MYCIL Powder	Anti-fungal, antibacterial medicated powder containing chlorphenesin 1% and zinc oxide 5%	Yes	No	No
43. NEO-NACLEX Tablets	Long-acting oral diuretic each tablet containing 2.5 mg bendrofluazide	Yes	No	No
44. OSTOCALCIUM Tablets	Calcium and vitamin D tablet (calcium phosphate 325 mg, calcium sodium lactate 162 mg, and vitamin D 500 units)	No	No	Yes
45. PARAPYRIN Tablets	Analgesic & antipyretic tablet containing paracetamol and aspirin	No	No	Yes
46. PIRITON Expectorant	Each teaspoonful (5 ml) contains chlorpheniramine maleate 2.5 mg, am-monium chloride 125 mg, sodium citrate 55 mg and glycerin.	Yes	No	Yes
47. PIRITON-G Linctus	Each teaspoonful (5 ml) contains chlorpheniramine maleate 2.5 mg, gualphenesin 100 mg, sodium citrate 55 mg, and glycerin	No	No	Yes

PRODUCT	DESCRIPTION	FORMULA-TION ON UK MARKET	FORMULA-TION ON WHO LIST	PRODUCT RECOMMENDED FOR WITH-DRAWAL, BANGLADESH EXPERT COMMITTEE MAY 1982
48. PIRITON Tablets	Antihistamine tablet containing chlorpheniramine maleate 4 mg	Yes	No	No
49. PLEXAN Injection	Injection of liver extract with added vitamin B12	No	No	Yes
50. PREPALIN	A sterile oily solution for injection containing 100,000 units of vitamin A per ml	No	No (on Bangladesh Essential Drug List)	No
51. PROBERON Injection	Vitamin B-complex injection	No	No	Yes
52. STIBATIN	A sterile solution of pentavalent sodium antimony (V) gluconate 100 mg per ml	No	Yes	No
53. VENTOLIN Tablets	Tablets containing 2 mg salbutamol sulphate	Yes	No	No
NEW PRODUCTS				
54. CEPOREX Capsules	A broad spectrum bacterial antibiotic containing 250 mg cephalexin monohydrate in each capsule	Yes	No	No
55. VIBELAN FORTE-C Capsules	A preparation of vitamin B-complex with therapeutic quantities of vitamin C in each capsule	No	No	Yes
56. VENTOLIN Elixir	An effective bronchodilator containing salutamol sulphate 1 mg and guaiphenesin 50 mg in each teaspoonful	Yes	Yes	No

(*From price list July 1981*)

* CALCI-OSTELIN *injection not on July 1981 Price List, but no evidence of withdrawal since March 1980 Medical List; included in May 1982 Review.*

267

APPENDIX III

FISONS (BANGLADESH) LIMITED PRODUCT RANGE

PRODUCT	DESCRIPTION	FORMULA-TION ON UK MARKET	FORMULA-TION ON WHO LIST	PRODUCT RECOMMENDED FOR WITH-DRAWAL, BANGLADESH EXPERT COMMITTEE MAY 1982
LIQUIDS				
1. DIGEPLEX	Digestive enzymes with vitamin B-complex	No	No	Yes
2. DIMYRIL	1so-aminile citrate(for irritating cough)	Yes	No	Yes
3. ENTERFRAM	Neomycin sulphate & kaolin (for infantile diarrhoea etc)	No	No	Yes
4. FIDAPLEX	Vitamin B-complex with sodium glycerophosphate and calcium glycerophosphate (avitaminosis convalescence and debility)	No	No	Yes
5. FULFORD'S GRIPE WATER	(For babies & young children)	Yes	No	Yes
6. HYPACID	Aluminium phosphate gel (For hyperacidity & peptic ulcer)	No	No	Yes
7. MINOLAD	Vits A, D, Lysine, Iron, Minerals, Choline, Methionine (a nutritional tonic for adults and children)	No	No	Yes
8. NEO-FERILEX	Iron choline citrate with Vit B-complex (for iron deficiency anaemia)	No	No	Yes
TABLETS				
9.- ANTISMAT	Ephedrine, Theophylline, Phenobarbitone and Aluminium hydroxide (for bronchial asthma)	No	No	No

PRODUCT	DESCRIPTION	FORMULA-TION ON UK MARKET	FORMULA-TION ON WHO LIST	PRODUCT RECOMMENDED FOR WITH-DRAWAL, BANGLADESH EXPERT COMMITTEE MAY 1982
10. CALCIPAN	Calcium Pantotherate (for burning feet syndrome, post-operative distension, paralyticileus, muscular cramps, and protective action against toxicity of streptomycin and di-hydrostreptomycin)	No	No	Yes
11. FICAL-D	Calcium lactate 150 mg Calcium gluconate 290 mg Calciferol (vitamin D 500 I.U) Calcium and vitamin D supplement)	No	No	Yes
12. FIDAPLEX	Vitamin B-complex Prophylaxis of Avitaminosis-B	No	No	Yes
13. FITAMOL	Paracetamol 500 mg	No	Yes	No
14. FISTREP	Streptomycin sulphate and Iodochlorhydroxy-quinoline (anti-dysentric/anti-diarrhoeal)	No	No	Yes
15. FOLFETAB	Ferrous fumarate and folic acid (for iron deficiency-anaemia)	No	No	No
16. FOLIC ACID	(For megaloblastic anaemia of pregnancy)	Yes	Yes	No
17. GENASPRIN	Acetysalicylic acid 300 mg	Yes	Yes	No
18. GENATOSAN	Multivitamins (Restores physical power, guards against disease, promotes appetite and growth)	No	No	Yes
19. HYPACID	Aluminium phosphate (for hyperacidity & pectic ulcer)	No	No	Yes
20. PEPS	Anti-cough lozenge	No	No	Yes

PRODUCT	DESCRIPTION	FORMULA-TION ON UK MARKET	FORMULA-TION ON WHO LIST	PRODUCT RECOMMENDED FOR WITH-DRAWAL, BANGLADESH EXPERT COMMITTEE MAY 1982
CAPSULES				
21. DECAPLEX FORTE	Ferrous fumarate, vitamin C,B1,B12 and folic acid (For iron deficiency anaemia)	No	No	Yes
22. DECATONE*	A geriatric preparation containing vitamins,iron, minerals,digestive enzymes and hormones.	No	No	Yes
23. FIDAPLEX-C	High potency vitamin B-complex with vitamin C & dried yeast	No	No	Yes
INJECTABLES				
24. CALCIPAN	Calcium pantothenate 100 mg/ml	No	No	No
25. FIDAPLEX	Vitamin B-complex with lignocaine hydrochloride	No	No	Yes
26. IMFERON	Iron dextran 50 mg	Yes	Yes	No
27. LIVEX B.C.	Liver extract with vitamin B-complex and lignocaine hydrochloride (for haemopoiesis)	Yes	No	Yes
OINTMENTS				
28. FRAMYCORT	Neomycin sulphate with hydrocortisone acetate	No	No (not with neomycin sulphate - but framycetin sulphate in U.K.)	Yes
29. ZAM-BUK	(Medicated oitment)	Yes	No	Yes
30. AURALGICIN	Ear drops. Chlorbutol, phenazone, ephedrine and potassium hydroxyquinoline	Yes	No	No

PRODUCT	DESCRIPTION	FORMULA-TION ON UK MARKET	FORMULA-TION ON WHO LIST	PRODUCT RECOMMENDED FOR WITH-DRAWAL, BANGLADESH EXPERT COMMITTEE MAY 1982
31. FRAMYGEN	Eye/ear drops. Neomycin, sulphate, ben-zalk chloride and benzyl alcohol	No	No	No
		(not with neomycin sulphate but framycetin sulphate in U.K.)		

(From product List September 1978 and Price List February 1981)

* DECATONE: *Although this is listed in Fisons (Bangladesh) February 1981 Institutional Price list and included in the May 1982 Review of Products on the market, a letter from Fisons UK to Professor Rawlins (21 February 1980) states that DECATONE was withdrawn from the Bangladesh market in June 1979.*

APPENDIX IV

DRAFT NATIONAL DRUG POLICY FOR BANGLADESH FROM EXPERT COMMITTEE REPORT. 11 MAY 1982.

To achieve the objectives of national drug policy and to provide guidelines for the formation of programme the following actions are to be taken:

Selection and provision of essential drugs:
3.1 The major strategy is to overcomne constraint of limited resources for the the option utilization. This also calls for the elimination of all unnecessary, useless drugs and drugs of doubtful efficacy from the market. A limited list of 150 essential drugs considered adequate for most therapeutic purposes shall be selected. Out of this about 45 essential drugs will be selected for the primary level of health care on the basis of priority health need, cost, safety and suitability of treatment of common disease and symptoms by up to Thana level health workers.

Besides, for the protection of the vast majority of people in the rural areas from hazards of undue prescribing in an attempt to give them relief by basic health workers it is essential to limit the essential drugs to 12 which are considered safe and adequate for common medical problems.

Besides there may be a list of another about 100 supplementary drugs needed for tertiary level of health care by specialists. The various brands of drugs in the market shall be evaluated annually on the basis of their usefulness, essentiality and cost-effectiveness in the light of up to date available information. In future, only products which are considered essential and relevant to health needs of the country and are consistent with this policy shall be licensed or registered. The selected essential drugs shall be given preferential treatment in terms of licensing, import authorization, duties and other financial benefits.

The selected 45 essential drugs for primary health care shall be allowed to be manufactured or sold only under their generic names. As soon as possible and not later than 1983, a National Formulary will be prepared and published, which shall include all the formulations that will be allowed for manufacture, import or sale in this country. Products such as liquid vitamin mixtures, multiple combinations of potent drugs, combination of antibiotics with other active drugs, alkali mixtures, gripe waters, cough mixtures, tonics, balms, digestive enzyme preparations, habit-forming drugs, vaporubs and other similar useless and non-essential products will be identified and their licensing/registration shall be cancelled so that such products are completely eliminated from Bangladesh.

DRUG ACT

3.2   The Drugs Act 1940 shall be revised or replaced by a new drug legislation incorporating provisions for:

i. a system of registration of all medicinal products including ayurvedic, unani and homeopathic medicines;

ii. enforcement of good manufacturing practices;

iii. full control of labelling, advertising;

iv. control of prices of finished drugs and pharmaceutical raw materials;

v. prescription control of toxic/poisonous and habit-forming drugs;

vi. summary trial for offences in special drug courts;

vii. heavy penalties including confiscation if equipment and properties for manufature and/or selling of spurious and sub-standard drugs;

viii. departmental adjudication for fine of up to taka 10,000/-;

ix. heavy penalties for possessing or selling of drugs stolen from government stores, hospitals and dispensaries;

x. regulation of technology transfer and licensing agreement with foreign collaborators;

xi. restriction of ownership of retail pharmacist to professional pharmacists only;

xii. control of manufacture and sale of unani, ayurvedic and homeopathic drugs;

xiii. the patent laws in respect of pharmaceutical substances shall be revised.

Product patent in respect of pharmaceutical substances shall not be allowed. Process patent may be allowed for a limited period of time if only the basic substance is manufactured within the country. The tariff structure in respect of pharmaceutical raw materials for selected essential drugs, quality control equipment and chemicals shall be revised. A drug technical advisory board consisting of representatives from the pharmaceutical profession, industry, Pharmacy dept. of the University, representations from the professional organisations, experts from the profession shall be constituted to review from time to time for the implementation of drug policy.

DRUG ADMINISTRATION

3.3   The Directorate of Drug Administration will be expanded and adequately staffed with experts in medical and pharmaceutical sciences. In view of the gross inadequacy of drug inspectors, all Thana Health Administrators shall be given a special course of training and be empowered to act as drug inspectors for the purpose, so that they can take meaningful sanctions against wholesalers, retailers and peddlers of drugs at Thana levels and below. All the government drug control laboratories should be brought under the control of Drug Administration. A properly staffed and equipped National Drug Control Laborartory with appellate facilities will be set up as early as possible, not later than

1985. Besides its function in respect of drug control and administration, the National Drug Control Administration Laboratory will devote itself to develop appropriate standards and specifications for unani and ayurvedic drugs. It will also help develop national formulations for unani and ayurvedic drugs.

The fees for licensing, registration and testing of drugs which are ridiculously low at present shall be enhanced. Licensing or registration fees for new products which are not included in the national list of essential drugs shall be very high (not less than taka 5000/-). The renewable fees of licensing, registration and testing shall be utilised for the expansion and development of drug administration and drug testing laboratories. No manufacturer will be allowed to produce drugs without adequate quality control facilities. However, the small national drug manufacturers may be allowed to establish quality control laboratories on a collective basis.

3.4 Local Production

The existing capacities of local pharmaceutical industries especially those owned by Bangladeshi nationals, shall be enhanced through liberal licensing for balancing and modernisation and by increasing entitlement for the import of raw materials. Government facilities for the economic and efficient production of essential drugs for primary health care, intravenous fluid and vaccines shall be expanded. Multinational companies will not be allowed to manufacture simple products like common analgesics, vitamins, antacids, etc. Such products will be exclusively manufactured by local firms. Local production of basic pharmaceuticals in bulk shall be promoted to attain self-reliance. To encourage such production, special benefits and protections will be provided to private investors. The public industrial sector shall also take appropriate measures for the local production of essential basic pharmaceuticals in bulk, including vital antibiotics.

3.5 Control of Prices

Government shall control the prices of finished drugs as well as those of pharmaceutical raw and packaging materials and intermediates. Level prices will be fixed for the 45 essential drugs for primary health care and their corresponding raw materials. It will be ensured that all raw and packaging materials of acceptable quality are procured from international sources at competitive prices only. The retail prices of finished drugs will be fixed on the basis of costing and reasonable profitability. Undue overhead expenditure shall be prevented. A maximum of 100% mark up for fast moving items and 150% for slow moving items over cost of raw materials shall be allowed.   .
In the case of injectable and sterile preparations, the mark-up may go up to 200%. No mark-up will be allowed on the cost of packaging materials, but actual cost on them will be added.
The agency responsible for drug control and administration shall be responsible for the control of pricing and their enforcement.

3.6 Distribution and Utilization

Retail sale of drugs and medicines shall be allowed only under the supervision of qualified pharmacists. As soon as possible, arrangement must be made to authorise the establishment of private retail pharmacies within the premises of every Government hospital up to the Thana Health Complex, where under the ownership (on lease) and management of qualified pharmacists, and under the supervision of hospital authorities, essential drugs will be made available for sale at fixed prices against prescriptions of qualified physicians.

3.7 Traditional Unani, Ayurvedic and Homeopathic system of medicine have a long tradition in many countries including Bangladesh. These systems are now exempted from the drug laws. Consequently unethical and not uncommonly harmful products proliferate and alcohol containing tonics are much abused.
Appropriate action requires to be taken for necessary training of their personnel, screening of the products and wherever possible identification of their active ingredients, and standardisation.
A National Pharmacopia of Traditional Medicine should be prepared.

INDEX

Index

Typeset by Compugraphic,

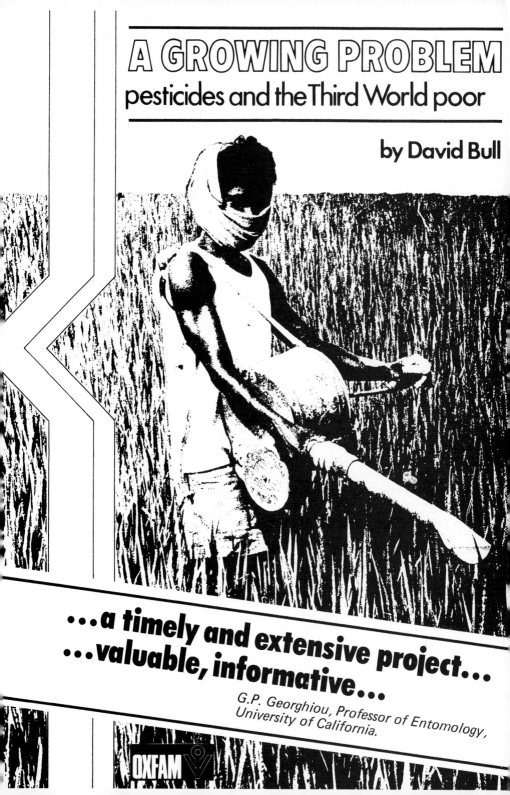

A GROWING PROBLEM
pesticides and the Third World poor

by David Bull

...a timely and extensive project...
...valuable, informative...

G.P. Georghiou, Professor of Entomology,
University of California.

OXFAM

Pesticides are a growing problem for the Third World poor.

They bring a promise of higher yields, more food for the hungry and freedom from the scourge of insect-borne disease. But they also threaten the health and livelihood of rural people.

- As pesticides kill off the natural enemies of pests and encourage the pests to develop resistance, so Third World farmers are faced with a treadmill of rising costs and deteriorating control.

- Anti-malaria campaigns suffer when agricultural pesticides accelerate the development of resistant mosquitoes.

- Poverty, illiteracy and heat mean farm labourers use very toxic pesticides under hopelessly unsafe conditions. Poisoning is widespread.

- Inadequate labelling and questionable marketing practices increase the dangers just where controls are lacking and extra care is most needed.

- Despite the hazards, pesticides restricted in the rich world continue to be exported to the poor without proper safeguards.

A Growing Problem investigates the alarming facts from the perspective of the poor. It suggests how to make the most of pesticides while minimising the dangers.

A Growing Problem describes initiatives under way to use and control pesticides for the benefit of the poor. It concludes with a series of practical suggestions for action by governments, industry and international organisations.

This thoroughly documented study is brought to life by evidence from OXFAM's first hand experience and contacts in the Third World. Real-life stories remind us of the human dimension.

A Growing Problem makes vital reading for all those interested in the struggles of the Third World poor and the plight of the world's environment.

A Growing Problem is essential reading for students, scientists and all those with a professional interest in pesticides, agriculture, health and ecology.

A Growing Problem — pesticides and the Third World poor, by David Bull. Publication: July 1982, £4.95 (plus p&p*).

A Growing Problem is published by OXFAM and distributed by TWP.

Trade enquiries to: Third World Publications, 151 Stratford Rd., Birmingham B11 1RD, UK.